INFECTION CONTROL
IN
LONG-TERM
CARE FACILITIES

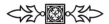

INFECTION CONTROL
IN
LONG–TERM
CARE FACILITIES

2ND EDITION

EDITED BY

Philip W. Smith, MD
Hospital Epidemiologist
Clarkson Hospital
President of the Board
Nebraska Infection Control Network
Consultant to the State of Nebraska
Department of Health for Infectious Diseases
Omaha, Nebraska

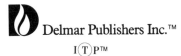
Delmar Publishers Inc.™
I(T)P™

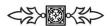

NOTICE TO THE READER

Publisher does not warrant or guarantee any of the products described herein or perform any independent analysis in connection with any of the product information contained herein. Publisher does not assume, and expressly disclaims, any obligation to obtain and include information other than that provided to it by the manufacturer.

The reader is expressly warned to consider and adopt all safety precautions that might be indicated by the activities described herein and to avoid all potential hazards. By following the instructions contained herein, the reader willingly assumes all risks in connection with such instructions.

The publisher makes no representations or warranties of any kind, including but not limited to, the warranties of fitness for particular purpose or merchantability, nor are any such representations implied with respect to the material set forth herein, and the publisher takes no responsibility with respect to such material. The publisher shall not be liable for any special, consequential or exemplary damages resulting, in whole or in part, from the readers' use of, or reliance upon, this material.

Cover Design by: *Timothy J. Conners*
Production Services: *TopDesk Publishers' Group*
Publishing Team: *Bill Burgower*, Senior Acquisitions Editor
Debra Flis, Assistant Editor
Mary Robinson, Project Editor
Mary Siener, Art & Design Coordinator
Barbara A. Bullock, Production Coordinator
David C. Gordon, Publisher

For information, address Delmar Publishers Inc.
3 Columbia Circle
Box 15015
Albany, NY 12212-5015

Printed in the United States of America
Published simultaneously in Canada
by Nelson Canada,
a division of the Thomson Corporation

10 9 8 7 6 5 4 3 2 1 XXX 99 98 97 96 95 94

ISBN 0-8273-5686 - 2
Library of Congress Catalog Card Number: 93 -73012

To the elderly we serve, who show us where we have been and where we will be.

CONTRIBUTORS

David W. Bentley, MD
Professor of Medicine and Head
  Division of Geriatrics/Gerontology
  SUNY School of Medicine and Biomedical Sciences
Chief, Geriatrics Section,
  Buffalo Veterans Administration Medical Center
Director, SUNY/Buffalo Multidisciplinary Center
  on Aging
  Buffalo, New York

Joyce M. Black, RNC, MSN
Assistant Professor of Adult Health and Illness
  University of Nebraska Medical Center
Editor, Plastic Surgical Nursing Journal
  Omaha, Nebraska

Steven B. Black, MD
Plastic Surgeon, Private Practice
Co-Medical Director
  Clarkson Hospital Center for Wound Healing
  Omaha, Nebraska

Mary C. Boehle, MT (ASCP), RS
Health Facilities Surveyor Consultant
  Bureau of Health Facilities Standards
  State of Nebraska Department of Health
  Grand Island, Nebraska

Kent B. Crossley, MD
Chief, Department of Medicine
  St. Paul–Ramsey Medical Center
Professor of Medicine
  University of Minnesota Medical School
  St. Paul, Minnesota

Pamela B. Daly, PhD
  University of Nebraska Medical Center
  Omaha, Nebraska

Richard A. Garibaldi, MD
Hospital Epidemiologist
Professor of Medicine
Department of Internal Medicine
University of Connecticut Health Center
Farmington, Connecticut

Nancy J. Haberstich, RN, CIC
Infection Control Nurse
  Lincoln General Hospital
  Lincoln, Nebraska

Virginia M. Helget, RN, MSN, CIC
Nurse Epidemiologist
  Clarkson Hospital
  Omaha, Nebraska

Linda A. Horning, RN, MSN, CIC
Nurse Epidemiologist
  Clarkson Hospital
  Omaha, Nebraska

Joseph M. Mylotte, MD
Associate Professor of Medicine
  State University of New York at Buffalo
Head, Infectious Diseases
  Buffalo General Hospital
  Buffalo, New York

Lindsay E. Nicolle, MD
Director, Infection Control Unit
  Health Sciences Centre
Associate Professor of Internal Medicine/Medical
  Microbiology
  University of Manitoba
  Winnipeg, Manitoba, Canada

Brenda A. Nurse, MD
Director, Department of Infectious
  Diseases and Epidemiology
  New Britain Memorial Hospital
  New Britain, Connecticut
Assistant Professor of Medicine
  University of Connecticut School of Medicine
  Farmington, Connecticut

Jane F. Potter, MD
Chief, Section of Geriatrics and Gerontology
  Department of Internal Medicine
  University of Nebraska Medical Center
  Omaha, Nebraska

Vicki G. Pritchard, RN, MSN, CIC
Infection Control Nurse
  Veterans Affairs Medical Center
  Chillicothe, Ohio

Jane S. Roccaforte, MD
Hospital Epidemiologist
  Immanuel Medical Center
  Omaha, Nebraska

Pat G. Rusnak, RN
Nurse Consultant

Treasurer of the Board
  Nebraska Infection Control Network
  Omaha, Nebraska

Philip W. Smith, MD
Hospital Epidemiologist
  Clarkson Hospital
President of the Board
  Nebraska Infection Control Network
Consultant to the State of Nebraska Department
  of Health for Infectious Diseases
  Omaha, Nebraslca

Judith K. Stern, MD
Geriatrician and Internist
  Omaha, Nebraska

PREFACE

T he field of infection in the long-term care facility has developed greatly since the first edition of this book was published ten years ago. Many studies have been published documenting the magnitude of infections and epidemics in this setting, infection control programs have become standard, and the unique concerns of infection control in the nursing home have been recognized.

The objective of this book is to delineate the concepts of diagnosis, transmission, and prevention of infection that are particularly applicable to the long-term care facility, and to present those concepts in a manner that will provide a thorough but practical background for the infection control practitioner. This book is intended for nursing home nurses, ancillary nursing home staff, long-term care administrators, geriatric program trainees, state surveyors, and physicians who practice in nursing homes.

The book is divided into sections for easy reference. Section I provides a background in aspects of infectious diseases relevant to the elderly person. Section II deals with infectious diseases that occur in the nursing home. The organization and major components of an infection control program for nursing homes are discussed in Section III, and Section IV covers specific measures to control and prevent infections in the long-term care facility.

The second edition of this text contains much updated information in all areas, and in addition, has several new features. All established chapters have been extensively revised, especially in the areas of isolation systems, infection definitions, pressure ulcers, and education. Certain topics such as methicillin-resistant *Staphylococcus aureus*, waste management, and resident health programs have been expanded considerably. The discussion of gastroenteritis has been expanded into a separate chapter. The problems of HIV infection, AIDS, and universal precautions have become significant for the nursing home and form the basis for a new chapter. The third new chapter addresses the unique infection control concerns of the long-term care facility employee.

The book would not be possible without the support of the editorial staff at Delmar Publishers, especially Bill Burgower and Debra Flis. I would like to acknowledge the valuable assistance of many reviewers, who provided thoughtful criticism of the contents of this book, and the outstanding secretarial assistance of Karen Evans. I thank my uncle, Philip Schumacher, who manages several outstanding nursing homes in Minnesota and who sparked my interest in the field. Finally, I wish to acknowledge the great support and assistance of my lovely wife, Sharon, and the inspiration of my three wonderful sons, Nathan, Alexander, and Matthew.

Philip W. Smith

CONTENTS

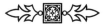

SECTION ONE

GENERAL BACKGROUND

CHAPTER 1

A FEW BASICS ABOUT INFECTIONS

Philip W. Smith

FACTORS INVOLVED IN INFECTION

Infection involves the interaction between a microorganism, the environment, and the host.

Microorganisms

Organisms that cause infectious diseases in humans form a large spectrum in terms of size and complexity. Viruses have a mean size of 0.1 μm (0.0000001 meter) and cannot be seen under the average laboratory microscope. Bacteria average about 1 μm in size and can be visualized by high-power microscopy. The largest agents that cause infection in humans are the helminths, or worms. Organisms are most often named by genus (e.g., *Staphylococcus*) and species (e.g., *aureus*).

Although we tend to associate microorganisms with disease, they are beneficial to humans in many ways. Bacteria found on the surface of the skin and mucous membranes, the normal bacterial flora, are very important because they inhibit the growth of potential pathogens. Bacteria are also involved in the metabolism of vitamin K in the human intestine.

Immunity

Immunity is resistance of the host to infection. Local defenses form the first barrier against potential invaders and are an important aspect of immunity. Examples of local defenses include intact skin, gastric acidity, and the normal bacterial flora of skin, mouth, gut, and vagina.

The normal host has several lines of defense against pathogenic microorganisms, including white blood cells, antibodies, and lymphocytes. These are reviewed in Chapter 2.

Pathogenesis of Infection

The interaction of the organism and the host has several outcomes. *Infection* may be defined as invasion of the host by microorganisms. *Colonization* is the coexistence of microorganisms and the host without injury to or reaction by the host. A person who is colonized with a particular organism may be referred to as a *carrier* of that organism.

Infection requires the replication of organisms in the tissues of the host. Whether or not infection develops depends upon the *virulence* (ability to produce disease) of the pathogen as well as host defenses against the pathogen. Related organisms may vary greatly in virulence. *Staphylococcus aureus* is a virulent organism and an important cause of infections, for example, whereas *Staphylococcus epidermidis* is a relatively benign organism that is part of normal skin flora.

Virulence is determined by several mechanisms. First, the organism may produce disease by direct invasion of tissues. Invasiveness of bacteria may be enhanced by capsules that resist ingestion by white blood cells (pneumococci) or by enzymes that promote the spread of organisms through connective tissue (staphylococci). A second mechanism involves injury of the host by production of toxins by invading organisms. Botulism, tetanus, diphtheria, and cholera are examples of toxin-related diseases. Finally, tissue damage may be caused by the response of the host to the organism. This mechanism is typified by the delayed hypersensitivity response of the host to infection with *Mycobacterium tuberculosis.*

Disease production also depends upon the portal of entry of the organism. For instance, *Legionella pneumophila* produces severe pneumonia when inhaled, but has little effect on the skin. *S. aureus* produces severe cutaneous infections, but rarely causes pharyngitis.

Infection requires an imbalance among the host, the environment, and the organism. *Immunity,* the resistance of the host to infection, is most important in determining host response. Specific immunity develops after exposure to a particular organism. A host that is not immune to a specific infectious disease is called *susceptible.*

Manifestations of Infection

The infected host may be asymptomatic or may develop clinical manifestations of infection. The most universal manifestation of infection is *fever,* which can be defined as an oral temperature above 99°F or 37.2°C. Rectal temperatures are 0.5°C higher. There are causes of fever other than infection, including neoplasms, autoimmune diseases, endocrine disturbances, vascular accidents, drugs, and neurologic disorders.

The host generally manifests organ-specific symptoms of infection. Urinary tract infections cause dysuria; cutaneous infections cause redness, warmth, and tenderness of the skin; infectious gastroenteritis results in diarrhea; and individuals with pneumonia manifest cough and shortness of breath. These symptoms provide a clue to the underlying cause of the infection.

Patients with severe or prolonged infection develop other generalized symptoms or signs, such as weakness, weight loss, fatigue, and anemia. The elderly may present with unusual symptoms, making the diagnosis of infection more difficult. For instance, the elderly may not develop the normal febrile response to bacterial sepsis but often present first with confusion or tachypnea.[1]

Diagnosis of Infection

The diagnosis of an infection may be made on clinical grounds or by laboratory tests. Clinical observation of signs and symptoms will reliably diagnose a number of infections, such as chickenpox. However, laboratory assistance is usually required to determine the specific cause of an infection. The organism may be identified either directly or indirectly (by measuring the host response to the organism).

There are several ways to directly identify a microorganism in the laboratory. The standard method is isolation and identification of an organism (bacteria and fungi) in an appropriate culture medium. Collection of specimens from normally sterile body fluids such as spinal fluid and blood should be preceded by cleansing of the skin with alcohol and iodine solution. Specimens that are contaminated by normal bacterial flora pose special problems. When culturing urine, for example, a clean-catch, quantitative midstream culture is necessary to distinguish contamination from infection. Other direct means of organism identification include direct visualization by staining techniques (e.g., acid-fast staining for diagnosis of tuberculosis) and detection of components or antigens of the organisms (e.g., enzyme immunoassay for hepatitis B surface antigen).

Alternatively, the laboratory may diagnose an infection indirectly by measurement of host response to a specific organism. Examples include detection of measles antibody by complement fixation technique and measurement of skin test reaction to a protein extract of *M. tuberculosis* (purified protein derivative, PPD). Serum antibody levels or titers against organisms can be measured by a variety of techniques. A single antibody titer is rarely diagnostic. Hence, every effort should be made to obtain two samples, preferably two to three weeks apart, to look for a diagnostic rise in antibody titer. A fourfold or greater rise in titer is generally considered to be significant.

BASIC MICROBIOLOGY

Viruses

Viruses are the smallest infectious agents. The basic structure of the virus is a central core of nucleic acid (DNA or RNA) wrapped in a protective protein coat. Some viruses also have an outer envelope. Replication requires the use of the host cell.

Viral infections are difficult to confirm microbiologically. Viruses grow only in tissue culture, a procedure that is quite expensive and technically difficult, and is available only at certain reference laboratories. Thus the diagnosis of viral infection frequently depends on measurement of host antibodies against the virus (see Table 1.1). Antibody testing for herpesvirus infections is often unsatisfactory, but fortunately these infections can usually be diagnosed clinically.

Bacteria

Unlike viruses, bacteria may survive and reproduce independent of the host cell. They have a rigid cell wall that surrounds the cell membrane and protects it from mechanical

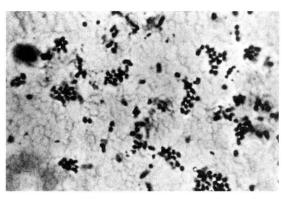

Figure 1.1 *Staphylococcus aureus in Gram stain of a wound*

damage. Some bacteria form endospores that are resistant to adverse environmental conditions: *Clostridium* and *Bacillus* species are the most important spore formers.

Bacteria are classified on the basis of shape, staining characteristics, and oxygen tolerance. Most bacteria are either round (cocci) or rod-shaped (bacilli). Staphylococci, for instance, form clusters of gram-positive cocci (Fig. 1.1). *Staphylococcus aureus* is the only staphylococcal species that gives a positive coagulase reaction. Aerobic bacteria grow in the presence of oxygen, whereas anaerobic bacteria are inhibited by oxygen. Bacteria are further subdivided on the basis of the Gram stain, which stains bacterial cell walls blue (gram-positive) or red (gram-negative). Some bacteria stain only with special stains such as the acid-fast stain (mycobacteria) or the Dieterle silver stain (*Legionella*). Aerobic bacteria are the most important clinically (Table 1.2).

Most bacterial infections are diagnosed by isolation of bacteria on appropriate culture media (Fig. 1.2). Aerobic bacteria can usually be isolated and identified in one to three days, anaerobic bacteria in three to six days, and mycobacteria in four to eight weeks. Legionnaires' disease is best diagnosed by testing for serum antibody or by direct fluorescent stain of bacteria in lung tissue. *Clostridium difficile* colitis is not diagnosed by stool culture but by stool assay for the toxin.

Fungi

Fungi are larger and more complex in structure than bacteria. They occur as single cells (yeasts) or multicellular organisms (molds). Some fungi cause endemic diseases in certain areas of the country, such as histoplasmosis in the

Table 1.1 *Mode of Diagnosis of Viral Infections*

MODE OF ORGANISM	DIAGNOSIS
Respiratory viruses	
Influenza	Cl, Ab, Cu
Parainfluenza	Ab
Respiratory syncytial virus (RSV)	Ab
Rhinovirus	Cl
Gastrointestinal viruses	
Enterovirus	Ab
Rotavirus	Ag, Ab
Norwalk virus	Ab
Hepatitis A	Ab
Hepatitis B	Ag
Miscellaneous viruses	
Herpes simplex	Cl, Cu
Herpes zoster	Cl
Rubella	Ab
Measles	Cl
Human Immunodeficiency Virus	Ab

KEY: Cl = clinical; Ag = antigen test; Ab = antibody test; Cu = cell culture

Mississippi Valley region and coccidioidomycosis in the southwestern United States. Cryptococcosis and aspergillosis occur primarily in the immunocompromised patient. *Candida* causes mucocutaneous infections, such as thrush, in patients receiving antibiotics or corticosteroids.

Like mycobacteria, fungi grow slowly in culture and usually require four to eight weeks for isolation and identification. Fungi may be seen in pathologic specimens by special staining (e.g., silver stain), and are usually diagnosed by culture. Oral candidiasis (thrush) is often diagnosed clinically.

Parasites

A number of parasites cause infectious diseases in humans. Protozoa are unicellular parasites; protozoa patho-

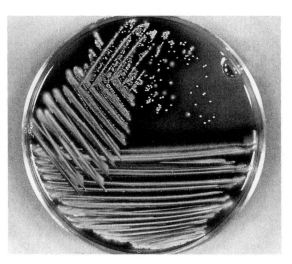

Figure 1.2 *S. aureus – culture on blood agar plate*

genic for humans cause giardiasis, amebiasis, and malaria. Helminths or worms that infect humans vary in size from 1 mm (*Heterophyes*) to 10 m or more (*Diphyllobothrium latum*). Insects that parasitize humans include mites (scabies), lice, fleas, and ticks.

Parasitic diseases of humans are generally diagnosed by direct visualization of the parasite, either with the naked eye or with a microscope.

Specimen Collection

The isolation and identification of organisms from clinical specimens require that a proper specimen be obtained and delivered promptly to the microbiology laboratory. Some organisms such as anaerobic bacteria are very fragile and will not survive delays in processing. Delay also permits the overgrowth of contaminating bacteria, which can invalidate a urine or sputum culture.

Different organisms require different collection techniques or culture media. Microbiologic techniques have been described in detail for various organisms.[2] Meticulous specimen collection is critical. The microbiology laboratory cannot compensate for a poorly collected sample.

Spinal fluid and blood are normally sterile. It is essential that cultures be collected aseptically, which is usually accomplished by cleansing the skin with alcohol

Table 1.2 *Bacterial Classification*

Aerobic	Anaerobic
Gram-positive	
Cocci	Cocci
Staphylococcus	Peptococcus
Streptococcus	Peptostreptococcus
Bacilli	Bacilli
Lactobacillus	Clostridium
Corynebacterium	Propionibacterium
Gram-negative	
Cocci	
Neisseria	
Bacilli	Bacilli
Escherichia	Bacteroides
Klebsiella	Fusobacterium
Proteus	
Pseudomonas	
Salmonella	
Shigella	
Hemophilus	
Acid-fast	
Bacilli	
Mycobacterium	

Source: Adapted from Smith PW: Infectious diseases, in Kochar MS and Kutty K (eds) Concise Textbook of General Medicine, 2nd ed. Norwalk, CT, Appleton & Lange, 1990. Used with permission.

and iodine solution prior to specimen collection. False-positive blood culture results occur most frequently with coagulase-negative staphylococci, such as *Staphylococcus epidermidis*, which reflects the role of these bacteria as predominant skin flora. Coagulase-negative staphylococci may cause infection, however, such as intravenous catheter-related bacteremia; infection rather than contamination is suggested by the presence of these bacteria in *more* than one blood culture.

All sputum specimens are contaminated by oral bacteria to some extent. *Streptococcus pneumoniae* and *Hemophilus influenzae* may be respiratory pathogens or normal pharyngeal flora. A percutaneous transtracheal aspiration bypasses oral flora and is mandatory if anaerobic bacteria are sought. The throat culture is not a substitute for sputum culture in the diagnosis of pneumonia. Only group A streptococci, *Corynebacterium diphtheriae*, and *Neisseria gonorrhoeae* are of diagnostic interest when present in a throat culture. Nasal cultures may be obtained to look for the *S. aureus* carrier state.

Urine cultures are contaminated with perineal bacteria, but quantitative midstream cultures distinguish contamination from infection. Lactobacilli and *Staphylococcus saprophyticus* are frequently contaminants, whereas *E. coli, Proteus mirabilis, Klebsiella, Pseudomonas*, enterococci, and *Candida* are usually pathogens. An improperly collected specimen is suggested by the presence of contaminants, of less than 10,000 bacteria per ml of urine, or of multiple bacterial isolates.

Open wounds and decubitus ulcers are usually contaminated with cutaneous organisms. For this reason, a surface swab of the lesion is of limited value and often yields multiple bacteria. A specimen is best obtained by subcutaneous needle aspiration or wound biopsy. Even a deep wound swab may be misleading; however, culture of a previously undrained abscess by needle aspiration or swab is appropriate and likely to reveal the causative organism. Some laboratories are able to perform quantitative cultures of wound biopsy specimens, an accurate way to distinguish infection from surface colonization.

Feces obviously contain large numbers of gut bacteria and should be cultured only for intestinal pathogens such as *Salmonella, Shigella*, and *Campylobacter*. Special media are required for isolation of these pathogens.

Stool may also be examined for parasites (such as *Giardia*) or assayed for *Clostridium difficile* toxin.

EPIDEMIOLOGY OF INFECTIOUS DISEASES

Definition of Terms in Epidemiology

Epidemiology has been defined as the dynamic study of the determinants, occurrence, and distribution of health and disease in a population.[3] There are a few background definitions and statistical calculations that are useful in the descriptive epidemiology of infections in nursing homes.

The *incidence rate* is the proportion of new cases of a disease occurring in a population in relation to the number of persons at risk for developing the disease:

$$\text{Incidence rate} = \frac{\text{Number of persons developing a disease}}{\text{Total number at risk}} \times 100$$

Incidence rates are usually stated in terms of a definite time period, such as one year. For example, if 200 people resided at a nursing home during a given year and 10 of them developed influenza, then the incidence rate for influenza during that year would be $(10 \div 200) \times 100 = 5\%$.

The *attack rate* is a type of incidence rate used to describe epidemics. It is appropriate when the population is at risk for a limited time period only and the study period incorporates the entire epidemic. If 40 residents ate a particular food and 25 developed diarrhea, the attack rate would be $(25 \div 40) \times 100 = 62.5\%$.

Another important epidemiologic rate is the *prevalence rate*, the proportion of persons with a disease at any given time relative to the total number of persons in the group:

$$\text{Prevalence rate} = \frac{\text{Number of persons with a disease}}{\text{Total number in the group}} \times 100$$

The prevalence rate provides a snapshot of a population relative to a disease at a certain point in time. For example, if a nursing home survey demonstrated that 30 residents had diarrhea on a particular day and there were 200 residents in the nursing home, then the prevalence rate of diarrhea in the nursing home at that time would be (30 ÷ 200) x 100 = 15%.

Infectious diseases may persist at a relatively constant level in the community (*endemic*) or may occur in significant excess of normal expectancy (*epidemic*). An infectious disease can be characterized by the number of existing cases in a population (prevalence), the number of new cases in a population (incidence), and the risk of transmission (contagiousness). These concepts are discussed further in Chapter 11.

Transmission of Infection

Transfer of an infectious agent may occur by either direct or indirect methods.[3] Direct contact between individuals is the method of spread of staphylococcal infections and syphilis. The fecal-oral route, a common mode of spread of infectious gastroenteritis, also involves direct-contact spread. Indirect spread involves an intermediate vehicle or vector (see Table 1.3). The list of common vehicles that have been implicated in the spread of infectious diseases is very long: Food, water, milk, blood products, intravenous fluids, drugs, medical equipment, and the hands of personnel may serve as vehicles of spread. Vector-borne spread of disease is relatively uncommon in the United States.

Airborne infectious agents may be spread on large droplets that are generated by talking and sneezing; measles, for example, is transmitted this way. Alternatively, airborne transmission may involve small-droplet nuclei or dust particles that remain suspended in the air for a prolonged period of time. A defective air-handling system may then result in widespread dissemination of the organism throughout the environment. For example, Legionnaires' disease has been transmitted by defective air-conditioning systems.

The spread of infectious diseases involves the following general sequence: *reservoir → means of transmission → host*. The reservoir may be humans (influenza), animals (tularemia), or the environment (Legionnaires' disease).

The most highly contagious diseases of humans are chickenpox, measles, influenza, rubella, mumps, and pneumonic plague. The risk of acquisition of disease by a nonimmune host after exposure is over 50% for these diseases. In contrast, a number of diseases that are widely feared are not highly contagious, including leprosy, meningococcal meningitis, diphtheria, tuberculosis, and AIDS.

Nosocomial Infections

Nosocomial infections, in reference to nursing homes, are those infections that develop in the nursing home or are produced by microorganisms acquired during residence in the nursing home. When describing infections quantitatively, raw numbers are often misleading, and one prefers to describe an infection rate which is the number of infections per unit of population per unit of time.[4]

The *nosocomial infection rate* is the proportion of nosocomial infections in a given period of time relative to the number of residents at risk; the latter is best reflected by the number of residents in the nursing home during the given time period (usually one month). Alternatively, the infection rate may be more accurately calculated by using resident-days for the measurement of number at risk (denominator).

For example, if a nursing home has an average census of 200 residents during a 30-day month and 20 nosocomial infections were diagnosed in residents during that time, then the monthly nosocomial infection rate is either

---

Table 1.3 *Transmission of Infection*

MEANS OF TRANSMISSION	EXAMPLE
Direct contact	
Surface contact	Staphylococci
Percutaneous inoculation	Hepatitis B
Fecal-oral spread	Hepatitis A
Common vehicle	
Food	Salmonellosis
Water	Giardiasis
Contaminated equipment	*Pseudomonas aeruginosa*
Insect vector	
Mosquito	St. Louis encephalitis
Airborne	
Common source	Legionnaires' disease
Person-to-person	Influenza

$$\frac{20 \text{ infections}}{200 \text{ residents}} \times 100 = 10\%$$

or

$$\frac{20 \text{ infections}}{200 \text{ residents x } 30 \text{ days}} \times 1000$$

$$= 3.3 \text{ nosocomial infections per 1000 resident-days}$$

Nosocomial infection rates are discussed further in Chapter 10, and Chapter 9 lists reference sources that expand upon the basic concepts covered in this chapter.

REFERENCES

1. Norman DC, Grahn D, Yoshikawa TT: Fever and aging. *J Am Geriatr Soc* 1985;33:859–63.
2. Balows A: Manual of Clinical Microbiology, 5th ed., Washington, DC American Society for Microbiology, 1991.
3. Brachman PS: Epidemiology of nosocomial infections, in Bennett JV, Brachman PS (eds): *Hospital Infections*, 2nd ed. Boston, Little, Brown, 1986;3–16.
4. Friedman GD: *Primer of Epidemiology*, 3rd ed. New York, McGraw-Hill, 1987.

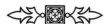

CHAPTER

IMMUNITY IN THE ELDERLY

Jane F. Potter

Immunity originally referred to the resistance of people to infection by bacteria and viruses. Severe immune deficiency diseases, such as AIDS, provide convincing evidence that an intact immune system is crucial for an individual's successful interaction with the environment. Although older people do not experience anything approaching the difficulty seen in AIDS patients, they clearly experience greater morbidity and mortality from infectious diseases.

Deficits in immune function and host defense mechanisms are easy to demonstrate in aged persons. However, as is true in other areas of clinical aging research, it is often difficult to be certain whether or not aging per se or other factors have the most important effect on immune function. In addition, most physiologic functions are more variable the older the age of the individuals studied. In fact, one finds highly immune competent individuals among the very elderly and much younger individuals with compromised levels of function.

Nevertheless, the incidence of infection, cancer, and autoimmune phenomenon increase dramatically with age. It is therefore helpful for clinicians to consider the average older person as less immune competent than a younger counterpart. The average older person who develops an infectious disease such as influenza has a greater risk of pneumonia and death. Death rates from many infectious diseases increase with age.

This chapter examines how normal immune function protects against disease, how age-related changes in the immune system impair the body's normal defense against infectious diseases, and how other common disorders of old age predispose the aged person to infection.

THE NORMAL IMMUNE SYSTEM

The immune system is essential to host defense, but it is not the only important element in this activity. Included in this brief discussion is a review of the basic elements that comprise the normal defense against infection. For a detailed description of the immune system, the reader is referred to recent texts.[1,2]

The major organs and cells involved in defense against infection and their functions are presented diagrammatically in Figure 2.1. On the first line of defense are *polymorphonuclear leukocytes*, as well as a variety of serum factors, natural killer cells, and monocytes. An intact and functioning first defense is critical, as development of an immune reaction takes time. The polymorphonuclear leukocyte (PMN) originates in the bone marrow and travels to sites of infection, where (by a process called *phagocytosis*) it ingests bacteria and cells that have been damaged by the infection. Once bacteria have been phagocytosed, they are killed by the PMNs' intracellular enzymes. When PMNs engulf large numbers of bacteria and necrotic tissue, they also eventually die. After several days, a cavity containing varying portions of necrotic tissue and dead PMNs (*pus*) is often

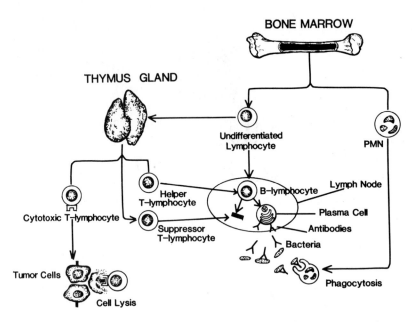

Figure 2.1 *Primary tissues and cells of the normal immune system. The bone marrow is the source of undifferentiated lymphocytes, polymorphonuclear leukocytes (PMNs), and macrophages (not shown). Undifferentiated lymphocytes travel to either the thymus gland where they are transformed into T cells or to lymph tissue where they become B cells. Under stimulation by antigens, cytotoxic T lymphocytes learn to recognize tumor cells (or cells transformed by infection) that they then destroy, a process called cell lysis. When antigens are detected by B lymphocytes, these cells change into plasma cells that produce antibodies capable of recognizing the antigen on the bacterial cell. Antibodies attach to the bacteria, which are then rendered susceptible to phagocytosis by PMNs.*

excavated in the inflamed tissues. Monocytes also capture organisms through phagocytosis, but they function much better if the organism has been coated with antibodies produced as part of the immune response (see below).

It may take several days to weeks to develop an effective immune response. Considerable harm can occur during this first exposure. However, if the individual survives, on subsequent exposure the same invading organism will be quickly stopped before much harm is done.

The tissues on which adequate immune function relies include the lymph nodes, bone marrow, spleen, tonsils, thymus, and localized lymph tissues in the gastrointestinal and respiratory tracts. These tissues provide cells that either control the immune response, provide cell-mediated immunity, or become antibody producing plasma cells.

The thymus gland, located in the base of the neck, is essential to development of an effective immune system early in life. This gland is large in the fetus and newborn and atrophies (or involutes) during midlife.

T-cells are so named because they depend on influences from the thymus for their development. The T-cell line is important in regulation and highly differentiated to do this job. Some subclasses of T-cells function to induce or help B-cells; others suppress the immune response. *B-cells* can also be subdivided into those whose primary purpose is to secrete immunoglobulin (antibodies) and others that provide memory for a time when the antigen is present again. As shown in Figure 2.1, interaction between the elements is either through direct contact or through factors secreted by the cells into the serum.

The immune system is activated by exposure to an invading agent (i.e., a bacteria or virus). The immune system recognizes a portion of the invading agent (the *antigen*) as foreign. The process whereby an antigen is recognized is

Table 2.1   *The Effect of Age on the Immune System*

IMMUNE SYSTEM	FUNCTION	AGE-RELATED CHANGE
Thymus gland	Transform undifferentiated lymphocytes into T-cells	Involution, decreased production of thymic hormones
B-lymphocyte	Produce antibodies	Decreased levels of specific antibody production, increased autoantibodies, increased incidence of monoclonal proteins
T-lymphocyte	Help or suppress B-cell function; cytotoxic reactions	Decreased mature T-cells, decreased proliferation to mitogen, diminished delayed hypersensitivity, decreased cell-mediated cytotoxicity
PMN	Phagocytosis	Decreased proportion with effective phagocytosis
Macrophage	Process antigen	Decreased fever response, decreased proliferation

fairly complex and may involve B-cells, T-cells, and macrophages. Once the original recognition of an antigen occurs, the continuing presence of antigen drives T- and B-cells in an immune response, which consists of T-cells helping to increase the activity of the response. In addition, B-cells move into an antibody synthesizing mode and are known as *plasma cells*. The plasma cells synthesize protein molecules known as *antibodies,* which are directed specifically against the invading organisms; the antibodies are then released from the plasma cell and attach to the invading bacteria. Presence of antibody on the organism facilitates elimination of the invading organism through phagocytosis. B-lymphocytes are stimulated to produce antibodies by most common pyogenic bacteria (see Fig. 2.1). Because B-lymphocytes express their effects through secretion of an active humor (antibodies), the function of these B-cells is referred to as *humoral immunity.* The response continues until the amount of antigen declines, at which time T-suppressor cells help to shut down the response. However,

memory B-cells are able to respond rapidly should that antigen reappear.

THE EFFECTS OF AGE ON HOST DEFENSES

Each of the defense mechanisms just described undergoes some degree of change related to age.[3] These are clinically important changes and very likely explain at least some of the increased morbidity and mortality from infectious disease experienced by older people. Changes in the immune system with age occur in both man and other species. These changes are so closely linked to aging that one theory suggests that they somehow regulate the aging process.[4]

The important changes that occur in cell-mediated immunity with age are summarized in Table 2.1. The number of mature T-cells declines with age, and those cells that remain are less responsive to invading organisms. Production of antibodies specific for the invading organism also declines as a function of age.

PMNs and Monocytes

The total number of white cells in the blood stream (PMNs, lymphocytes, etc.) is relatively constant for a given individual and does not change with age. However, it has been observed that the white blood cell count declines in the two or three years immediately prior to death. This decline occurs before any overt sign of illness can be detected.[5]

Although not technically part of the immune system, the PMNs are critical first-line defenders against infection. The numbers of PMNs and their ability to chemically kill ingested organisms does not change with age; however, the number that are able to phagocytose organisms does decline with age.[6] Whether or not this is a clinically relevant change is uncertain. Changes in monocyte function with age are less well studied. In those laboratory studies that have been done, there is not uniformity of opinion on what, if any, changes occur.[7] The fact that many older people have a decreased fever response (a monocyte-mediated phenomenon) and the fact that monocytes tend not to proliferate as well in the laboratory suggest that there are important age-associated changes in this cell system.[3]

T-Lymphocytes

There is a progressive involution of the thymus gland after puberty. Therefore, the observation that aging is associated with both thymus involution and the development of important defects in the thymus dependent (T-cell) lymphocyte system has led to speculation that these two phenomena are related.[7]

With age there is a decline in the number of mature T-lymphocytes.[8] A major job of the T-lymphocyte is to get an immune response going by causing other lymphocytes to proliferate. In the laboratory this process is measured as the T-cell response to a special type of foreign protein called a *mitogen*. One of the most marked changes in immune response with age is the reduced ability of lymphocytes from old humans to proliferate in response to a mitogen. Other studies suggest that the lack of responsiveness is a result of the T-cell producing fewer of the necessary molecular messengers. Learning precisely where the problem

lies may some day lead to therapies directed at the underlying defect.

There appears to be an age-related defect in the ability to shut down immune reactions. Whether this is due to a change in the number or the activity of regulatory T-cells is still an area of study. These changes are likely responsible for the increase in antibodies directed against self (autoantibodies) seen in older persons (see autoimmunity, following).

Delayed hypersensitivity is a reaction by T-cells to an antigen injected into the skin and requires prior exposure to that antigen. Activity of T-cells can also be measured by skin tests to common antigens. A skin test reaction to the antigen is assessed as an area of induration around the injection site. Active T-cells are necessary for development of a positive skin test (delayed hypersensitivity). Early clinical studies (which often involved nursing home patients) suggested that those persons reacted to fewer skin test antigens (e.g., mumps, *Candida*, or purified protein derivative-[PPD]) than younger people.[7] More recent studies of healthier older persons suggest that skin reactivity to common antigens is maintained in old age, although the area of induration from a positive test does decline as a function of age. False-negative skin test reactivity to tuberculosis is quite uncommon even among nursing home residents, a finding that differs from earlier studies.[9]

B-lymphocytes

When older people are experimentally injected with an antigen from *Salmonella* (a common causative organism for diarrhea), antibodies specific for that organism are produced at a lower level than in younger people.[10] Lower levels of specific antibody response to other antigens have been seen as well,[11] which suggests that older people have impaired ability to defend themselves against infection with certain organisms. The antibody response is most impaired the first time the older individual is exposed to an antigen. Antibody production is better and more like that seen in younger persons on the second or subsequent exposures. The etiology of this age-related reduction in specific antibody production is less clear. Whatever the mechanism, there is an apparent increase in susceptibility of older persons to infection with pyogenic bacteria and a higher mortality when such infections occur.

Common disorders of B-cells seen in elderly persons involve excess production of antibodies. These disorders probably result from some loss of regulatory control of terminal B-cell differentiation. The most lethal example of this process is the disease multiple myeloma. In this disorder, the person produces one specific portion of an antibody at very high levels and shuts off production of normal antibodies. Fortunately, multiple myeloma is rare; however, production of lesser amounts of excess antibody (monoclonal proteins) is quite common. This condition is referred to as benign monoclonal gammopathy or monoclonal gammopathy of uncertain significance.[12] About 10% of cases progress to a cancerous process, usually during the first year after diagnosis. There is also some risk that high levels of these monoclonal proteins can shut off immunoglobulin production.

Autoimmunity

Normally, the immune system only produces antibodies or sensitized lymphocytes against undesirable invaders such as bacteria or cancer cells. The immune system recognizes normal cells and protects them from attack by T-cells and antibodies. When the system for recognition of normal cells breaks down, T-cells and antibodies (*autoantibodies*) begin to attack the body's own cells. The disorders wherein the immune system reacts against the body's own cells are called *autoimmune* phenomena. Autoantibodies directed at thyroid, gastric, and smooth muscle cells and at cell nuclei increase with age and are present in 50% of older people.[7] In some cases, these autoantibodies may lead to problems, as for example when the gastric cells are destroyed and the stomach no longer produces acid, or when the thyroid gland is damaged and hypothyroidism occurs. However, more often than not, the presence of autoantibodies is asymptomatic, and studies have shown that autoantibodies do not increase mortality above that expected.[7]

A special type of autoantibody, called an anti-idiotype antibody, is directed at another antibody. These act as signals to help shut off the production of antibodies and also are felt to have some role in autoimmune disease.[13] Anti-idiotype antibodies are increased in aged persons,[14] however, their role and significance have yet to be defined with certainty.

Immunization

A person's first exposure to an infectious agent is the most damaging and may result in serious injury to the infected tissue or in death. On subsequent exposure to the same infectious agent, the immune system responds more quickly to control the infection. Unfortunately, many viruses (e.g., influenza) and bacteria (e.g., *Streptococcus pneumoniae*) come in many different strains, and the individual must be exposed to each strain in order to develop immunity to that disease.

Immunity to some infectious agents can be induced by exposing an individual to very small amounts of antigen (a vaccine), a process called *immunization*. The antigen (usually a protein from a bacteria or virus) stimulates either B- or T-cells in a manner similar to that seen when a person is infected with the live organism. The immunity induced by immunization is usually not as long-lasting as that resulting from active infection, and repeat immunization may be necessary.

Legitimate concern could be expressed regarding the use of vaccines in older people because of the age-related changes in immune system function. The antibody response to many antigens decreases with age, and T-cell responses are generally decreased, both of which could impair the older person's ability to respond to a vaccine.[15] As a practical matter, vaccinations are probably better given when the immune response is more intact (i.e., at a younger age). This also explains why many studies show suboptimal response to influenza and pneumococcal vaccines. Work is being done to improve the results of vaccination in the elderly, which may eventually lead to special doses, boosting schedules, or immune enhancers to achieve a better response and greater protection. The vaccinations of importance for the elderly are discussed in Chapter 17.

UNDERLYING DISEASES AND DISORDERS THAT PREDISPOSE TO INFECTION

Disease is not a normal part of aging, but many diseases become increasingly prevalent with age, a fact that cannot be forgotten when dealing with the older population. In this section, consideration is given to age-related changes in physiology and disorders that interact with the changes in immune function and predispose persons to development of infectious diseases in old age. The conditions of importance here are either local disorders (see Table 2.2), which lead to infection at a single site or in a single organ

✦

Table 2.2   *Common Afflictions of Elderly People Associated with Impaired Local Resistance to Infection*

ORGAN SYSTEM	CONDITION COMMON IN ELDERLY PEOPLE
Gastrointestinal	Poor oral hygiene and dentition, lack of gastric acid
Skin	Skin thinning, ulceration, frequent trauma and superficial wounds
Nervous	Peripheral neuropathy, stroke
Urinary	Foley catheters, urinary retention
Respiratory	Abdominal breathing, decreased air exchange
Heart	Heart failure during stress

system, or systemic factors (see Table 2.3), which increase a person's susceptibility to a variety of different infections.

Local Factors

Oral Hygiene

Oral and dental problems are the rule rather than the exception in the elderly institutionalized population (16). Local infection of the gums (periodontal disease) can progress to localized abscess. Bacteria from dental infections or loose teeth may be aspirated to cause pneumonia or lung abscess. Poor oral hygiene (usually in combination with dehydration)

Table 2.3   *Systemic Factors That Predispose to Infections in Elderly People*

Diabetes mellitus
Calcified heart valves
Dehydration
Immobility
Hospitalization
Diminished pain sensitivity and atypical symptoms
Decreased mental status
Tumors
Malnutrition
Drugs

in a debilitated patient can precipitate parotid gland infection. Measures to prevent these problems include careful oral hygiene, regular dental care, appropriate treatment of periodontal infection, extraction of loose, nonfunctional teeth, and conscientious hydration.[16,17]

Gastric Acid

The stomach is lined with cells (gastric parietal cells) that secrete acid. Acid production aids in digestion and also kills bacteria that are swallowed along with food. Aging results in a loss of gastric acid production due to a decline in parietal cell mass.[18] By 70 years of age, 30% of people have lost the ability to secrete stomach acid and, although it does not cause important problems with digestion, this allows bacteria to enter the upper part of the gut and initiate infection. As an example, *Salmonella* is a bacterium that is a common cause of epidemic diarrheal illness in institutions. In order to be infected with *Salmonella*, a person with normal stomach acid must ingest between 100,000 and 1,000,000 organisms.[19] When fewer organisms are ingested, they will be killed by the stomach acid. Persons who do not produce gastric acid will be infected when exposed to far fewer organisms. For reasons that are not clear, there is an association between gastric resection and reactivation of previously inactive tuberculosis.

Skin Ulcers

The rate at which the skin ages is directly related to the amount of ultraviolet (UV) light exposure.[20] People who have worked outdoors will experience premature aging of their skin. As the skin ages, both dermal and epidermal layers become thinner, skin collagen loses strength, and skin elasticity is decreased. Even without extensive UV light exposure, these same changes occur as a part of normal aging. For these reasons skin tears more easily in old age, increasing the chance for skin infection. Thinning of the skin is one reason why older people are predisposed to decubitus ulcers, which can then become a site for local or systemic spread of infection (see Chapter 7). Care must be taken to handle fragile, aged skin carefully, to keep skin lesions clean and dry, and to give tetanus toxoid at appropriate intervals.

Skin ulcers also develop because of disease in either the arteries or veins. With age, veins become less elastic and enlarge in diameter, and venous valves are less effective at preventing back flow of blood. As a consequence, blood pools in the lower extremities, tissues swell, and blistering and skin breakdown follow. Venous stasis ulcers characteristically occur on the inner aspect of the ankle and, like any ulcer, can become infected. Both treatment and prevention require regular elevation of the extremities during the day as well as at night. Arteriosclerosis occurs to some extent in all older people. Severe vascular disease, however, rarely occurs in the absence of smoking, hypertension and/or lifelong lipid disorders. Vascular disease in the peripheral arteries leads to low blood flow and low oxygen levels in the skin. In the presence of ischemia, minor breaks in the skin and skin infection can threaten loss of that limb. Infection-fighting cells and antibodies reach these tissues in suboptimal quantities. Signs of poor blood flow are coolness of the extremity, decreased or absent pulses, lack of hair, and thick, overgrown toenails. When injury occurs to the feet or lower leg of patients with these physical findings, additional caution should be exercised. Prompt medical attention should be obtained if redness, warmth, or swelling develop, indicating the onset of infection.

A final contributing factor to skin breakdown and skin infection is nervous system disease. Peripheral nerve damage occurs from a variety of toxins (e.g., alcohol abuse), vitamin deficiency (e.g., vitamin B_{12}), or diabetes mellitus. Central nervous system damage most commonly occurs from strokes, but also from head trauma or spinal cord injury. Patients with these disorders lose sensation and are unaware of developing pressure sores. The only effective preventative measures are frequent rotation of the patient and frequent observation of body parts at risk.

Urinary Tract

The urinary tract is a very common site of infection in elderly people. A variety of conditions make the urinary tract susceptible to infections, including prostatic enlargement, urethral stricture, and neurogenic bladder. In elderly men, the prostate is often at fault; this gland is often enlarged in old age, sometimes due to cancer, but much more frequently due to benign growth (hyperplasia). When the prostate reaches sufficient size, it blocks the free flow of urine and a stagnant pool of urine develops. Bacteria migrate up the urethra and enter the bladder. Because the bladder does not completely empty, the urine becomes infected. A narrowing of the blocked urethra (stricture) can develop in both men and women and cause urinary tract infection by the same mechanism as prostatic obstruction. In women, the loss of estrogen at menopause results in thinning of the urethral epithelium and loss of protection against bacteria that migrate from the perineum to the urethra and bladder.

A third problem that predisposes to bladder infection is degeneration of the nerves that produce bladder emptying (neurogenic bladder). Bladder catheters provide a direct route for spread of infection from the collection bag into the bladder and/or prostate gland. A detailed discussion of urinary tract infection is given in Chapter 6.

Pulmonary Function

The respiratory tract is one of the two most common sites of serious infection in older persons. Several important age-related changes in the lungs and chest wall predispose older people to chest infections. In order to defend against infection, the lungs must take in and release air efficiently. Movement of the rib cage during inspiration draws air into the lungs, and rib cage mobility decreases as people grow older.[21] The older person compensates to a degree for the loss of rib cage mobility by using abdominal muscles.[22] However, when the older patient is put to bed or confined to a wheelchair, the abdominal muscles are no longer effective in expanding the lungs. Unless an older person comes to a standing position, the lungs do not expand well, atelectasis develops, and bacteria or viruses can set up infection. Important measures to prevent pneumonia are having the older person assume an upright posture and encouraging the patient to cough and breathe deeply. Bed rest is to be avoided, as this is even more deleterious to the aged respiratory system.

Not only are the lungs of older people less efficient at intake of air, they are also less efficient at air release. Movement of air out of the lungs normally occurs because elastic tissue in the lung springs back, forcing air out of the lung. There is an age-related loss of lung elastic tissue,[23] so many of the airways in the lower poles of the lung are closed during most or all of the respiratory cycle. This accounts for the fact that an 80-year-old person has 50% more air left in the lung at the end of expiration than a 25-year-old.[24] Air trapped in the lung exchanges with inspired air very slowly and is lower in oxygen content. The increase in the amount of air trapped in the lung is a primary reason why blood oxygen decreases with age. Normally this lower blood oxygen is well tolerated by the older person, but it does lower the reserve oxygen available should pneumonia develop. Lower blood oxygen in combination with immune system abnormalities may account for the increased mortality seen in older patients with pneumonia.

A final aging change that increases risk of lung infection is decreased mucociliary clearance. Mucus normally moves up the respiratory tract, carrying with it bacteria, viruses, and particulate matter. The speed of movement of mucus up the tract is slower in older persons, a fact that likely predisposes to infection.

Circulation

Aging is associated with structural and functional changes at most levels of the vascular system.[25] The arterial wall becomes less compliant, systolic blood pressure rises somewhat, and the myocardium hypertrophies. Very healthy and carefully selected older persons are able to achieve high levels of cardiac output during exercise. Less select (more typical) older persons experience a decline in cardiac output during exercise (a type of stress). This later observation probably explains why some older persons, without known or clinically apparent heart disease, develop heart failure during stress from fever, surgery, and so on. In addition to what may be a normal aging predisposition to heart failure, a relatively high proportion of persons have heart disease and chronic congestive failure. Heart failure increases in prevalence with age and affects between four and ten times more people over 75 years old than those aged between 45 and 65 years.[26,27] People with heart failure are particularly prone to infections of the lower respiratory tract, possibly due to defects in oxygenation and perfusion of the edematous lung.

Systemic Factors

In addition to local disorders, certain diseases, drugs, and common problems predispose older people to a variety of infections. These systemic factors interact with impaired immune function and local disorders to further increase a person's risk for infection.

Diabetes

Diabetes mellitus is an extremely common disorder of old age. Using conservative criteria for the diagnosis of diabetes, between 6% and 20% of people over 65 years old suffer from this disorder.[28] The diabetic has an increased risk of infection for a variety of reasons. The immune system cells of diabetics do not efficiently phagocytose infectious particles due to a defect in T-lymphocyte function.[29] In addition, high glucose levels in tissues create a rich breeding ground for microorganisms. Diabetics have an accelerated form of vascular disease and are at particular risk for infection in the lower extremities. In addition, the diabetic state is associated with infection in soft tissues, the oral cavity, sinuses, kidney, meninges, bone, joints, and a variety of other sites.[30]

Heart Disease

Some abnormality of the heart is found at autopsy in 75% of people over 75 years of age.[31] Certain types of heart disease occur almost exclusively in older people. Of these, calcification of the mitral and aortic heart valves are the most common.[26] Calcium is deposited in the heart valves after years of wear and tear from constant opening and closing. Valves that do not move normally are further damaged, and when bacteria are present in the bloodstream (bacteremia), those damaged valves become infected (bacterial endocarditis). Calcification of the aortic and mitral valves is one reason why older people account for a high percentage of all cases of bacterial endocarditis.[27]

Dehydration

The patient who becomes dehydrated is at risk for infections in any of the body's normal secretory or excretory sites. The lung's bronchial tree normally secretes a small amount of mucus that then moves upward along the bronchi to remove inspired bacteria and particles. In a similar manner, free flow of urine limits the amount of bacterial growth in a urinary tract with a low-grade infection. In the absence of obstruction, the parotid gland remains free of infection as long as adequate hydration insures a free flow of saliva. In any of these systems, dehydration decreases secretions and allows infection to develop.

Immobility

The immobile patient is predisposed to infection because of changes induced in the skin, veins, and lungs. Perhaps the most frequent problem in such patients is development of pressure sores over bony prominences such as the buttocks, elbows, and feet. A second very common problem is stasis edema in the lower extremities. Normal venous return from the legs occurs when muscles contract and force blood upward toward the heart. Immobile muscles do not perform this important pumping action, blood pools in veins, and fluid seeps from the engorged veins into the surrounding tissues. Most immobile patients will have some degree of edema in their legs. This type of edema is not the result of an excess in total body fluid and should not be treated with diuretics. To prevent edema from leading to skin breakdown, the primary treatment is elevation of the legs and use of elastic stockings.

Effects of Hospitalization

Twenty percent of people over 65 are hospitalized each year,[32] and this figure is very likely higher for the more disabled residents of long-term care facilities. Hospitalization in acute care facilities predisposes to infection in several important ways. Antibiotics, which are commonly used during hospitalization, destroy the normal bacteria that live in and on the body and allow those bacteria to be replaced with antibiotic-resistant and infection-producing bacteria. Intravenous catheters and solutions become infected and seed bacteria directly into the bloodstream. Finally, proximity to other infected patients increases the possibility that infection will be transmitted to the uninfected person. As increasingly ill patients who require complex treatments are cared for in nursing facilities, these same factors are becoming important in development and spread of infection. This problem is examined in detail in Chapter 4.

Symptoms in the Elderly

Diminished pain sensitivity, atypical symptoms, and decreased mental status can hamper diagnosis while a disease is at an early stage and before serious infection develops. In clinical settings, older persons report less pain.[33] Symptoms in the elderly are often different than in young people, and, as a rule, symptoms in older people are less specific.[34] Between 75% and 78% of residents in long-term care facilities are demented[35] and therefore have some difficulty describing symptoms. Not infrequently, the only sign of illness in the resident is a further decrease in mental status. It is obviously important that the staff of long-term care facilities report such changes and obtain a medical evaluation for the resident.

Malignancy

One half of all cancers develop after 65 years of age.[36] Each of the major classes of malignancies produce specific defects that predispose to infection. Treatment of cancer can also increase infectious complications in these patients.[37]

Nutrition

Excluding the immune dysfunction of old age, malnutrition is probably the most common cause of impaired immunity in adults. Malnutrition is very common in both hospitalized and institutionalized elderly persons.[38] Identification of the malnourished patient and classification as to the type of malnutrition present can be carried out by obtaining a nutritional history, body measurements, and a few simple laboratory tests. There are basically two types of malnutrition. In malnutrition with calorie deficiency but adequate protein intake (sometimes called *marasmus*), patients are underweight and have low fat stores, decreased muscle mass, and normal levels of serum proteins. In the second type, malnutrition with protein deficiency but adequate caloric intake (sometimes called *kwashiorkor*), patients have normal or even increased body weight, decreased skeletal muscle protein, and decreased serum protein levels (see Table 2.4).

Weight loss is present in both types of malnutrition. Even a small weight loss is important when it occurs over a short period of time.[39] Loss of 2% of body weight over two weeks' time, or 10% in six months, leads to a malnourished

Table 2.4 *Detection and Classification of Malnutrition in the Elderly Patient*

TEST	NORMAL	MALNUTRITION OF	
		CALORIES	PROTEIN
Body mass index (BMI)[a]			
Male or female	24.9–28.9	↓	− → ↓
Over 60 years			
Triceps skinfold thickness (mm)[b]			
Male	> 5.0	↓	− → ↑
Female	>12.0	↓	− → ↑
Arm muscle circumference (cm)[b]			
Male	>20.5	↓	↓
Female	>19.5	↓	↓
Serum albumin (g/dl)	> 3.5	→ −	↓

[a] Age-specific Gerontology Research Center recommendations. [43]

[b] Lower 5th percentile values for individuals aged 65–74 years in the 1970 U.S. DHHS health and nutrition examination survey. [46]

state. Table 2.4 summarizes the other important measurements in the detection and classification of malnourished patients. The body mass index (BMI) is an index of body weight that has been adjusted for the fact that taller people weigh more. The body mass index is calculated by dividing the patient's weight in kilograms by the square of the height in meters (weight/height²). If the person is unable to stand, there are techniques for using arm length, ankle–knee height or wing span to estimate full height.[40]

Several studies suggest that higher body mass is not detrimental and in fact may be beneficial to older persons.[41,42] The recommended normal/acceptable range of BMI in Table 2.4 are based on data from persons of both sexes aged 60–69 years.[43] Although information on persons older than 70 is more limited, there is no reason to think that it is lower (thinner) than this range.

A second important parameter of nutritional state is the triceps skinfold thickness, which correlates fairly well with total body fat stores. This measurement, which can be done by most dieticians, is performed by measuring the thickness of the fat overlying the midpoint of the upper arm. The triceps skinfold thickness in women and the subscapular skinfold thickness in men provide estimates of the total amount of fat in the body. Midarm muscle circumference is an index of muscle mass that predicts mortality in the elderly.[44] This parameter is calculated by subtracting one half the triceps's skinfold thickness from the total arm circumference.[45,46]

The patient who is consuming inadequate amounts of protein will mobilize protein from the skeletal muscle in order to maintain serum protein at normal levels. Once the skeletal muscle protein stores have been exhausted, serum protein will also fall. Skeletal protein can also be burned as energy and will be utilized during times of low caloric intake. Serum albumin is the laboratory test most commonly used to evaluate the level of serum protein. A serum albumin below 3.5 is abnormal and in the absence of liver disease usually indicates a state of protein malnutrition. Once albumin falls below 3.5, the state of protein nutrition is advanced. The immune malfunction that occurs in malnourished patients depends on whether calories or protein are in short supply. Malnutrition produces many of the same changes in immune function seen with aging. The immune defects of malnutrition involve lymphocytes and polymorphonuclear leukocytes.[47]

Drugs

An important factor that alters immune function in the elderly is the use of multiple medications.[48] Those drugs that impinge on immune function most directly are those that are designed to do so, such as steroids and antineoplastic agents. These drugs are powerful modulators of the immune response. Steroids cause a redistribution of lymphocytes from the circulation into other body compartments, which renders the cells less accessible to sites of infection and immune reactivity. The effect of steroids on PMNs is to prevent these cells from migrating out of the vascular system into sites of inflammation and infection. In addition to the effect on the migration of immunologically active cells, steroids also reduce the functional activity of those cells. Almost every step of the immune process is affected, including antigen processing, phagocytosis, and cytotoxic T-cell function. Almost all cancer chemotherapeutic agents nonspecifically lower the immune response. This is accomplished by a direct attack on all immunologically active cells.

Certain drugs such as aspirin, common nonsteroidal anti-inflammatory agents, theophylline, and propranolol alter laboratory tests of immune function. However, there is no evidence that these drugs alter the course of infectious diseases.

SUMMARY

The three major classes of cells involved in defense against infection are macrophages, lymphocytes, and polymorphonuclear leukocytes (PMNs). These cells interact with one another to control the first infection with a given organism and to retain a memory (immunity) that prevents future infection with the same organism.

There is some decline in immune function with age, especially in antibody production and cell-mediated immunity. Even though antibody response to vaccination is often lower in older people, sufficient levels of antibodies are generally attained to achieve protection from disease.

Some age-related changes in physiology and many diseases and drugs interact with immune system deficits to further predispose the aged person to the development of infections. The physiologic changes of concern are reduc- ed gastric acid production, dermal atrophy, venous dilation, decreased rib cage mobility, reduced mucociliary clearance, and thinning of the urethral epithelium. Pathologic changes that predispose infection include loss of sensory function, urinary retention, and calcification of heart valves. Diabetes mellitus, malnutrition, tumors, and drugs all interact directly with one or more of the immune system's cells to predispose elderly people to a wide variety of infections. Either under- or overhydration predisposes to infection by impairing the normal mechanisms for clearing bacteria from the body's secretory and excretory sites. Decreased mental status is common in residents of long-term care facilities and, in combination with the atypical symptoms of many diseases in old age, often impairs our ability to diagnose infectious diseases at an early stage.

REFERENCES

1. Kuby J (ed): *Immunology*, New York, W.H. Freeman, 1992.

2. Roitt IM, Brostoff J, Male DK (eds): *Immunology*, New York, Gower, 1989.

3. Adler WH, Nagel JE: Clinical immunology, in Hazzard WR, Andres R, Bierman EL, Blass JP (eds): *Principles of Geriatric Medicine and Gerontology*, 2nd ed. New York, McGraw-Hill, pp 60–71, 1990.

4. Walford RL, Gottesman SRS, Weindruch RH, et al: Immunopathology of aging, in Eisdorfer C (ed): *Annual Review of Gerontology and Geriatrics*. New York, Springer, 1981, p 3.

5. Bender BS, Nagel JE, Adler WH, et al: Absolute peripheral blood lymphocyte count and subsequent mortality in elderly men: The Baltimore Longitudinal Study of Aging. *J Am Geriatr Soc* 1986;34:649–654.

6. Nagel JE, Pyle RS, Chrest FJ, et al: Oxidative metabolism and bacteriocidal capacity of polymorphonuclear leukocytes from normal young and aged adults. *J Gerontol* 1986;37:529–534.

7. Hausman DB, Weksler ME: Changes in the immune response with age, in Fitch CE, Schneider EL (eds): *Handbook of the Biology of Aging*, New York, Van Nostrand Rehold,1985.

8. Jensen TL, Hallgren HM, Yasmineh WG, et al: Do immature T-cells accumulate in advanced age? *Mech Ageing Devel* 1986;33:237–245.

9. Stead WW, Lofgren JP, Warren E, et al: Tuberculosis as an endemic and nosocomial infection among the elderly in nursing homes. *N Engl J Med* 1985;312:1483–1487.

10. Antonaci S, Gallitelli M, Garofalo AR, et al: Functional properties of Salmonella minnesota Rb-bound and Rb-unbound cell fractions in elderly donors. *Diagn Clin Immunol* 1987;5(1):1–7.

11. Whisler RL, Williams, JW, Newhouse YG: Human B cell proliferative responses during aging: Reduced RNA synthesis and DNA replication after signal transduction by surface immunoglobulins compared to B cell antigenic determinants CD20 and CD40. *Mech Ageing Devel* 1991;61(2):209–222.

12. Zhu JZ, Juo TT, Wang HR: Analysis of 128 cases of multiple myeloma and 31 cases of monoclonal gammapathies of undetermined significance. *Chung Hua Nei Ko Tsa Chih* 1989;28(8):463–465.

13. Shoenfeld Y, Schwartz RS: Immunologic and genetic factors in autoimmune diseases. *N Engl J Med* 1984;311:1019–1029.

14. Garratty G. Effect of cell-bound proteins on the in vivo survival of circulating blood cells. *Gerontology* 1991;37(1–3):68–94.

15. Gross PA, Quinnan GV, Weksler ME, et al: Immunization of elderly people with high doses of influenza vaccine. *J Am Geriatr Soc* 1988;36:209–212.

16. Berkey DB, Berg RG, Ettinger RL, Meskin LH. Research review of oral health status and service use among institutionalized older adults in the United States and Canada. *Spec Care Dentist* 1991;11(4):131–136.

17. Dolan TA, Monopoli MP, Kaurich MJ, et al: Geriatric grand rounds: Oral diseases in older adults. *J Am Geriatr Soc* 1990;38:1239–1250.

18. Nelson JB, Castell DO: Aging of the gastrointestinal system, in Hazzard WR, Andres R, Bierman EL, et al (eds): *Principles of Geriatric Medicine and Gerontology*, 2nd ed. New York, McGraw-Hill, 1990, p 596.

19. Hood EW, Johnson WD: Nontyphoidal salmonellosis, in Hoeprich PD (ed): *Infectious Diseases*, New York, Harper & Row, 1972, pp 583–591.

20. Dalziel KL: Aspects of cutaneous ageing. *Clin Exp Dermatol* 1991;16(5):315–323.

21. Mittman C, Edelman HN, Norris AH, et al: Relationship between chest wall and pulmonary compliance and age. *J Appl Physiol* 1965;20:1211–1216.

22. Rizzato G, Marrazini L: Thoracoabdominal mechanics in elderly men. *J Appl Physiol* 1970;28:457–460.

23. Turner JM, Mead J, Wohl ME: Elasticity of human lungs in relation to age. *J Appl Physiol* 1968;25:664–671.

24. Jones RL, Overton TR, Hammerlindl DM, et al: Effects of age on regional residual volume. *J Appl Physiol* 1978;44(2):195–199.

25. Lakatta EG: Changes in cardiovascular function with aging. *Eur Heart J* 1992;11 (suppl C):22–29.

26. Chakko S, Kessler KM: Changes with aging as reflected in noninvasive cardiac studies. *Cardiovasc Clin* 1992;22(2):35–47.

27. Wenger NK, O'Rourke RA, Marcus FI: The care of elderly patients with cardiovascular disease. *Ann Intern Med* 1988;109(5):425–428.

28. Harris MI: Epidemiology of diabetes mellitus among elderly in the United States. *Clin Geriatr Med* 1990;6:703–719.

29. Kolterman OG, Olefsky JM, Jurahara C, et al: A defect in cell-mediated immune function in insulin-resistant diabetic and obese subject. *J Lab Clin Med* 1980;96:535–543.

30. Froom J: Diabetes mellitus in the elderly. *Clin Geriatr Med* 1990;6:691–693.

31. Noble RJ, Rothbaum DA: History and physical examination, in Noble RJ, Rothbaum DA (eds): *Geriatric Cardiology*. Philadelphia, Davis, 1981, pp 55–63.

32. Coroni-Huntley J, Brock DB, Ostfeld AM, et al (eds): *Established Populations for Epidemiologic Studies of the Elderly*. NIH Publication No. 86-2443, Resource Data Book U.S. Department of Health and Human Services, Public Health Service, 1986, p 214.

33. Crook J, Rideout E, Browne G: The prevalence of pain complaints in a general population. *Pain* 1984;18:299.

34. Eberle CM, Besdine RW. Disease in old age, in Fulmer TT, Walker MK (eds): *Critical Care Nursing of the Elderly*. Springer, New York, 1992, pp 48–60.

35. Truax BT: Selected neurological problems in the nursing home, in Katz P, Calkins E (eds): *Principles and Practice of Nursing Home Care*. Springer, New York, 1989, p 358.

36. Baranovsky A, Myers MH: Cancer incidence and survival in patients 65 years of age and older. *CA* 1986;36:26.

37. Gallis HA: Infections in elderly cancer patients. *Clin Geriatr Med* 1987;3:549–560.

38. Lipschitz DA: Malnutrition in the elderly. *Semin Dermatol* 1991;10(4):273–281.

39. Blackburn GL, Harvey KB: Nutritional assessment as a routine in clinical medicine. *Postgrad Med* 1982;71:46–63.

40. Mitchell C, Lipschitz D: Arm length measurement as an alternative to height in nutritional assessment of the elderly. *J Parenter Enteral Nutr* 1982;6:226.

41. Potter JF, Schafer DF, Bohi RL: In-hospital mortality as a function of body mass index: An age-dependent variable. *J Gerontol* 1988;43:M59–63.

42. Tuomilehto J: Body mass index and prognosis in elderly hypertensive patients: A report from the European Working Party on High Blood Pressure in the Elderly. *Am J Med* 1991;90(3A):34S–41S.

43. Andres R, Elahi D, Tobin JD, et al: Impact of age and weight standards. *Ann Intern Med* 1985;103:1030–1033.

44. Friedman PJ, et al: Prospective trial of a new diagnostic criterion for severe wasting malnutrition in the elderly. *Age Ageing* 1985;14:149.

45. Vague J, Boyer J, Jubelin J, et al: Adipomuscular ratio in human subjects, in Vague J, Denton RM (eds): *Physiopathology of Adipose Tissue*, Proceedings of the Third International Meeting of Endocrinologists, Amsterdam, Excerpta Medica Foundation, 1969, pp 360–386.

46. *Skinfolds, Body Girths, Biacromial Diameter, and Selected Anthropometric Indices of Adults, United States, 1960–1962*, Publication No. 1000, Series 11, No. 35. U.S. Department of Health, Education, and Welfare, National Center for Health Statistics, 1970.

47. Lipschitz DA: Nutrition, aging, and the immunohematopoeitic system. *Clin Geriatr Med* 1987;3(2):319–328.

48. Hadden JW: Immunopharmacology and immunotoxicology. *Adv Exp Med Biol* 1991;288:1–11

CHAPTER

INFECTIONS IN
THE ELDERLY

Brenda A. Nurse and Richard A. Garibaldi

It is a common assumption that susceptibility to infection increases as we grow older. Although this statement is probably true, specific data to document its validity are difficult to find. There is little disagreement, however, that clinicians are frequently faced with diagnostic and therapeutic problems in managing infections in the elderly. Infections are often the terminal event in the life of an elderly patient with multiple, chronic medical problems. This chapter reviews the pathophysiology of infections in the elderly, outlines why infections are so difficult to diagnose and treat in this population, and describes some of the latest approaches to managing infections at specific sites.

PATHOPHYSIOLOGY

The data that the aging process alone makes us more prone to infection are controversial. Even though there are subtle age-related changes in the immune system (see Chapter 2), these changes are not sufficient to explain the increased risk for infection.[1]

Despite the relative preservation of immune function in the elderly, there is little doubt that physiologic changes associated with aging and the presence of comorbid chronic or acute diseases combine to impair host defenses and increase susceptibility to infection. For instance, even

seemingly healthy elderly persons may be at increased risk for pneumonia because of a diminished gag reflex, a less effective cough, and age-related decreases in mucociliary clearance mechanisms. Elderly women are susceptible to urinary tract infection (UTI) because of postmenopausal estrogen deficiency, changes in vaginal and periurethral colonization, and lax pelvic support structures. Other common conditions such as chronic constipation or the presence of cysto- or rectocele may further increase the risk of UTI by causing partial urinary obstruction and impaired bladder emptying. A similar problem is seen in males with age-related prostatic hypertrophy. Physiologic and pathologic deterioration in other organ systems predispose to focal infections at other sites. For instance, diminished skin elasticity and loss of subcutaneous fat make the elderly more susceptible to pressure sores and skin infections; gastric achlorhydria predisposes to diarrhea caused by bacterial pathogens; age-related aortic valvular calcification increases the risk for infective endocarditis.

In addition to the physiologic changes associated with aging, the presence of acute or chronic underlying diseases further increases the likelihood of infection. Those who smoke or have chronic pulmonary disease or congestive heart failure are at increased risk for pneumonia because of defects in the clearance of microorganisms from the respiratory tract. The risk of aspiration pneumonia is increased in patients with neurologic or esophageal disease as well as in those who use alcohol or sleeping pills. Any disease that obstructs urinary outflow results in incomplete bladde® emptying and an increased risk of urinary tract infection. This includes conditions and medications that decrease bladder tone as well as diseases that obstruct urinary flow on a mechanical basis. Finally, many medications that are commonly prescribed for the elderly, including tricyclic antidepressants, other anticholinergic drugs, antacids, H2 blockers, and steroids, have side effects that may impair specific host defenses and predispose to infection. Antibiotics that are prescribed as therapy or as prophylaxis for infection alter normal flora in the mouth, GI tract, and vagina, and select for bacteria that are antibiotic-resistant.

Elderly patients with increasing levels of debility due to chronic underlying diseases, particularly those who are institutionalized in nursing homes or hospitals, are at even higher risk of infection. These patients are often incontinent of stool or urine, nonambulatory, poorly responsive, and managed with invasive therapies. Female patients who are incontinent of feces will have increased perineal and periurethral colonization with enteric bacteria and are at increased risk for UTI. Nonambulatory incontinent patients frequently develop bedsores that can become secondarily infected. These patients often have alterations in mental function and are prone to aspiration pneumonia. Many of them are treated with indwelling urethral catheters because they are incontinent of urine; if feeding is also a problem, they may receive nutritional support through a feeding tube. These invasive therapies bypass normal host defenses and predispose to urinary tract infection and aspiration pneumonia, respectively.

Because of their underlying diseases and general levels of debility, elderly patients are more likely to develop infections that are severe and life-threatening. The familiar adage that pneumonia is the "old man's friend" still rings true today. Pneumonia continues to rank among the top five leading causes of death in the elderly in the United States. Elderly patients who develop pneumonia are more likely than younger patients to require hospitalization, to have prolonged hospital stays, and to have fatal outcomes.[2] The increased mortality associated with infections in the elderly is largely due to the impact of debilitating, comorbid diseases. Difficulties in diagnosis and complications of therapies also increase the morbidity and mortality of infections in the elderly.

CLINICAL ASPECTS OF INFECTIONS IN THE ELDERLY

Infections in the elderly usually present with typical, focal signs and symptoms that are similar to those that characterize infections in younger populations. However, infections in the elderly may also present with extremely subtle, nonfocal, or atypical findings. For instance, it is not uncommon for pneumonia to present without cough, sputum production, or fever in elderly patients. Urinary tract infection may be present without dysuria or polyuria; meningitis may occur without neck stiffness; intestinal perforation may present without pain or tenderness; and bacteremia may develop without fever. The only clue suggesting infection in these patients may be an unexplained decrease in appetite, increase in forgetfulness, or decreased responsiveness. Thus, the clinician or nursing staff must be aware of the patient's usual functional status and be alert to the development of infection when changes are noted.

Identifying infection in the elderly is even more difficult because suggestive clues may be hidden by the presence of underlying conditions that alter or obscure the signs or symptoms of local inflammation. For instance, it may be extremely difficult to diagnose pneumonia in a patient with chronic bronchitis and constant sputum production. Urinary tract infection may not be considered in the differential diagnosis of a febrile patient in whom focal complaints are obscured by the presence of an indwelling urethral catheter. The diagnosis of any infection is made more difficult when patients cannot communicate symptoms because they are confused, forgetful, or mute.

Even laboratory tests cannot be relied on to differentiate a new infection from a chronic underlying condition. Purulent sputum with a positive culture does not differentiate chronic bronchitis from acute pneumonia. Neither pyuria nor a positive urine culture is diagnostic of UTI; positive urine cultures are seen in as many as 25% of asymptomatic, noncatheterized elderly female residents of nursing homes.[3] Leukocytosis is not a constant finding in elderly patients with either focal or systemic infections; in fact, acute granulocytopenia is an important sign of impending sepsis in an elderly patient. Thus, the diagnosis of infection in the elderly requires a thorough evaluation of the patient, knowledge of the underlying conditions that are present, a careful physical examination to detect subtle signs of infection, and a critical review of available laboratory studies.

Even then, clinical intuition and judgment may be the only way in which suggestive clues for infection are identified and the decision to prescribe antibiotics is made. The use of empiric antibiotics is often indicated because early intervention may be lifesaving.

The treatment of infections in the elderly is also fraught with difficulties. Selection of an appropriate agent may have to be modified by the setting in which infection occurs, because antibiotic-resistant infections are more likely in institutional or hospital environments. The dosage of the antibiotic must take into account physiologic and pathologic changes in organ function. The possibility of drug interactions must be considered because many of these patients are also receiving medications for other chronic diseases. With noninstitutionalized patients, compliance may be a problem, not only because they might be forgetful, but also because they may be confused about the instructions for taking their antibiotics, especially when they are taking several other medications.

Table 3.1 *Infections of Importance in the Elderly*

SITE	INFECTION
Genitourinary tract	Urinary tract infection
	Asymptomatic bacteriuria
	Symptomatic urinary tract infection
Respiratory tract	Pneumonia
Gastrointestinal tract	Biliary tract infection
	Diverticulitis
	Hepatic abscess
	Appendicitis
	Diarrhea
Skin	Bacterial infections (e.g., *Staphylococcus, Streptococcus, Pseudomonas*)
	Viral infections (e.g., Herpes zoster)
Heart	Endocarditis
Central nervous system	Bacterial meningitis

Infections are difficult problems for the elderly and for the clinicians who care for them. Infections have serious clinical outcomes and are often directly responsible for the death of the patient. They can be difficult to identify and problematic to treat. The following sections deal with some of the more common types of focal infection that affect the elderly (see Table 3.1). These sections outline in greater detail the specific risk factors, diagnostic considerations, and therapeutic strategies that are available to the clinician.

URINARY TRACT INFECTIONS

Elderly men and women are susceptible to bacteriuria and urinary tract infection because of physiologic changes associated with aging, underlying diseases, and increasing debility. With advancing age, changes occur in the urinary tract that predispose to infection. In men, there is a predictable occurrence of prostatic hypertrophy that may obstruct urinary outflow. In women, postmenopausal estrogen deficiency promotes bacterial colonization with potential urinary pathogens. The likelihood of infection in women is further increased when there is poor perineal hygiene or fecal incontinence resulting in high levels of perineal colonization with enteric organisms. In addition, in elderly women, conditions that impair urine flow—such as cystoceles, rectoceles, atonic bladders, genitourinary tumors or bladder calculi—also predispose to infection. Certain medications, including those with anticholinergic side effects, may also impair bladder function. Once bacteria gain entry into the bladder, colonization of the urine is likely to occur, particularly if there is incomplete bladder emptying. Elderly patients frequently have impairments of other physiologic mechanisms that normally are able to maintain urine sterility. They may be unable to dilute, concentrate, or acidify urine to levels that are antibacterial; their urine flow may be diminished. All of these factors increase the likelihood of urinary tract infection in the elderly.

Pathophysiology

Perhaps the single most important risk factor for urinary colonization and infection in the elderly, or any patient, is the presence of an indwelling urethral catheter. It has been shown that the risk of developing bacteriuria is between 1%

and 20% when a catheter is inserted and immediately removed; the more debilitated the patient, the higher the likelihood of bacteriuria.[4] The indwelling catheter serves as a conduit for bacteria to pass into the bladder.

There are no good prospective, cross-sectional epidemiologic studies that have defined the actual incidence of urinary tract infection in the elderly in general. The rate of infection is determined by the presence and severity of risk factors that predispose to infection in the population under surveillance. Prevalence surveys have shown that the rate of bacteriuria in ambulatory, elderly women increases from approximately 10% in 60-year-olds up to 15% to 25% in 80-year-olds. The prevalence of bacteriuria in ambulatory, elderly men rises from less than 5% to approximately 10% over the same age range. For catheterized men and women, the incidence of bacteriuria is approximately 5% for each day of catheterization; the rate of bacteriuria for those who are catheterized for more than one month is virtually 100%.[5]

Diagnosis

The diagnosis of urinary tract infection in the elderly is frequently problematic. Sometimes, infection presents with nonspecific or atypical findings. The cardinal symptoms of dysuria, local pain, urinary frequency, and fever may be absent. Instead, infection may present as the new onset of incontinence, mental confusion, or unexplained loss of appetite. Many elderly patients are unable to communicate complaints accurately. Those with urinary catheters have no awareness of burning or frequency. For these, the diagnosis of UTI is made only after excluding other possibilities and obtaining appropriate cultures that define the urinary tract as the likely source of infection.

The laboratory identification of UTI in the elderly may also be confusing. Findings such as a positive urine culture, bacterial colony counts of greater than 10^5 cfu/ml (colony-forming units per milliliter of urine), or the presence of white blood cells in the urine do not establish the diagnosis of infection. The diagnosis of UTI in the elderly must rely on both objective laboratory findings and clinical judgment including the exclusion of other possible causes of infection on the basis of clinical and laboratory findings.

Asymptomatic Bacteriuria

As many as 30% of elderly, noncatheterized women and 10% of elderly, noncatheterized men have asymptomatic bacteriuria. Most studies of the long-term consequences of asymptomatic bacteriuria in noncatheterized patients have shown no increased incidence of symptomatic infection or decreased survival in untreated patients compared with treated controls.[6–8] Thus, it is not recommended to obtain routine cultures from elderly patients to identify asymptomatic bacteriuria or to treat asymptomatic bacteriuria with antibiotics when it is found.

For those with indwelling urethral catheters, bacteriuria is a predictable occurrence; the prevalence of bacteriuria increases with increasing days of catheterization. Symptomatic infection, bladder calculi, and urosepsis are well-known complications of urethral catheterization. For hospitalized patients with temporary indwelling catheters averaging two to three days, the cumulative incidence of bacteriuria is between 5% and 15%.[5] Approximately 10% of patients with catheter-associated bacteriuria will develop symptomatic infection, and 1% will become bacteremic.[9] In one study of chronically catheterized patients with bacteriuria, the incidence of fever was only one episode per 100 catheter days; in this study, febrile episodes that were identified could not always be related to urinary tract infection.[10]

Symptomatic Urinary Tract Infection

For most elderly, urinary tract infections present with signs, symptoms, and laboratory findings similar to those in younger patients. Focal symptoms such as dysuria, frequency, and local pain, with or without fever, should suggest the diagnosis of UTI and prompt appropriate evaluation and treatment. For elderly women, *Escherichia coli* is responsible for between 75% and 85% of episodes of symptomatic UTI. Most other infections are caused by other enterobacteriaceae or enterococci. Infections with *Pseudomonas aeruginosa, Serratia marcescens,* or *Providencia stuartii* are usually limited to patients who have received prior antibiotics, are institutionalized, or are being treated with indwelling urethral catheters. For men, *E. coli* is also a common cause of UTI. However, enterococci are much more prevalent in men than in women, perhaps because men with enlarged prostates are often catheterized to treat urinary obstruction.

Treatment

Antibiotic therapy is not recommended for patients with asymptomatic bacteriuria; patients with signs and symptoms of urinary tract infection should be treated with antibiotics. For women with first-time urinary tract infections, *E. coli* are assumed to be the cause of infection and treatment with oral trimethoprim sulfamethoxazole or ampicillin is usually sufficient; many clinicians favor a three- to seven-day course of therapy.

Residents in nursing homes with catheter-associated urinary tract infection pose a difficult management problem. They are likely to be colonized with multiple bacterial species that are resistant to commonly used antibiotics. If possible, the indwelling catheter should be removed, or at least changed, during the course of therapy. Often, the catheter itself is the site of incrustations and glycocalyx formation that can become a nidus for recurrent catheter-associated infection.

Prevention

Strategies to prevent urinary tract infection in the elderly are similar to those that are recommended to prevent infection in younger populations. Underlying diseases should be treated, and anatomic abnormalities that predispose to infection should be corrected whenever possible. Efforts should be made to remove indwelling urethral catheters if possible. UTIs are discussed further in Chapter 6.

RESPIRATORY TRACT INFECTIONS

Respiratory tract infections are an important cause of morbidity in the elderly. Influenza and pneumonia combined are a leading cause of death in this age group and the fourth leading cause of death overall. Also of note is the predisposition in the geriatric patient to develop secondary complications of pneumonia such as bacteremia and meningitis. Some pathogens, such as *Streptococcus pneumoniae*, can take on a more virulent course in the elderly with a higher rate of secondary bacteremia and mortality. Finally, nosocomial pneumonias with gram-negative organisms and *Staphylococcus aureus* are more commonly seen in the elderly and are associated with significant morbidity and mortality.

Pathophysiology

There are age-related changes in normal pulmonary defenses that predispose the elderly to infection, especially of the lower respiratory tract.[11] With normal aging, there

is an increase in the anterosuperior chest diameter as well as a decrease in elastic tissue around alveoli and alveolar ducts. In addition, age-related weakening of respiratory muscles and a less vigorous cough result in a decreased ability to clear secretions. Mucociliary function has also been shown to become less efficient in the elderly, with a noted decrease in tracheal mucus velocity. Although it is still not clear whether these findings are indicative of abnormal ciliary function or a change in the viscoelastic properties of mucus, the final result is a relative inability to achieve effective clearance of aspirated material.

Underlying diseases that can be commonly found in the elderly can increase their risk for pulmonary infection. Patients with abnormal pulmonary function status, such as chronic obstructive pulmonary disease and chronic bronchitis, have altered pulmonary inflammatory responses and damaged clearance mechanisms. Smoking can have an adverse effect on macrophage and mucociliary function. Patients with cancer are predisposed to infection for a number of reasons including bronchial obstruction, malnutrition, bone marrow invasion, and defects in white blood cell number and function. Risk of aspiration pneumonia increases with underlying neurologic disease, esophageal disease, and excessive alcohol use. Medications can add to the risk of respiratory infection as well. Tranquilizers and sedatives can increase aspiration risk; steroids and immunosuppressives can increase risk of infections as well as interfere with its normal containment and resolution. Recent or recurrent use of broad-spectrum antibiotics in institutionalized patients can alter the causes of infection due to colonization with more resistant bacteria, especially with gram-negative bacilli and methicillin-resistant *S. aureus* (MRSA).

Diagnosis

The "usual" signs and symptoms of lower respiratory tract infections occur frequently in the elderly. These include fever, chills, cough, sputum production, shortness of breath, and elevated peripheral white blood count. However, clinical suspicion must remain high for those who do not have a classic presentation. Sometimes the only hint of clinical infection is lethargy, mental status changes, anorexia, worsening congestive heart failure, or change from baseline respiratory status. Physical examination in this age group may be difficult because they are unable to cooperate fully by taking deep breaths. Even in ideal situations, rales may not be heard. In patients with underlying pulmonary disease, a change from baseline may be difficult to discern.

Diagnosis of pneumonia is aided and usually confirmed with the chest x-ray; however, baseline abnormalities in a patient with known cardiac and pulmonary abnormalities may make interpretation impossible. Every effort should be made to obtain an adequate sputum specimen for Gram stain with culture and sensitivity. However, in a weak, uncooperative, or dehydrated patient, expectorated specimens will be difficult to obtain. In those situations, nasotracheal aspiration may give the best results. Sputum Gram stain should be performed to quantify the number of polymorphonuclear (white blood) cells per high-power field and identify predominant bacteria. A specimen with less than 25 white blood cells or more than 10 epithelial cells per high-power field usually suggests oropharyngeal contamination and questions the reliability of the culture results.[12]

Nosocomial pneumonia in institutionalized patients can be among the most difficult to treat, given the more resistant bacteria and the multiplicity of organisms found in culture. Gram-negative bacteria, such as *Klebsiella pneumoniae, E. coli* and *Proteus species*, and gram-positives, such as *S. aureus* (methicillin sensitive), are common isolates in nursing home patients. Over the years, methicillin-resistant *S. aureus* (MRSA) has become endemic in some long-term care facilities and has complicated antibiotic management in this setting. Patients intubated or receiving inhalation therapy are at increased risk of pneumonia with water-based organisms such as *Pseudomonas aeruginosa, Serratia marcescens*, and *Legionella pneumophila*.

Initial antibiotic therapy for respiratory tract infections in nursing home residents should be broad enough to cover gram-negative bacilli and *S. aureus*. The final choice of antimicrobial agent should be guided by the results of cultures and antimicrobial susceptibility testing. Respiratory infections are discussed further in Chapter 5.

GASTROINTESTINAL INFECTIONS

Infections of the gastrointestinal (GI) tract are an important cause of morbidity and mortality in the elderly. Given the frequent cryptic presentation and subtle physical findings that can occur with GI infection in the elderly, a high index of suspicion is critical in evaluating fever and clinical status change in these patients.

Biliary Tract Infection

The biliary tract is one of the more common abdominal foci of infection in this age group. In fact, the elderly are at high risk for some of the less common complications of biliary tract infection, including ascending cholangitis and empyema of the gallbladder. In these patients, gallstones obstructing the cystic duct are most frequently the direct cause, with resultant trapping of bile acids causing inflammation and secondary infection. Unrelieved cystic duct obstruction can lead to compromise of venous, arterial, and lymphatic flow, necrosis with gallbladder perforation, peritonitis, and secondary intra-abdominal abscess formation.

Classic signs and symptoms of acute cholecystitis seen in all age groups include right upper quadrant pain accompanied by fever, chills, nausea, and vomiting. However, in as many as one third of elderly patients who are evaluated for cholecystitis, these classic findings are absent.

Appropriate workup to evaluate a patient for biliary tract disease includes a complete blood count with differential, blood cultures, and liver function tests, including calculation of total/direct bilirubin and alkaline phosphatase. Abdominal ultrasound is the most sensitive and practical diagnostic procedure to confirm the presence of gallstones and evaluate possible ductal obstruction.

Antibiotic therapy of biliary tract sepsis should be broad enough to cover the bacteria most frequently identified. These organisms would include gram-negative bacilli, such as *E. coli, Enterobacter species*, enterococci, and anaerobes. In conjunction with antibiotics, adequate hydration must be maintained during restricted oral intake. Once stable, the patient can be evaluated for surgical intervention: cholecystectomy for the more stable patients, and cholecystotomy drainage for those less able to tolerate a longer surgical procedure. Other alternatives, such as laparoscopic surgery and percutaneous dissolution of gallstones with ether derivatives are presently being evaluated for patients in whom surgery is contraindicated.

Diverticulitis

The risk of diverticular disease increases as an individual ages. This association is due to the aging process itself, as well as decreased intake of dietary fiber. The incidence of diverticulosis is 30% in those 60 years of age and over and as high as 50% in persons over the age of 80. Most diverticula are the "pulsion" type, with pockets of colonic mucosa bulging through the muscularis layers of bowel wall and extending into pericolic fat. Diverticulitis develops when fecal material obstructs the diverticular lumen, resulting in irritation, inflammation, erosion and leakage, often with perforation into the pericolic fat.[13]

The most frequent complaint of patients with diverticulitis is lower abdominal pain, which is often accompanied by fever, chills, and constipation. Physical examination includes a tender, palpable lower quadrant mass with rectal tenderness and diminished bowel sounds. However, as with other infections in this age group, signs and symptoms may be quite misleading. Typical signs and symptoms may be absent. Nausea and vomiting with nonlocalized abdominal pain may be the only focal clues of a GI source of infection. Bacterial pathogens implicated in diverticulitis include the normal flora of the large intestine, including gram negative bacilli, gram-positive cocci, and anaerobes such as *Bacteroides fragilis.*

Management of patients with diverticulitis depends very much on the severity of presentation. Frequently, they can be managed medically with bowel rest and adequate hydration. In more severe cases, where medical management is still indicated, broad spectrum antibiotic therapy, effective against polymicrobial enteric bacteria, is warranted. Those patients who do not respond to conservative medical management or who show signs of clinical decompensation, including perforation or abscess formation, must be treated surgically.

Hepatic Abscess

As many as 30% of cases of liver abscess occur in adults over the age of 60.[14] The source of this infection is most frequently secondary to prior biliary tract surgery, episodes of cholecystitis, or malignancy involving the biliary tree or pancreas. The clinical presentation of liver abscess can be quite subtle and lack the classic signs of right upper quadrant abdominal pain, fever, chills, malaise, and anorexia. Some elderly patients will manifest atypical abdominal pain, mental status changes, and nonspecific symptoms; others continue to have good appetite despite hepatic dysfunction. Workup should include a complete blood count with differential, which usually shows a leukocytosis, and liver function tests, which may have elevations of both serum alkaline phosphatase and bilirubin levels. Diagnosis is usually confirmed by a noninvasive abdominal imaging study such as abdominal ultrasound, computerized tomography (CT scan), or gallium scan.

With advances in management techniques since the 1970s, liver abscess can now usually be managed by a percutaneous drainage procedure based on abscess size and location. Surgical management is reserved for those patients with abscesses that are multiple, multichambered, or inaccessible to a percutaneous catheter. Antimicrobial therapy should be broad spectrum to cover the most likely bacterial pathogens; these include enteric gram-negatives such as *E. coli, Klebsiella, Proteus* and *Enterobacter species,* and anaerobes such as *Bacteroides fragilis.*

Appendicitis

Although less commonly a cause of intra-abdominal sepsis in the elderly, appendicitis does occur in this age group and should be included in the differential diagnosis of intra-abdominal sepsis. Normal aging changes of the appendix include narrowing and obliteration of the lumen, mucosal thickening, and arterial sclerosis, which can result in vascular thrombosis, gangrene, and perforation. Symptoms of acute appendicitis include nausea, vomiting, abdominal pain, and anorexia. However, abdominal guarding and rebound are present in only 50% to 75% of elderly individuals with appendicitis.[15] Treatment of acute appendicitis includes supportive care, intravenous antibiotics directed against enteric pathogens, and surgery.

Diarrhea

Normal changes in the aging gut may predispose the elderly to diarrheal infection. Underlying diseases that delay intestinal motility and cause atrophy of gastric acid secreting cells make this age group more susceptible to intestinal pathogens that cause diarrhea. Administration of antacids, drugs that delay intestinal transport, and antibiotics further increase susceptibility to infection. Diarrhea in the elderly can be self-limiting or can lead to severe enteritis with bacteremia that can be life-threatening. Infectious gastroenteritis is discussed in Chapter 8.

Gastrointestinal infections can be grouped into three clinical syndromes: acute food poisoning, noninvasive diarrhea, and invasive diarrhea. Bacterial agents responsible for food poisoning include enterotoxin-producing *S. aureus*, (with an incubation period of one to six hours), *Clostridium perfringens* (with an incubation period of 48 to 72 hours), *Clostridium botulinum*, *Vibrio parahemolyticus*, and *Bacillus cereus*. Typical clinical findings include nausea and vomiting (mediated by enterotoxins) and diarrhea that is watery without abdominal pain, systemic symptoms, and fever.

Viruses, bacteria, and parasites can cause noninvasive diarrhea. The most commonly occurring viral causes are norwalk agent, rotavirus, and enteroviruses, all of which have been implicated in cluster outbreaks in nursing homes. Other agents in this category include enterotoxigenic *E. coli*, *Vibrio species*, and parasites such as *Giardia lamblia* and *Cryptosporidia*. Symptoms include loose or watery diarrhea without systemic symptoms, fever, or abdominal pain.

Invasive diarrhea caused by *Salmonella*, *Shigella*, and *Campylobacter species* can result in the most serious problems in the elderly. The spectrum of infection with these bacteria can range from localized gastroenteritis to bacteremia with sepsis and death. The clinical presentation includes abdominal discomfort, fever, and bloody diarrhea. Management includes supportive care with maintenance of adequate hydration and electrolyte balance. Antidiarrheal agents should be avoided when these bacteria are isolated from culture because they can result in prolongation of clinical symptoms and increased likelihood of tissue invasion with bacteria.[16] The majority of episodes of diarrhea caused by these agents are self-limited and do not warrant antibiotic therapy; in fact, antibiotics are known to prolong the carrier state with *Salmonella*. However, antibiotics are recommended for the management of severely ill patients who have profuse diarrhea, dehydration, positive blood cultures, or evidence of systemic toxicity. The decision to treat with antibiotics should be based on the severity of the clinical presentation and the presence of other underlying diseases. Erythromycin is the drug of choice for *Campylobacter* infections, whereas trimethoprim sulfamethoxazole or a quinolone is used for *Salmonella* and *Shigella*.

Clostridium difficile is another important entity responsible for diarrhea, especially in chronic care settings. Infection with this organism occurs as a complication of antibiotic therapy and causes a toxin-mediated pseudomembranous colitis. Although this complication has been reported with most antibiotics now available for use, the highest incidence has been reported with beta-lactam agents in the penicillin and cephalosporin classes and with clindamycin, the drug with which the entity was first described.

Patients with pseudomembranous colitis present with diarrhea and low-grade fever. On occasion, temperatures as high as 102°F can be seen with an impressive peripheral leukocytosis. Frequent and careful physical examination of the abdomen is warranted to evaluate and rule out toxic megacolon, a potentially life-threatening complication. Pseudomembranous colitis is treated by stopping the offending antimicrobial agent and giving oral metronidazole or oral vancomycin. Pseudomembranous colitis is discussed further in Chapter 8.

SKIN INFECTIONS

The skin is the largest organ system of the body, and it, too, undergoes normal changes of aging over time. The epidermis becomes dryer, thinner, and more fragile, with fewer blood vessels. Impaired collagen synthesis and decreased vascularity lead to poor wound healing. Loss of the protection that intact integument normally gives leads to a higher risk of various skin diseases, minor skin tears, and the like, as well as pressure sores and, overall, an increased risk of infection. Underlying medical conditions, malnutrition, immobility, incontinence, and medications such as corticosteroids increase the risk of breakdown and secondary infection. Elderly diabetic patients are prone to peripheral vascular disease and foot ulcers. These small ulcers can become infected with both aerobic and anaerobic bacteria and serve as a source of secondary bacteremia.

The most frequently occurring bacterial skin infections involve *S. aureus* and group A streptococci. Differentiation between clinical infections with *S. aureus* and streptococci can sometimes be difficult. The range of infections seen with these organisms is varied, including cellulitis, erysipelas, toxic shock syndrome, bullous impetigo, pustules, folliculitis, and abscesses.

Pseudomonas aeruginosa can also cause skin infections in the elderly that range from simple chronic folliculitis to a fulminant cellulitis. Ecthyma gangrenosum is a dermatologic manifestation of life-threatening *Pseudomonas* infection in compromised patients who are malnourished, have diabetes mellitus or cancer, or are on chemotherapy. *Pseudomonas* pyoderma can develop at pressure ulcer sites and ischemic ulcers of the leg.

Pressure Sores

Pressure sores or decubitus ulcers are a problem in the institutionalized elderly. Risk is highest among those who are immobilized, incontinent, and malnourished (see Chapter 7). Antibiotic treatment of pressure ulcers, per se, is not indicated unless they are complicated and there is no other source of fever. Careful evaluation includes examination of the wound for surrounding cellulitis as well as evaluating the extent of the wound itself to rule out the presence of a deep abscess or possible bone involvement if the skin is undermined or the ulcer is found to be extending within fascial planes. In the latter situation, in addition to antibiotic therapy, surgical management with incision, drainage, and debridement is necessary. Even with optimal management, wound healing in these patients can be quite poor. Thus, there is an increased incidence of morbidity and mortality from sepsis.

Herpes Zoster

The viral skin infection that occurs most frequently in the elderly is herpes zoster (shingles). Zoster peaks in incidence between ages 50 and 70 and is caused by a reactivation of varicella (chicken pox) virus found in the dorsal root ganglion. Although many factors have been postulated as causes for reactivation, including stress, trauma, and immunosuppressive agents, none has been proven. Although a depressed cell-mediated immune system is very likely involved, its degree of involvement is not clear. In fact, the majority of individuals who develop zoster are quite healthy.

The diagnosis of zoster skin infections is not difficult, given its usual dermatomal distribution of erythematous papules that progress to vesicles within 12 to 48 hours. A few lesions may be seen outside of the dermatome; however, more than 10 to 15 lesions outside of the dermatome suggest possible early dissemination. High-dose acyclovir, available in oral and IV forms, can decrease the

duration of viral shedding and hasten the healing process; however, it may not prevent postherpetic neuralgia, an extremely problematic complication of herpes zoster in the elderly.[17] Supportive treatment for the patient consists of adequate analgesia and care of the wounds to prevent secondary bacterial infection.

OTHER INFECTIONS IN THE ELDERLY

Endocarditis

Although once considered a disease of the young, the incidence of endocarditis in the elderly has continued to increase over the years. The explanation for the increase in cases is not clear but may be explained by the increase in the number of elderly individuals in the population, the longer life span of individuals with degenerative valvular heart disease, and the increased chance of hospitalization as an individual ages, with all of the associated risks for nosocomial infection that entails.[18]

Degenerative or arteriosclerotic changes of the heart valves is the most important predisposing factor for endocarditis in the elderly. The valves most frequently involved are the aortic valve, where calcification or a congenital bicuspid valve are frequently found, and the mitral valve. Some studies suggest that aortic valve involvement is most frequent; others have found the aortic and mitral valves are equally affected. In recent years, there has been an increased incidence of nosocomial tricuspid valve endocarditis directly related to infected indwelling central venous catheters.[19]

The presentation of endocarditis in older patients is, in many ways, similar to that seen in younger age groups. Fever and murmurs that are new or have changed are almost always present. However, as in other infectious processes in this age group, a high index of suspicion is necessary to make the diagnosis, because murmurs, especially isolated aortic stenosis and mitral regurgitation, are more common in the elderly. The clinician must also be cautious in the evaluation of seemingly innocent flow murmurs in the presence of fever in this population. Changes in the central nervous system, such as new onset stroke, hemiplegia, or meningitis, may be the initial presentation and are seen in 20% to 40% of elderly endocarditis patients.[20] Musculoskeletal manifestations are also common with endocarditis; arthralgias and back pain associated with fever are frequently presenting symptoms.[21]

A variety of bacteria cause endocarditis in the elderly. Gram-positive cocci, such as viridans streptococci are associated with a less acute presentation, with low-grade temperatures, malaise, and weight loss persisting over weeks to months. Group D streptococci (enterococci) also cause endocarditis that is frequently secondary to either a gastrointestinal focus or a genitourinary source. Nonenterococcal group D streptococci, such as *Streptococcus bovis*, may also cause endocarditis. Identification of this organism in blood cultures warrants a complete workup of the lower GI tract with long-term follow-up because of the organism's high incidence of association with carcinoma of the colon. *S. aureus* can be a causative agent of endocarditis in the elderly that results in a particularly invasive destruction of heart valves and a high mortality rate. Coagulase-negative staphylococci can cause endocarditis in patients with prosthetic heart valves; they have also been identified on native valves in patients who have had central, as well as peripheral, venous catheters.[22]

Blood cultures are essential for the diagnosis of endocarditis. Taking two to three sets of blood cultures optimally separated in time over 20 to 30 minutes has a 96% chance of recovery of the responsible microorganism. Echocardiography, particularly transesophageal echocardiography, is an adjunctive test that can evaluate the heart valves for bacterial vegetations. The sensitivity for detecting vegetations on valves is anywhere from 40% to 60% for the two-dimensional method. The echocardiogram by itself rarely makes the diagnosis of endocarditis, but it may be helpful in predicting clinical outcome and possibly the need for surgery based on vegetation number, size, and location.[23]

Antimicrobial treatment of endocarditis is based on optimal choice as suggested by final bacterial culture results. Streptococci are best treated with penicillin G, based on MICs (minimal inhibitory concentrations). Enterococci require ampicillin or penicillin G with an aminoglycoside added for synergy; careful follow-up of the patient's renal function and aminoglycoside peak and trough levels are mandatory. *S. aureus* is best treated by a semisynthetic penicillin such as oxacillin or nafcillin; in situations where MRSA is identified, vancomycin is the drug of choice. Optimal treatment of coagulase negative staphy-

lococci is determined by final sensitivities; some of these bacteria, especially those acquired nosocomially, can be quite resistant and may require vancomycin for effective treatment.

Bacterial Meningitis

Meningitis remains a relatively uncommon infection in the elderly, but delays in the recognition of this diagnosis contribute to a high frequency of morbidity and mortality. *S. pneumoniae* and *Neisseria meningitidis* are the most common pathogens. Pneumococcal meningitis is frequently a secondary complication of pneumococcal pneumonia; it is also seen with otitis media, mastoiditis, and fractures of the skull. In patients who have been chronically ill with elevated sedimentation rates and anemia, multiple myeloma should be considered in the differential diagnosis. Although *Neisseria meningitidis* is more commonly seen in younger age groups, it accounts for approximately 16% of meningitis cases seen in the elderly.[24]

Haemophilus influenzae, once thought only to be a disease of young children, is being reported in higher numbers of elderly patients with meningitis. Bacterial meningitis in the elderly can also be caused by more unusual pathogens such as *S. aureus*, gram-negative bacilli, and *Listeria monocytogenes*. The gram-negative infections are frequently seen with bacteremic seeding from distant sites such as the urinary tract but are also associated with trauma and neurosurgical procedures. *Listeria* infections are most frequently reported in patients with underlying chronic diseases such as alcoholism, connective tissue disease, chronic renal failure, and cancer.

The most frequent symptoms of meningitis for all age groups are headache, nausea, vomiting, and fever. Physical examination reveals signs of meningeal irritation with marked nuchal rigidity. However, in some older individuals, these classic signs and symptoms may never appear. Evaluation can be problematic in those patients with underlying chronic diseases, neurologic abnormalities, and cervical arthritis, where signs and symptoms can be masked. A high index of suspicion is therefore indicated in this age group, and early consideration of performing a lumbar puncture is critical to establish the correct diagnosis as soon as possible.

Examination of the cerebrospinal fluid (CSF) in a patient with meningitis usually shows an increased number of polymorphonuclear leukocytes, elevated protein, and low glucose levels. Gram stain with culture and sensitivities are critical factors in the workup. Additional tests such as sputum, blood, and urine cultures and chest x-ray should be done to help identify the possible source of primary infection.

Survival is improved with the prompt initiation of antibiotic therapy with an agent that crosses the blood/brain barrier and covers the most likely bacterial pathogens. High-dose penicillin G remains the antibiotic of choice against bacteria such as *S. pneumoniae* and *N. meningitidis. Listeria* infections and beta-lactamase-negative *Haemophilus influenzae* are best treated with high-dose ampicillin, whereas semisynthetic penicillins, such as oxacillin, are the drugs of choice for infections caused by *S. aureus.* Where MRSA is a known endemic problem, vancomycin is the recommended drug of choice. Third-generation cephalosporins, such as cefotaxime or ceftazidime, are the agents of choice for beta-lactamase-positive *H. influenzae* and gram-negative bacilli, given their ability to cross the blood/brain barrier and their low incidence of toxicity. The final antibiotic choice should be guided by culture results and sensitivities.

Despite appropriate antibiotic therapy, morbidity and mortality from bacterial meningitis remain high in the elderly. Some neurologic sequelae such as deafness, cranial nerve palsies, hemiparesis, and dementia are common, especially with pneumococcal meningitis.

Fever of Unknown Origin

Fever of unknown origin (FUO) can occur in all age groups, although the differential diagnosis is somewhat different for the elderly. It is defined in clinical situations in which patients have intermittent temperature elevations of 100 to 101°F. or more over a three-week or longer period of time when appropriate noninvasive workup fails to find a cause.

The differential diagnosis of FUO for any age group is quite broad. In the elderly, diagnoses of inflammatory bowel disease and systemic lupus erythematosis are less frequent, and diagnoses such as renal cell carcinoma and pancreatic and primary neoplastic processes that result in metastatic liver disease are more common than in younger patients. Lymphoma should be kept in the differential diagnosis as well, when fever and enlarged liver or spleen and retroperitoneal lymph nodes are present. Hematologic malignancy such as leukemia may cause FUO as well.[25]

Occult abscesses can also be the cause of FUO. The possibility of intra-abdominal abscess may be difficult to evaluate based on history and physical examination alone. Neoplastic or inflammatory disease of the liver, biliary tract, or kidneys can give rise to abscess formation. The elderly can also develop cryptogenetic liver abscess without a clearly recognizable precipitating event such as colonic infection, biliary tract disease, or blunt trauma.

Other infectious causes of FUO in the elderly include tuberculosis, endocarditis, and bloodborne viral infections. Miliary tuberculosis should always be considered as a cause of FUO in any age group. The diagnosis is supported by hepatomegaly, splenomegaly, cough, and weight loss. Isolated tuberculous involvement of the GU tract, bones/joints, or lymph nodes are rare causes of FUO. Subacute bacterial endocarditis can be an important cause of FUO in the elderly. Subtle findings such as an innocent flow murmur and neurologic changes can make the diagnosis elusive to the clinician. Viral illnesses such as cytomegalovirus (CMV) need to be considered as well. CMV can cause nonspecific signs and symptoms with prolonged fever and should be considered in patients who have received blood anywhere from three to six weeks earlier.

Noninfectious etiologies can cause FUO as well; collagen vascular diseases need to be considered. Giant cell arteritis is the most common collagen vascular disease in this age group and can present with weight loss, weakness, prolonged fever, headache, jaw claudication, changes in vision, and temporal artery tenderness. However, it is important to remember that the patient may present with all, some, or only a few of these signs and symptoms. Polyarteritis nodosa is another collagen vascular disease that can present with fever, abdominal pain, anorexia, weight loss, nausea and vomiting. Almost half of these patients will have arthralgias; arthritis, when present, is nondeforming and asymmetric.

For patients where daily careful follow-up documents temperature elevation, appropriate initial tests include a complete blood count with differential, erythrocyte sedimentation rate (ESR), urinalysis with culture and sensitivity, stool test for blood, antinuclear antibody (ANA), and liver aminotransferases and alkaline phosphatase. Serologic tests for hepatitis B (hepatitis B surface antigen), syphilis (VDRL and fluorescent antibody test), and serum protein electrophoresis may be helpful as well. All patients with FUO should have a chest x-ray to rule out miliary tuberculosis, emboli from a cardiac origin, and occult malignancy.

Two to three sets of blood cultures should be obtained, ideally separated by 20 to 30 minutes to rule out subacute bacterial endocarditis. Obtaining 10 to 15 ml of blood to store in the laboratory may be invaluable if a specific need for testing arises or if serum is needed for an acute phase titer.[25]

Imaging tests such as computerized tomography (CT) scan can rule out abscesses at many locations—including the liver, perinephric space, and gut—as well as tumors such as hypernephroma; it can also identify the presence of enlarged lymph nodes. Echocardiography can evaluate heart valves for vegetations.

More noninvasive studies may be indicated if all other tests are negative. Barium enema and sigmoidoscopy may rule out colon carcinoma; bone marrow examination can diagnose leukemia, preleukemic states, lymphoma, metastatic disease, and granulomas to rule out miliary tuberculosis. Liver biopsy is usually reserved for patients with liver function test abnormalities of unknown etiology and when it can be safely done can confirm diagnoses such as cirrhosis, metastatic disease, and hepatoma. If temporal arteritis is in the differential, temporal artery biopsy is indicated; more than one biopsy may be required to make the diagnosis.[26]

PREVENTION OF INFECTIONS IN THE ELDERLY

The diagnosis and management of infections in the elderly can be difficult. Even when the diagnosis is made in a timely manner and an appropriate antibiotic started, elderly patients have a higher morbidity and mortality rate thanyounger patients. Attempts to avoid infection should be initiated where possible.

Underlying disease processes should be treated to help maintain the patient's clinical stability as much as possible and to avoid the need for acute hospitalization. Invasive catheters should be avoided unless absolutely necessary. If they are utilized, appropriate care should be used in their maintenance and they should be discontinued when no longer needed. In patients with underlying cardiac/valvular abnormalities, accepted antibiotic prophylaxis guidelines should be followed prior to dental work and invasive gastrointestinal/genitourinary procedures.

Finally, vaccinations to prevent disease should be aggressively offered to patients in this age group. Pneumococcal vaccine (23 valent) should be offered to all patients 65 years of age or older to prevent serious infections with *Streptococcus pneumoniae*. There are no recommendations at this time to revaccinate or give booster vaccinations to those who have already received the vaccine. Influenza vaccine, effective against strains of influenza A and B should be offered to elderly patients annually; the only contraindication to its use is an allergy to eggs. In those patients unable to take the vaccine and those unvaccinated patients exposed to, or infected with, influenza A, amantadine can be given for prophylaxis and treatment. If administered, the dosage of amantadine in the elderly should be reduced to 50 mg a day to avoid neurologic complications such as lethargy and confusion. Vaccinations in the elderly are discussed further in Chapter 17.

REFERENCES

1. Saltzman RL, Peterson PK: Immunodeficiency of the elderly. *Rev Infect Dis* 1987;9:1127–1138.
2. Garibaldi RA, Nurse BA: Infections in the elderly. *Am J Med* 1987;81:53–58.
3. Boscia JA, Kobasa WD, Knight RA, et al: Epidemiology of bacteriuria in an elderly ambulatory population. *Am J Med* 1986;80:208–214.
4. Kunin CM: *Detection, Prevention and Management of Urinary Tract Infections*, 2nd ed. Philadelphia, Lea & Febiger 1974, pp 144–146.
5. Garibaldi RA, Burke JP, Dickman ML, et al: Factors predisposing to bacteriuria during indwelling urethral catheterization. *N Engl J Med* 1974;291:215–219.
6. Boscia JA, Kobasa WD, Abrutyn E, et al: Lack of association between bacteriuria and symptoms in the elderly. *Am J Med* 1986;81:979–982.
7. Nicolle LE, Mayhew WJ, Bryan L: Prospective randomized comparison of therapy and no therapy for asymptomatic bacteriuria in institutionalized elderly women. *Am J Med* 1987;83:27–32.
8. Nicolle LE, Henderson E, Bjornson J, et al: The association of bacteriuria with resident characteristics and survival in

elderly institutionalized men. *Ann Intern Med* 1987;106:682–686.

9. Garibaldi RA, Mooney BR, Epstein BJ, et al: An evaluation of daily bacteriologic monitoring to identify preventable episodes of catheter-associated urinary tract infection. *Infect Control* 1982;3:466–470.

10. Warren JW, Damron D, Tenney JH, et al: Fever, bacteriuria, and death complications of bacteriuria in women with long-term urethral catheters. *J Infect Dis* 1987;155:1151–1158.

11. Verghese A, Berk S: Bacterial pneumonia in the elderly. *Medicine* 1983;62:271–285.

12. Garibaldi RA, Neuhaus EH, Nurse BA: Infections in the elderly, in Rowe JW, Besdine RS (eds): *Geriatric Medicine*, 2nd ed. Boston, Little, Brown, 1988, pp 302–323.

13. Parks TG: Natural history of diverticular disease of the colon. *Clin Gastroenterol* 1975;4:53.

14. Rubin RH, Swartz MN, Malt R: Hepatic abscess changes in clinical, bacteriologic and therapeutic aspects. *Am J Med* 1974;57:601.

15. Glew RH: Abdominal Infections, in Gleckman RA, Gatz NM (eds): *Infections in the Elderly*. Boston, Little, Brown, 1983:177–206.

16. Raudin JI, Guerrant RL: Infectious diarrhea in the elderly. *Geriatrics* 1983;38:95.

17. Smith LG, Sensakovic JW: Skin and soft tissue infections, in Cunha BA, (ed): *Infectious Diseases in the Elderly*. Littleton, Massachusetts PSG Publishing, 1988:243–253.

18. Friedland G, Von Reyn CF, Levy B, et al: Nosocomial endocarditis. *Infection Control* 1984;5:284–288.

19. Robbins N, Demaria A, Millder MH: Infective endocarditis in the elderly. *South Med J* 1980;73:1335–1338.

20. Pruitt AA, Rubin RH, Karchmer AW, et al: Neurologic complications of bacterial endocarditis. *Medicine* 1978;57:329–343.

21. Churchill MA, Geraci JE, Hunder GC: Musculoskeletal manifestations of bacterial endocarditis. *Ann Intern Med* 1977;87:754–759.

22. Kauffman CA, Terpenning MS: Endocarditis: Problems emerge as our population ages. *Contemp Intern Med* 1989:25–30.

23. Lutas EM, Robert TB, Devereux RB, et al: Relation between the presence of echocardiographic vegetations and the complication rate in infective endocarditis. *Am Heart J* 1986;112:107–113.

24 Bryan CS: Update on serious infections in the elderly. *Consultant* 1989:42–55.

25. Gantz NM, Gleckman RA: FUO in the elderly. *Contemp Intern Med* 1989:16–22.

26. Strampfer MJ, Cunha BA: Fever of unknown origin, in Cunha BA (ed): *Infectious Diseases in the Elderly*. Littleton, Massachusetts PSG Publishing, 1988:243–253.

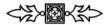

SECTION TWO

NURSING HOME INFECTIONS

CHAPTER

NOSOCOMIAL INFECTIONS IN NURSING HOMES

Philip W. Smith

OVERVIEW OF NOSOCOMIAL INFECTIONS

The term *nosocomial* derives from the Greek *nosos* meaning disease and *komeo* meaning to care for. It has generally been applied to hospitals, in which context nosocomial infections are those infections that develop within a hospital or are produced by microorganisms acquired during hospitalization.[1] The term may also be applied to infections that develop in a nursing home or long term care facility (LTCF).

Hospitals and LTCFs share a number of similar factors that predispose patients to nosocomial infections. In both settings, patients with weakened defenses against infection are clustered together, and contact with potential pathogens is frequent. There is a chain of infection consisting of the three interlocking elements necessary for a nosocomial infection: a reservoir of pathogenic organisms, a means of transmission, and a susceptible host (see Fig. 4.1).

Two types of nosocomial infection may develop. The organisms that cause *endogenous* infections are part of the resident's own normal bacterial flora, such as *Escherichia*

coli, *Klebsiella*, *Proteus* and group D enterococci in the gut, *Staphylococcus aureus* in the nares, and *Staphylococcus epidermidis* on the skin. In *exogenous* infections, the causative organisms are not part of the resident's normal flora, but spread from the external environment. For example, *Pseudomonas* may originate from water or equipment, and *Mycobacterium tuberculosis* may spread from residents with pulmonary tuberculosis. Most nursing home infections are of endogenous origin.

The presence of nosocomial infection does not necessarily imply that the hospital or the LTCF was in any way negligent. Although nosocomial infections can be minimized by a good infection control program, a certain number of nosocomial infections is inevitable. Nosocomial infections may be either *endemic*, occurring at a relatively constant level, or *epidemic*, occurring at greater than expected frequency. Most infections in hospitals and LTCFs are endemic, although epidemics attract a great deal of attention (see Chapter 11). Geographic and temporal clustering of infections suggest an epidemic.

Hospital-Associated Infections

Nosocomial or hospital-associated infections develop in 5% to 10% of all hospitalized patients. In the United States as a whole, this results in about two to three million cases per year.[2] The consequences of nosocomial infection are serious in terms of morbidity, mortality, and cost. The mortality of nosocomial infections is approximately

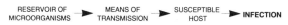

DEVELOPMENT OF NOSOCOMIAL INFECTION

RESERVOIR OF MICROORGANISMS → MEANS OF TRANSMISSION → SUSCEPTIBLE HOST → **INFECTION**

Figure 4.1 *Development of nursing home nosocomial infections*

1%, and the morbidity, as reflected by prolongation of hospital stay, is quite significant.[3,4]

Why do hospital-associated infections occur? The first link in the chain of infection is the organism. *Staphylococcus aureus, E. coli, Pseudomonas aeruginosa*, enterococci, *Klebsiella species*, and *Proteus species* are the leading causes of nosocomial infection in hospitals. In addition to these bacteria, a number of new organisms have been found to be nosocomial pathogens, including *Legionella pneumophila* (the agent causing Legionnaires' disease), *Clostridium difficile* (which causes antibiotic-associated enterocolitis), and atypical mycobacteria.[5] The hospital abounds with microorganisms that cause nosocomial infection. The patient serves as a reservoir of endogenous bacteria; the environment and hospital personnel are reservoirs of exogenous organisms.

The second link in the chain of infection is a means of transmission. Endogenous bacteria do not require a vehicle for transmission to the patient. Exogenous bacteria may be spread by personnel or equipment to the patient, most often via the hands as a final common pathway. This process is potentially preventable and emphasizes the importance of handwashing in the hospital setting. In general, gram-positive infections are transmitted by contact. Personnel with dermatitis or boils have served as sources of epidemics of streptococcal or staphylococcal infections. Gram-negative infections, on the other hand, are often associated with the hospital environment: examples include intravenous fluids, intravenous catheters, respiratory therapy equipment, room humidifiers, hand lotion, prosthetic implants, sinks, foods, surgical instruments, endoscopes, air-conditioning systems, scales, thermometers, and flowers.

The final link in the chain of infection is the susceptible host. What determines whether the patient will be infected or merely colonized by an organism? The patient in the hospital is much less able to defend against pathogens than the healthy individual in the community. A variety of treatments breach local defenses, the body's first line of defense against infection. Intravenous cannulas, urinary catheters, nasotracheal tubes, endotracheal tubes, endoscopy, and surgery bypass local defenses of the skin, urinary tract, intestine, or respiratory tract. In addition, many of the diseases that afflict hospitalized patients impair host defenses against infection (see Chapter 2).

The urinary tract is the leading site of hospital-associated infection, accounting for about 40% of all nosocomial infections, usually following urinary tract catheterization. Nosocomial pneumonia occurs primarily in patients who have nasotracheal or endotracheal tubes in place, are receiving assisted ventilation, are immunosuppressed, have underlying chronic obstructive pulmonary disease, or have undergone surgery. Surgical wound infections cause significant morbidity and mortality in postoperative patients. Nosocomial gastroenteritis is a particular problem on pediatric wards.

Urinary tract infections, wound infections, and pneumonias are generally endemic or sporadic. *E. coli*, enterococci, *Staphylococcus aureus, Pseudomonas, Proteus*, and *Klebsiella* cause most endemic nosocomial infections. Most epidemic nosocomial infections involve the gastrointestinal tract, skin, or bloodstream. The leading causes of epidemic infections are *S. aureus, Salmonella*, hepatitis B, *Aspergillus, Legionella*, atypical Mycobacteria, and aerobic gram-negative bacteria like *Pseudomonas*. Several comprehensive reviews of hospital nosocomial infections are available to the reader.[1,6,7]

Knowledge of infection patterns in hospitals is important to the LTCF practitioner because there is a dynamic equilibrium between the reservoirs of infectious agents in LTCFs and those in hospitals due to transfer of patients between these institutions. Many LTCF admissions are transferred from hospitals, and a significant number of LTCF infections, especially those that occur shortly after admission to the LTCF, are associated with pathogens that more closely reflect usual hospital bacteria rather than LTCF flora.[8]

Causes of Nursing Home–Associated Infections

There are many similarities between hospital and nursing home nosocomial infections in terms of risk factors and types of infections acquired, but several major differences exist (see Table 4.1). First of all, hospitals and LTCFs have different high-risk areas: In the hospital, the patients at greatest risk are immunosuppressed (e.g., cancer patients, renal transplant recipients), postoperative and intensive care patients, and those receiving ventilatory support. Infections are increased by drug or radiation therapy, intravenous catheters, and invasive procedures. In the nursing home, the population is elderly, but less

Table 4.1 *Leading Nosocomial Infections*

NURSING HOMES	HOSPITALS
Urinary tract infection	Urinary tract infection
Infected pressure ulcers	Wound infection
Pneumonia/influenza	Pneumonia
Diarrhea	Bacteremia
Conjunctivitis	

acutely ill. They are impaired by a variety of underlying diseases, immobilization, and urinary catheterization.

Second, the focus of hospitals and LTCFs is different. The hospital focuses on acute care, emphasizing early discharge. Usually, efforts are made to evaluate and treat the patient to the limit of modern technology. There is a general urgency about the patient stay that is not noted in the LTCF setting. The LTCF, on the other hand, is geared to long-term care, with a greater emphasis being placed on the social and psychological aspects of care. Unlike the temporary hospital bed, the nursing home room is a living arrangement for the resident that serves as a home. Resident resistance to infection generally declines during the nursing home stay; the focus is comfort rather than recovery.

Third, ancillary and support services differ greatly between the two types of institutions. LTCFs have lower nurse-to-patient ratios, less physician availability, less elaborate laboratory and support services, and more modest financial resources.

Reservoirs of Infection

In LTCFs, as in hospitals, there is a chain of events that leads to nosocomial infection (see Fig. 4.1). The first element is a *reservoir* of infection. Residents themselves can be reservoirs of infection; many are colonized or infected with potentially pathogenic organisms. Pressure ulcers and urinary catheters, for example, are usually colonized with bacteria. *Staphylococcus aureus* skin colonization or *Pseudomonas* colonization of the perineum can occur. Antibiotic therapy may encourage colonization with antibiotic-resistant bacteria. Finally, an infected resident may serve as a reservoir of infectious organisms (e.g., tuberculosis or salmonellosis).

Organisms may also be found in the environment. Almost any part of the LTCF environment may serve as a reservoir of pathogenic organisms, although this is less of a hazard than the hospital environment. Possible reservoirs include food, air-conditioning systems, thermometers, bathtubs, humidifiers, linen, dust, and even employees. Bacteria are the most significant microorganisms in the LTCF reservoir. As a general rule, gram-negative bacteria such as *Pseudomonas* are the most important organisms in the inanimate environmental reservoir. Gram-positive staphylococci and streptococci are usually found on personnel. The LTCF reservoir is discussed at greater length in Chapters 16 and 18.

Means of Transmission

The second step in the development of infection is a *means of transmission*. Physicians, nurses, and other personnel go from room to room, thereby serving as potential vectors of infectious diseases. Hands are the most important pathway for spread of infection in the hospital and certainly play a similar role in the LTCF. In LTCFs, as in hospitals, residents are in close proximity to each other, which makes transmission more likely. Resident factors encouraging transmission of infection include incontinence and shared activities. The LTCF must also deal with the ambulatory resident who may serve as the source for spread of an infectious disease (e.g., tuberculosis or salmonellosis). Parts of the environment that contact multiple residents may spread organisms (e.g., personnel, food, bathtubs, bedpans, and other equipment).

Spread of organisms may be encouraged by poor handwashing, improper handling of food, poor aseptic technique with resident care, or lack of educational and training programs for the health care worker. LTCFs frequently lack rooms specifically designed for isolation and sinks that are located in close proximity to the rooms, thereby discouraging handwashing.[9] Other factors that contribute to the spread of infection in some LTCFs include the high percentage of nonprofessional staff, high resident/staff ratios, inconsistent immunization practices, work policies that penalize staff for taking sick leave, rapid turnover of employees, and lack of uniform policies and procedures relating to infection control.[10]

Cross-infection in the LTCF setting is most dramatically exemplified by outbreaks of infection. In Garibaldi's study, clustering of infections according to site was frequently observed and accounted for more than 20% of all infections identified. Clusters of upper respiratory tract infections, diarrhea, conjunctivitis, and urinary tract infections were found, which suggested that epidemics of infection occurred frequently.[10] LTCF epidemics are discussed in Chapter 11 and measures to control transmission in Chapter 19.

Host Factors

The third link in the chain of infection is host resistance to infection. Not all persons who have contact with potentially pathogenic organisms become infected; the resident may simply be colonized by a microorganism. The body resists infection with the help of immune defenses. The elderly have impaired resistance to infection because of deficiencies in immune defenses that occur with aging and because of other medical problems that afflict them (see Table 4.2 and Chapters 2 and 3).

A LTCF resident may have additional host defense problems. The majority of residents have multiple underlying chronic diseases,[10,11] and many have indwelling urinary catheters or pressure ulcers that breach local defenses. Therapeutic drugs that residents receive may contribute to the problem. Antibiotics impair the protective function of normal bacterial flora, sedatives depress the cough reflex, and anticholinergics dry respiratory secretions and decrease

Table 4.2   *Important LTCF Infection Risk Factors*

Infection	Predisposing Factor
Urinary tract infection	Indwelling bladder catheter
	Urinary incontinence
	Diabetes mellitus
Pneumonia	Altered mental status
	Cerebrovascular accidents
	Tube feeding
Cutaneous infection	Pressure ulcers
	Incontinence
	Immobilization

bladder contractility. These effects in turn predispose to respiratory and genitourinary tract infections. Immobilization and incontinence predispose to pressure ulcers and urinary tract infections. Surveys have described host factors that are strongly associated with infections in the LTCF, including indwelling urinary catheters (urinary tract infection), incontinence (infected pressure sores), diabetes mellitus, and a number of other underlying diseases. Host factors are discussed in Chapter 17.

General Factors

A number of factors inherent in the nursing home care delivery system affect nosocomial infections. The majority of primary care physicians have not received formal training in geriatric medicine or long-term care, and physician visits to nursing home residents are often brief and superficial.[12]

Many LTCFs do not provide services required by the physician to give optimal medical care to the resident. Services such as urinalysis, chest x-ray, or common blood studies[13] are often beyond the financial scope of the facility. There is a wide variation in incidence of urinary catheterization and in approach to such problems as removal of catheters through policies and procedures.[14] Finally, many facilities do not perform systematic surveillance for infection, routinely monitor resident care practices, or conduct training programs in infection control techniques on a regular basis (see Chapter 9). The designated infection control practitioner frequently has limited time available and other responsibilities as well.

These features of LTCF care may contribute to delays in the diagnosis and treatment of individual infections in residents. They may also affect prevention of infection in the LTCF community.

Frequency of Nursing Home–Associated Infections

There are a number of surveys of LTCF infections, and available studies suggest that nosocomial infections are as prevalent in these institutions as in hospitals. A discussion of the methods used to gather data on nosocomial infections in LTCFs can be found in Chapter 10.

Approximately 15 surveys of LTCF nosocomial infections,[9–10,15–30] both incidence and prevalence studies, have been published since 1980 (see Table 4.3). The incidence rate is most commonly reported as infections per 100 resident months, or infection rate %. The studies found

Table 4.3 *Nursing Home Infections—Surveys*

AUTHOR	REFERENCE	TYPE OF STUDY	NI RATE
Magnussen	9	Incidence	18.2%
Garibaldi	10	Prevalence	16.2%
Gambert	15	Incidence	15.9%
Nicolle	16	Incidence	16.1%
Farber	17	Incidence	20.1%
Standfast	18	Prevalence	32.7%
Setia	19	Prevalence	12.0%
Price	20	Prevalence	5.4%
Franson	21	Prevalence	12.5%
Scheckler	22	Incidence	10.7%
Alvarez	24	Prevalence	6.6%
Jacobson	25	Prevalence	22.0%
Steinmiller	27	Prevalence	9.8%
Magaziner	28	Prevalence	4.4%

nosocomial infection prevalence rates ranging from 4.4% to 32.7% (infections per 100 resident months) and incidence rates ranging from 10.7% to 20.1%. Several studies analyzed infection rates as infections per 1000 resident days,[17,21,23–26,29–30] and results ranged from 1.8 to 7.1 infections per 1000 resident days (see Table 4.4).

It is interesting to note that the rate of 5% to 10% is similar to the acute care hospital rate of 5% to 10% (in this case, 5 to 10 infections/100 discharges), and the rate of 3 to 7 infections per 1000 resident days is comparable to the acute care hospital rate of 6 infections per 1000 patient days.[31] The 5% to 10% rate, when annualized, yields an infection rate of about one infection per resident per year. The CDC estimates 1.5 million infections per year in the United States,[2] and there are about 1.5 million nursing home residents in the United States, resulting in a crude but similar estimate of one infection per resident per year, on the average.

Rates differ from study to study because of variations in data collection methods, definitions of infections, host status, and level of nursing intensity. Severity of illness would be expected to vary widely, for instance, between a free-standing rural facility and a long-term care unit attached to a VA hospital. Some surveys used the medical record as the only source for infection data.[11] Although this technique is

standard in hospitals, the nursing home medical record is felt to be much less complete and accurate.[14] Most studies used a variation of the standard CDC hospital surveillance infection definitions as study definitions.[32]

Although infections vary from institution to institution, the leading nosocomial infections in the LTCF overall are (1) urinary tract infection, (2) respiratory tract infection, (3) skin and soft tissue infection (especially infected pres-

Table 4.4 *Nursing Home Infections per 1000 Days*

AUTHOR	REFERENCE	NI RATE/1000 DAYS
Farber	17	6.7
Franson	21	4.6
Vlahov	23	3.6–3.8
Alvarez	24	3.86
Jacobson	25	2.6
Hoffman	26	4.6
Darnowski	29	1.8
Jackson	30	7.1

sure ulcers), and (4) infectious gastroenteritis. Many other LTCF nosocomial infections have been described, including herpes simplex infections, scabies, conjunctivitis, herpes zoster, bacteremia, and infections due to antibiotic-resistant bacteria.

A majority of nursing home–acquired infections arise endogenously from the resident's own bacteria, which become pathogenic because of indwelling urinary catheters, abraded skin, or depressed immunity. A significant percentage of infections occur by cross-infection; epidemic infections accounted for over 20% of nosocomial infections in nursing homes in the Utah survey, for example.[10]

The importance of LTCF nosocomial infections lies not just in their frequency. Nosocomial infections cause symptomatic complications ranging from fever to septic shock and death. The morbidity of nosocomial infections may profoundly affect the resident. Anyone who has cared for a person with an infected pressure ulcer, for instance, is impressed with pain, the tissue destruction, and the chronicity of this nosocomial infection. Finally, nosocomial infections threaten not just the afflicted resident, but also other residents and personnel. The potential for spread is always present.

SPECIFIC INFECTIONS OF IMPORTANCE IN NURSING HOMES

In this section, the infections that occur in LTCF residents will be identified, with emphasis on epidemiology, diagnosis, prevention, and treatment. The most important infections in nursing homes (urinary tract infections, infected pressure ulcers, pulmonary infections, and gastroenteritis) are reviewed in depth in the following four chapters.

Urinary Tract Infection

Urinary tract infection is the leading nosocomial infection seen in nursing homes.[8] By far the most important factor predisposing to urinary tract infection in the institutionalized elderly is the presence of an indwelling urinary catheter. Hence, control measures should be directed toward prevention of contamination of the catheter system.

Urinary tract infections occur predominantly with gram-negative aerobic bacteria, many of which are normal gut flora (*E. coli, Proteus species*). Even though endogenous bacteria account for the majority of cases, cross-infection is also a risk in nursing homes; the urinary tract is a major site of epidemic, gram-negative antibiotic-resistant infections. A full discussion of urinary tract infection is presented in Chapter 6.

Bacterial Skin and Soft Tissue Infections

Infected Pressure Ulcers

Decubitus ulcer, or pressure ulcer, infection has been a major nosocomial infection in LTCF surveys. The majority of organisms that colonize the ulcer and cause secondary complicating infections of soft tissue or bone are endogenous bacteria, such as enteric gram-negative bacilli, anaerobic gut bacteria, and *Staphylococcus aureus*. A complete discussion of pressure ulcers is found in Chapter 7.

Cellulitis and skin abscess

Other cutaneous infections may be seen in the LTCF (see Table 4.5). Most uncomplicated infections of skin and soft tissues are caused by gram-positive cocci, specifically group A streptococci and *S. aureus*.

Streptococci are bacteria that produce disease on the basis of invasiveness and toxin production. *Erysipelas* is a rapidly spreading superficial infection caused by group A streptococci. The patient is usually febrile. Physical examination reveals lymphangitis and a painful, advancing, red raised area of dermal inflammation. Prompt therapy is

Table 4.5 *Cutaneous Infections in the Nursing Home*

Infected pressure ulcers
Erysipelas
Cellulitis
Cutaneous abscesses
Herpes simplex infections
Herpes zoster
Scabies

important, especially for facial infections. Penicillin is the drug of choice.

Cellulitis, infection of the skin that extends deeper than erysipelas to involve subcutaneous tissues, is almost always caused by group A streptococci or *S. aureus*. Streptococcal cellulitis is more rapidly progressive. Local heat, swelling, and tenderness are seen. Antibiotic therapy of cellulitis is important.[33]

Staphylococci appear as clusters of gram-positive cocci when viewed microscopically (see Fig. 1.1). *S. aureus* is a virulent bacterium capable of producing a variety of extracellular toxins and enzymes. It may be carried in the moist areas of the skin (nares, axilla, rectum) without causing disease, but the skin and soft tissues are frequent sites of staphylococcal infection. *S. aureus* is the leading cause of furuncles, carbuncles, cellulitis, and wound infection. A *furuncle*, or *boil*, is a localized cutaneous infection that begins as an infection of a hair follicle and evolves to a pustule. A *carbuncle* is a deeper and more destructive abscess that extends into the subcutaneous tissue. Furuncles generally resolve without therapy, but carbuncles and abscesses require surgical drainage. Antibiotic therapy is required for cellulitis and extensive abscesses.

The diagnosis of specific infectious skin lesions is by culture, if infected fluid is available. Both staphylococci and streptococci grow readily on standard bacterial media (see Fig. 1.2). A swab of involved skin, however, seldom provides useful information; the correct diagnostic approach involves aspiration of fluid or pus for culture. Streptococci remain extremely sensitive to penicillin, whereas most staphylococci encountered in the nursing home are resistant to penicillin. Antistaphylococcal penicillins, such as oxacillin or nafcillin, are the antibiotics of choice for serious staphylococcal infections. Cephalosporins are alternatives for the penicillin-allergic resident. Methicillin-resistant *S. aureus* (MRSA) needs to be treated with intravenous vancomycin.

Preventive aspects must be addressed. Cellulitis usually poses little hazard for cross-contamination in the LTCF. However, an infected wound or pressure ulcer that drains pus containing *S. aureus* or group A streptococci poses a serious threat and requires appropriate isolation. MRSA requires more stringent isolation.

The institutional reservoir of staphylococcal and streptococcal bacteria is people. This means an infected resident, an infected staff member, or a person who is an asymptomatic carrier of the potentially hazardous organism. The approach to the carrier state in personnel is discussed in Chapter 16.

Other Cutaneous Infections

Herpesvirus Infections

Herpesviruses are DNA viruses that tend to persist in the host and produce recurrent infections. The two most important viruses in this group are herpes simplex virus and varicella-zoster virus. Herpesviruses are spread by direct contact. Herpes simplex type 1 usually causes disease above the waist, primarily the mouth and lips, and is generally acquired during the first decades of life. Herpes simplex type 2 involves areas below the waist, primarily genital sites, and is usually transmitted sexually. The varicella-zoster virus causes chickenpox in children. The virus survives in dorsal nerves and reactivates years later to produce herpes zoster (shingles).

Herpes simplex vesicles (blisters) are characteristically painful and evolve from vesicles to ulcers. Herpes simplex type 1 virus is responsible for ulcerative gingivostomatitis (cold sores). Herpetic vesicles or ulcers occur most frequently on the lips, but may be seen anywhere on the skin, and usually last 7 to 10 days.

Herpes lesions tend to recur. Recurrences may be spontaneous or may follow stress. Primary infections are more severe than recurrent infections; fever and lymphadenopathy are typical clinical manifestations. Extensive, widespread skin lesions occasionally develop in persons with atopic dermatitis, eczema, or abnormal immunity.

The incidence of *herpes zoster* peaks at ages 50 to 80. The vesicles resemble chickenpox, evolving from macules to papules to vesicles, but occur in a dermatomal distribution. Herpes zoster is usually unilateral and most commonly affects the thoracic dermatomes. Local paresthesias or pain may precede the rash. The complication of severe, long-lasting pain (postherpetic neuralgia) is seen most commonly in the elderly.

The diagnosis of cold sores and herpes zoster is primarily clinical, because herpesvirus are not routinely cultured and antibody studies are not helpful. Acyclovir therapy is indicated in severe cases of herpes simplex and herpes zoster, but will not prevent recurrences. Corticosteroid therapy should be avoided. The lesions should be kept dry and clean to prevent secondary bacterial infection.

Nosocomial transmission of the herpesvirus requires direct contact and is relatively uncommon. A special nosocomial hazard is herpetic whitlow, a herpes simplex infection of the digit that occurs primarily in medical personnel.[34] The cutaneous lesions of herpes simplex or herpes zoster remain infectious until the lesions are dry and crusted. Most authorities recommend secretion precautions for localized herpes simplex and localized herpes zoster. Strict isolation is suggested for disseminated herpes infections because of the possibility of airborne transmission (see Chapter 19).

Scabies

Scabies, a disease of the skin produced by the mite *Sarcoptes scabiei*, can be a problem in the LTCF.[33,35–37] The mite burrows into the skin, deposits its eggs, and causes a pruritic skin eruption with characteristic scaling and crusting. A symmetrical eruption is seen most commonly in the axillary region, around the waist, between the fingers, on the inner thighs, and on the backs of the arms and legs. In the nursing home resident, scabies may be limited to sites in contact with the sheets. Because of mental status and immune problems, residents may be heavily infected before the diagnosis is suspected.

The disease is spread by direct contact or through objects such as bedding and clothing. Outbreaks often involve both residents and staff because of extensive hands-on care. If a number of residents and staff members complain of a pruritic eruption, scabies is a likely diagnosis.

The diagnosis is made by placing a drop of mineral oil on the lesion and scraping with a sharp scalpel blade. The mite or its eggs may be seen under low-power microscopy. Because there are a number of conditions that mimic the itching dermatitis of scabies, making a specific diagnosis by scraping is imperative.

Infected individuals should be treated with 5% permethrin or 1% lindane (Kwell) lotion, which are applied to the entire body from the neck down, left on overnight for 8 to 12 hours, and thoroughly washed off. A repeat application may be needed one to two weeks later, especially in heavily infested cases. Permethrin appears to be as effective as lindane and is not associated with any potential neurotoxicity.[37] Treatment will generally make the resident noninfectious in 24 hours. A thorough cleaning of the environment is also indicated; laundering and heat drying of clothing and bedding is usually sufficient to kill mites in exfoliated scales. All infected residents should be treated at the same time. If the outbreak continues, *all* residents and staff may need to be treated simultaneously.

Respiratory Infections

Pneumonia, Influenza and Tuberculosis

A number of respiratory infections are of importance in the LTCF. Pneumonia, tuberculosis, and influenza are discussed in depth in Chapter 5. Pneumococcal pneumonia is the leading cause of pneumonia in the elderly, although LTCF residents are also at increased risk for aspiration pneumonia.

Outbreaks of tuberculosis in LTCFs are common. Both residents and personnel may be involved in such outbreaks, and the infection may cause serious morbidity or even death. Control measures include adequate screening of personnel and residents for tuberculosis. Because tuberculosis is spread by the airborne route, it is also important to institute appropriate isolation measures for residents who have active disease.

Influenza is a very contagious disease spread from person to person by respiratory aerosol. The virus causes epidemics of respiratory disease. Influenza deaths occur predominantly among the elderly and the chronically ill. Influenza outbreaks in LTCFs are not uncommon and may have a significant impact on a facility's population. Control of influenza outbreaks in LTCFs is analyzed in more depth in Chapter 11.

Other Viral Respiratory Tract Infections

A number of other viral respiratory tract infections are important. Upper respiratory infection (URI), especially the common cold, is the most common infectious human disease. The illness is quite contagious, with peak incidence in the winter months. Nasal congestion, rhinorrhea, headache, and low-grade fever are the primary symptoms. URIs are caused by many agents, especially rhinoviruses. Antibiotics have no place in the treatment of this self-limited viral illness. There is evidence to suggest that transmission of rhinovirus infection is as efficient by hand contact as it is by the aerosol route, and good handwashing is most important in preventing spread of URIs.

Outbreaks of respiratory syncytial virus (RSV) and parainfluenza respiratory disease have been reported in nursing homes.[38–40] RSV appears to be spread by the aerosol route. Most residents have fever, cough, and rhinorrhea; pneumonia may occasionally develop. Parainfluenza is a virus that may cause URI, bronchitis, and occasionally pneumonia. In nursing home outbreaks, case clustering in living units and dining areas suggested person-to-person spread. The illness occurred in both employees and residents, suggesting that employees may be an important transmission line.[40] Diagnosis of these viral illnesses can be made by measuring a rise in serum antibody level.

Other respiratory infections reported in the LTCF setting include *Hemophilus influenzae*,[41] psittacosis,[42] pertussis,[43] coronavirus, and adenovirus.[44] These respiratory agents may occur in outbreaks.

Gastroenteritis

Gastroenteritis is quite common in the LTCF. *Salmonella* is the leading cause of confirmed foodborne outbreaks, but *Staphylococcus aureus* and *Clostridium perfringens* outbreaks are not rare.

Viral gastroenteritis is a very common, usually self-limited infectious disease that causes diarrhea and occasionally low-grade fever. Rotavirus, Norwalk virus, and enteroviruses are the usual causes of viral gastroenteritis. Outbreaks are propagated primarily by person-to-person transmission. Gastrointestinal and abdominal infections are covered in detail in Chapter 8, and gastrointestinal outbreaks are discussed in Chapter 11.

Miscellaneous Nosocomial Infections in the Nursing Home

Conjunctivitis

Conjunctivitis was found in 3.4% of the residents surveyed by Garibaldi.[10] Clustering of cases suggested cross-infection or epidemics of conjunctivitis. Persons with conjunctivitis classically have a red and painful eye associated with a scratchy foreign body sensation. Most epidemic conjunctivitis is viral in origin. Nosocomial outbreaks have occurred with a number of viruses, especially adenovirus and Coxsackievirus.[45,46] Transmission is usually person-to-person, although transmission of adenovirus has been associated with medical instruments.

Conjunctivitis may involve both residents and staff at a facility. Appropriate isolation precautions are recommended for residents with conjunctivitis. The resident is not required to be in a private room, but the staff should practice careful handwashing and special handling of infected secretions and dressings. Others have recommended steril-

ization of instruments between uses, heating instruments in a bath at 75°C for 10 minutes, or immersing instruments in a 1% to 2% solution of sodium hypochlorite.[47]

Bacteremia

Nosocomial bacteremia (bacteria in the bloodstream) is relatively uncommon in LTCFs compared to hospitals, but is seen with some frequency due to the increased acuity of illness in these residents and the common use of long-term, indwelling central intravenous (IV) devices.[48–50]

Bacteremias may be primary, in which case they generally originate from contaminated IV devices, or they may be secondary to other infections such as wound infection, intra-abdominal infection, urinary tract infection, or pneumonia. Bacteria causing IV-related bacteremia may originate from the patient's skin, the hands of personnel, or the intravenous fluid or apparatus.

Guidelines have been published for minimizing intravenous-related nosocomial infections,[51] including minimizing IV catheter use, changing the IV catheter frequently, inserting the IV catheter with proper aseptic technique, changing the infusion apparatus every 48 hours, changing IV bottles at least every 24 hours, and suspecting that the IV catheter may be the source of infection in any resident with such a catheter who develops fever.

Fever

Fever is an important sign of infection and an important clue to infection in all surveillance systems (see Chapter 10). There is evidence that the elderly do not develop the same febrile response to an infection as young patients (see Chapter 3), yet fever is noted in most significant infectious episodes.

Several studies have looked specifically at the significance and treatment of febrile episodes in the LTCF. In one study, lower respiratory tract infections were the most common cause of fever and there was a 16% mortality associated with febrile episodes, although many residents recovered without specific therapy.[52] Franson noted that residents in community-based nursing homes were less likely to have evaluation and therapy than patients in hospital-based nursing facilities.[53] Residents with severe underlying diseases may not receive aggressive antibiotic therapy; for less severely afflicted residents, appropriate diagnosis and therapy improved survival.[54]

OTHER EXTENDED CARE FACILITIES

The term *long-term care facility* is generally used interchangeably with the term *nursing home*, a facility that provides skilled nursing or intermediate care for residents, usually the elderly. Other extended care facilities not dealing primarily with the elderly include rehabilitation facilities, spinal injury units, institutions for the mentally retarded, psychiatric hospitals, and even some correctional facilities. The general principles covered in this book apply to most long-term care facilities, but some facilities have specific problems.

Hepatitis is a particular concern in the *institution for the mentally retarded* (IMR). Hepatitis B is a concern because of the problem of biting human carriers,[55] Down's syndrome, and crowding.[55,56] Spread of hepatitis A may readily occur in a situation where fecal hygiene is poor. Similar transmission of other fecal agents such as helminths has been described.[57,58] Respiratory outbreaks in this setting are also commonly reported,[59-62] and diseases such as tuberculosis (airborne) and HIV infection (bloodborne) need to be addressed by policies and procedures in any IMR.

Because of similar hygienic problems, fecal-oral spread of infectious diseases is a major concern in *psychiatric hospitals* and reports of viral gastroenteritis, *Shigella* and salmonellosis can be found.[63-65] Infection control programs also need to be concerned with hepatitis B, tuberculosis, and HIV infection. Reported infection rates are somewhat lower than those observed for nursing homes caring for the elderly, which may reflect less intensive surveillance or the younger average age of residents.[66]

Rehabilitation facilities and spinal injury units tend to have very long stay residents who are at risk of developing pressure ulcers. Many of them require long-term indwelling urinary catheters. Commonly reported infections include urinary tract infections and pressure ulcers infected with MRSA or other pathogens.[67,68] Rehabilitation patients have been shown to be at high risk of acquiring infections associated with chronic urinary catheterization or skin breakdown.[69]

REFERENCES

1. Brachman PS: Epidemiology of nosocomial infections, in Bennett JV, Brachman PS (eds): *Hospital Infections*, 2nd Ed. Boston, Little, Brown, 1986, p 3–16.
2. Haley RW, Culver DH, White JW, et al: The nationwide nosocomial infection rate—a new need for vital statistics. *Am J Epidemiol* 1985;121:159–167.
3. Freeman J, Rosner BA, McGowan JG Jr: Adverse effects of nosocomial infection. *J Infect Dis* 1979;140:732–740.
4. Green MS, Rubinstein E, Amit P: Estimating the effects of nosocomial infections on length of hospitalization. *J Infect Dis* 1982;145:667–672.
5. Fraser DW: Bacteria newly recognized as nosocomial pathogens. *Am J Med* 1982;70:432–437.
6. Wenzel RP (ed): *Prevention and Control of Nosocomial Infections*. Baltimore, MD, Williams & Wilkins, 1987.
7. Mayhall G (ed): *Hospital Epidemiology and Infection Control*, Baltimore, MD, Williams & Wilkins, (in press).
8. Sherman FT, Tucci V, Libow LS, et al: Nosocomial urinary-tract infections in a skilled nursing facility. *J Am Geriatr Soc* 1980;28:456–461.
9. Magnussen MH, Robb SS: Nosocomial infections in a long-term care facility. *Am J Infect Control* 1980;8:12–17.
10. Garibaldi RA, Brodine S, Matsumiya S: Infections among patients in nursing homes: Policies, prevalence, and problems. *N Engl J Med* 1981;305:731–735.
11. Cohen ED, Hierholzer WJ Jr, Schilling CR, et al: Nosocomial infection in skilled nursing facilities: A preliminary survey. *Public Health Rep* 1979;94:162–166.
12. Ouslander JG: Medical care given in the nursing home. *JAMA* 1989;262:2582–2590.
13. Brown MN, Cornwell J, Weist JK: Reducing the risks to the institutionalized elderly: I. Depersonalization, negative relocation effects, and medical care deficiencies. *J Gerontol Nurs* 1981;7:401–404.
14. Zimmer JG: Medical care evaluation studies in long-term care facilities. *J Am Geriatr Soc* 1979;27:62–72.
15. Gambert SR, Duthie EH Jr, Priefer B, et al: Bacterial infections in a hospital-based skilled nursing facility. *J Chron Dis* 1982;35:781–786.
16. Nicolle LE, McIntyre M, Zacharias H, et al: Twelve month surveillance of infections in institutionalized elderly men. *J Am Geriatr Soc* 1984;32:513–519.
17. Farber BF, Brennen C, Puntereri AJ, et al: A prospective study of nosocomial infections in a chronic care facility. *J Am Geriatr Soc* 1984;32:499–502.
18. Standfast SJ, Michelsen PB, Baltch AL, et al: A prevalence survey of infections in a combined acute and long-term care hospital. *Infect Control* 1984;5:177–184.
19. Setia U, Serventi I, Lorenz P: Nosocomial infections among patients in a long-term care facility: Spectrum, preva-

lence and risk factors. *Am J Infect Control* 1985;13:57–62.

20. Price LE, Sarubbi FA Jr, Rutala WA: Infection control programs in twelve North Carolina extended care facilities. *Infect Control* 1985;6:437–441.

21. Franson TR, Duthie GH Jr, Cooper JE, et al: Prevalence survey of infections and their predisposing factors at a hospital-based nursing home care unit. *J Am Geriatr Soc* 1986;34:95–100.

22. Scheckler WE, Peterson PJ: Infections and infection control among residents of eight rural Wisconsin nursing homes. *Arch Intern Med* 1986;146:1981–1984.

23. Vlahov D, Tenney JH, Cervino KW, et al: Routine surveillance for infections in nursing homes: experience in two facilities. *Am J Infect Control* 1987;15:47–53.

24. Alvarez S, Shell CG, Woolley TW, et al: Nosocomial infections in long-term facilities. *J Gerontol* 1988;43:M9–17.

25. Jacobson C, Strausbaugh LJ: Incidence and impact of infection in a nursing home care unit. *Am J Infect Control* 1990;18:151–159.

26. Hoffman N, Jenkins R, Putney K: Nosocomial infection rates during a one-year period in a nursing home care unit of a Veterans' Administration hospital. *Am J Infect Control* 1990;18:53–66.

27. Steinmiller AM, Robb SS, Muder RR: Prevalence of nosocomial infection in long-term-care Veterans Administration medical centers. *Am J Infect Control* 1991;19:143–146.

28. Magaziner J, Tenney JH, DeForge B, et al: Prevalence and characteristics of nursing home–acquired infections in the aged. *J Am Geriatr Soc* 1991;39:1071–1078.

29. Darnowski SB, Gordon M, Simor AE: Two years of infection surveillance in a geriatric long-term facility. *Am J Infect Control* 1991;19:185–190.

30. Jackson MM, Fierer J, Barrett-Connor E, et al: Intensive surveillance for infections in a three-year study of nursing home patients. *Am J Epidemiol* 1992;135:685–696.

31. Culver DH, Banerjee SN, Martone WJ, et al: *Analysis of NNIS Surveillance Component Data: Oct 1986–May 1988.* Preliminary report, Atlanta, GA, Centers for Disease Control: National Nosocomial Infection Surveillance System, August 1988.

32. Garner JS, Jarvis WR, Emori TG, et al: CDC definitions for nosocomial infections, 1988. *Am J Infect Control* 1988;16:128–140.

33. Smith PW: Approach to nursing home patients with skin and soft tissue infections, in Duma RJ (ed): *Recognition and Management of Nursing Home Infections*, Bethesda, MD, National Foundation for Infectious Diseases, 1992.

34. Greaves WL, Kaiser AB, Alford RH, et al: The problem of herpetic whitlow among hospital personnel. *Infect Control* 1980;1:381–385.

35. Scabies in institutions. *J Iowa Med Soc* 1981;71:78–79.

36. Burkhart CG: Scabies: An epidemiologic reassessment. *Ann Intern Med* 1983;98:498–503.

37. Degelau J: Scabies in long-term care facilities. *Infect Control Hosp Epidemiol* 1992;13:421–425.

38. Mathur U, Bentley DW, Hall CB: Concurrent respiratory

syncytial virus and influenza A infections in the institutionalized elderly and chronically ill. *Ann Intern Med* 1980;93(pt 1):49–52.

39. Garvie DG, Gray J: Outbreak of respiratory syncytial virus infection in the elderly. *Br Med J* 1980;281:1253–1254.

40. Center for Disease Control: Parainfluenza outbreaks in extended care facilities—United States. *MMWR* 1978;27:475–476.

41. Smith PF, Stricof RL, Shayegani M, et al: Cluster of Haemophilus influenzae type B infections in adults. *JAMA* 1988;260:1446–1449.

42. Robson D, Frederick H, Speerman G, et al: Avian psittacosis outbreak in a geriatric wing of a tertiary care hospital (abstract). Association for Practitioners in Infection Control 16th Annual Conference, Reno, NV, 1989.

43. Addiss DG, Davis JP, Meade BD, et al: A pertussis outbreak in a Wisconsin nursing home. *J Infect Dis* 1991;164:704–710.

44. Falsey AR: Noninfluenza respiratory virus infection in long-term care facilities. *Infect Control Hosp Epidemiol* 1991;12:602–608.

45. Christopher S, Theograj S, Godbole S, et al: An epidemic of acute hemorrhagic conjunctivitis due to coxsackievirus A-24. *J Infect Dis* 1982;146:16–19.

46. Warren D, Nelson KE, Farrar JA, et al: A large outbreak of epidemic keratoconjunctivitis: problems in controlling nosocomial spread. *J Infect Dis* 1989;160:938–943.

47. Kennlyside RA, Hierholzer JC, D'Angelo LJ: Keratoconjunctivitis associated with adenovirus type 37: An extended outbreak in an ophthalmologist's office. *J Infect Dis* 1983;147:191–198.

48. Setia V, Serventi I, Lorenz P: Bacteremia in a long-term care facility—spectrum and mortality. *Arch Intern Med* 1984;144:1633–1635.

49. Rudman D, Hontanosas A, Cohen Z, et al: Clinical correlates of bacteremia in a Veterans Administration extended care facility. *J Am Geriatr Soc* 1988;36:726–732.

50. Muder RR, Brennen C, Wagener MM, et al: Bacteremia in a long-term facility: A five year prospective study of 163 consecutive episodes. *Clin Infect Dis* 1992;14:647–654.

51. Simmons BP, Hooton TM, Wong ES, et al: Guidelines for prevention of intravascular infections. *Infect Control* 1982;3:61–72.

52. Finnegan TP, Austin TW, Cape RDT: A 12-month fever surveillance study in a Veterans' long-stay institution. *J Am Geriatr Soc* 1985;33:590–594.

53. Franson TR, Schicker JM, LeClair SM, et al: Documentation and evaluation of fevers in hospital-based and community-based nursing homes. *Infect Control Hosp Epidemiol* 1988;9:447–450.

54. Fabiszewski KJ, Volicer B, Volicer L: Effect of antibiotic treatment on outcome of fevers in institutionalized Alzheimer patients. *JAMA* 1990;263:3168–3172.

55. Van Ditzhuljsen JM, De Witte E, Van Loon AM, et al: Hepatitis B virus infection in an institution for the mentally retarded. *Am J Epidemiol* 1988;128:629–638.

56. Cancio-Bello TP, de Medina M, Shorey J, et al: An institu-

tional outbreak of hepatitis B related to a human biting carrier. *J Infect Dis* 1982;146:652–656.

57. Braun TI, Fekete T, Lynch A: Strongyloidiasis in an institution for mentally retarded adults. *Arch Intern Med* 1988;148:634–636.

58. Allen KD, Green HT: An outbreak of *Trichuris trichiura* in a mental handicap hospital. *J Hosp Infect* 1989;13:161–166.

59. Atkinson WL, Arden NH, Patriarca PA, et al: Amantadine prophylaxis during an institutional outbreak of type A (H1N1) influenza. *Arch Intern Med* 1986;146:1751–1756.

60. Steketee RW, Wassilak SGF, Adkins WN, et al: Evidence for a high attack rate and efficacy of erythromycin prophylaxis in a pertussis outbreak in a facility for the developmentally disabled. *J Infect Dis* 1988;157:434–440.

61. Jackson BM, Smith JD, Sikes RK: Parainfluenza outbreak in a retardation facility. *Am J Infect Control* 1990;18:128–129.

62. Finger R, Anderson LJ, Dicker RC, et al: Epidemic infections caused by respiratory syncytial virus in institutionalized young adults. *J Infect Dis* 1987;155:1335–1339.

63. Mitchell E, O'Mahony M, McKeith I, et al: An outbreak of viral gastroenteritis in a psychiatric hospital. *J Hosp Infect* 1989;14:1–8.

64. Hunter PR, Hutchins PG: Outbreak of Shigella sonnei dysentery in a long stay psychogeriatric ward. *J Hosp Infect* 1987;10:73–76.

65. Meara J, Mayon-White R, Johnston H: Salmonellosis in a psychogeriatric ward: Problems of infection control. *J Hosp Infect* 1988;11:86–90.

66. Loving P, Porter S, Stuifbergen A, et al: Surveillance of nosocomial infections in private psychiatric hospitals: An exploratory study. *Am J Infect Control* 1992;20:149–155.

67. Flaherty PJ, Liljestrand JS, O'Brien TF: Urinary tract infections in an American rehabilitation hospital. *J Hosp Infect* 1984;5(suppl A):75–80.

68. Aeilts GD, Sapico FL, Canawati HN, et al: Methicillin-resistant Staphylococcus aureus colonization and infection in a rehabilitation facility. *J Clin Microbiol* 1982;16:218–223.

69. Nicolle LE, Buffet L, Alfieri N, et al: Nosocomial infections on a rehabilitation unit in an acute care hospital. *Infect Control Hosp Epidemiol* 1988;9:553–558.

CHAPTER

PULMONARY INFECTIONS: INFLUENZA, PNEUMONIA, AND TUBERCULOSIS

Joseph M. Mylotte and David W. Bentley

This chapter focuses on three infections that cause significant morbidity and mortality among residents of long-term care facilities (LTCFs): influenza, bacterial pneumonia, and tuberculosis. The major objectives are to (1) understand the epidemiology and pathogenesis of these infections and the relevance in their control and prevention, (2) describe the clinical presentation of these infections and the practical laboratory and diagnostic approaches, and (3) recommend appropriate treatment and preventive strategies for LTCFs.

INFLUENZA

Epidemiology

The predominant influenza viruses that circulate in the community (and in LTCFs) are several types of influenza A and influenza B. Unpredictable independent antigenic "drifts" or "shifts" of the H (hemagglutinin) protein and the N (neuraminidase) protein lead to outbreaks and epidemics, which require yearly vaccination. Although the rates of community-acquired influenza virus infection in older persons are relatively low (<5%), the rates for residents in LTCFs with sporadic cases (13%) and in the presence of LTCF outbreaks (21%–33%) are substantial. In addition, complications associated with underlying chronic conditions, especially cardiopulmonary diseases, occur frequently in this high-risk population, including hospitalization (3.5%–6.6%) and death (1.1%–4.5%) Outbreaks, defined as an overall attack rate of at least 10% among residents in any nursing home, can occur in more than 50% of a community's LTCFs.[1]

Pathogenesis

Infection is the result of transfer of virus-containing respiratory secretions via small-particle aerosols from infected persons who are sneezing, coughing or talking vigorously to a susceptible person. Neutralizing, hemagglutination-inhibiting (HAI) and complement-fixing (CF) antibodies (all primarily IgG antibodies) begin to develop in the serum by 14 days and reach peak titers by four to six weeks following infection. The severity of illness correlates temporally with quantities of virus shed in respiratory secretions. Although there is no exact correlation, protection against infection (or amelioration of disease severity) is associated with the presence of substantial levels of antibody, which develop two to four weeks after infection.[2]

Clinical Features

Uncomplicated influenza is characterized by the abrupt onset of a febrile systemic illness. Frequently an unexplained fever (37.7°C, 100°F) may be the first sign noted. Other early features include chills (rigors) or chilliness, headache, myalgia, and malaise, although these may be difficult to identify in the cognitively impaired resident. Local respiratory signs and symptoms (e.g., cough, nasal obstruction and sore throat) predominate over the next three to five days and can persist for two to four weeks along with malaise. Ocular symptoms and signs (e.g., photophobia, tearing and painful eye movements) may be helpful in distinguishing milder cases of influenza from other respiratory viral infections. Gastrointestinal signs and symptoms (e.g., nausea, vomiting, diarrhea and abdominal cramps) are present rarely. The clinical suspicion of influenza infection in the individual resident is easier with the knowledge that an influenza virus outbreak is occurring in the community and multiple residents on the same nursing unit have a similar influenza-like illness (I-LI).

The most frequent complication of influenza is bacterial pneumonia. This occurs generally during the third to tenth day of the illness, often following signs of initial improvement. Clinical manifestations are as noted in the pneumonia section following. The etiologic agents are usually mixed flora, *S. pneumoniae* and *H. influenzae*, although *S. aureus* (both methicillin-sensitive and methicillin-resistant) pneumonia may be problematic. Primary influenza viral pneumonia is caused by progressive involvement of the lung parenchyma with influenza virus. Clinical manifestations include continuation of the classical influenza syndrome with relentless progression of dyspnea, cough, and hypoxia, and a chest radiograph suggesting pulmonary edema. Fortunately this appears to be uncommon in residents in LTCFs. A frequent complication is tracheobronchitis, which is characterized by a persistent irritative productive cough with moderate to profuse mucopurulent sputum that is occasionally blood-streaked. Acute exacerbations of chronic bronchitis are also frequent in residents with chronic obstructive pulmonary disease (COPD).

Diagnosis

Although residents in LTCFs with influenza may not develop fever or have sufficient clinical complaints,[3] a practical case definition for I-LI is an acute febrile illness with a temperature of 37.7°C (100°F) or higher and one or more respiratory signs—e.g., cough, sore throat, or nasal congestion (coryza). It is important to make a laboratory diagnosis of influenza as the suspected respiratory viral pathogen

because the management of the infected resident (and any related outbreaks) will require a substantially different approach if the pathogen is not influenza virus.[4] Therefore, infection control programs in LTCFs should identify a reliable local certified laboratory, usually in a tertiary care hospital or a laboratory under contract to the State Department of Health, to which viral cultures and serologic studies can be sent.

Influenza virus can be isolated from naso-oropharyngeal swabs or sputum samples. A convenient culture technique in LTCFs is to use one swab for both nasal turbinates and a second swab for a vigorous throat culture. Both swabs are placed in refrigerated viral transport media and carried on ice within one or two hours to the virus laboratory. Over half of positive cultures can be detected within three days of inoculation and the remainder by five to seven days. Direct detection of influenza viral antigen in clinical samples, either by immunofluorescence or enzyme immunoassay, is a research tool that when commercially available will serve as a rapid diagnostic test for influenza. Although not helpful during the acute illness, acute and convalescent (21 days after onset of I-LI) sera may be obtained for CF antibody studies.

Treatment

For the individual resident with an I-LI, nonspecific supportive symptomatic treatment should include bed rest and fluids. Antipyretics and analgesics may be helpful if fever or headache and myalgias are bothersome. Cough suppressants and nasal decongestants should be used cautiously because of the adverse reactions of elderly residents. More intensive use of bronchodilator therapy may be helpful in residents with COPD.

Amantadine hydrochloride (Symmetrel®) was licensed in 1976 as an antiviral compound for the treatment (and prevention) of upper respiratory tract infections caused by all strains of type A (but not type B) influenza viruses. The most safe and effective dose for elderly residents is unknown. The usual recommended dose for adults is 200 mg orally for one dose, then 100 mg twice per day thereafter. Because amantadine is primarily cleared by the kidney and renal function declines with age, the manufacturer's package insert recommends reducing the dosage to 100 mg per day for older persons, although this regimen has not been associated with a reduction in efficacy.[5] Residents with impaired renal function require further reduction in dose.[6]

Amantadine side eff cts can occur in up to 33% of recipients and are most frequently related to its action on the central nervous system.[7] Particularly bothersome side effects for the LTCF resident are confusion, anxiety, insomnia, depression, dizziness, and ataxia. Other difficulties noted are gastrointestinal (anorexia and nausea) and anticholinergic (dry mouth, constipation, and urinary retention) side effects. Seizures occur with increased frequency, especially in residents with active preexisting major motor seizure disorders. Approximately 3% of elderly persons who receive amantadine fall each month as a result of drug-induced dizziness or postural hypotension.[8] Falls are especially problematic for frail nursing home residents during prophylaxis (see below) and can occur at rates of 6.4 falls per 1,000 residents/day.[9]

Double-blinded placebo-controlled therapeutic efficacy trials in LTCF residents demonstrate in the amantadine-treated group (dose 100 mg twice per day) lower mean temperatures (1–2°F) than in the placebo-treated group in the first 70 hours of illness.[10] Therapeutic efficacy trials with rimantadine hydrochloride, an analog of amantadine under study, demonstrate similar effects.[11] There are no data on the efficacy of amantadine therapy in preventing complications of influenza A among this high-risk population.

Treatment with amantadine can be recommended when influenza A viral infections are documented in the community or LTCF and the acutely ill resident is identified as (1) a high-risk resident with active cardiopulmonary conditions and a febrile I-LI of less than 24 to 48 hours duration or (2) a resident with suspected primary influenzal pneumonia. The dosage is as noted and is continued for 48 hours after resolution of symptoms for a maximum of 7 to 10 days. Whether amantadine is effective when treatment is started beyond the first 48 hours of illness is not known.

Prevention

Influenza prevention measures are listed in Table 5.1. Inactivated influenza virus vaccines have been the principal means for preventing influenza since the late 1940s. In general, the vaccine has contained both type A and B virus strains representing influenza viruses believed likely to circulate in the upcoming winter. Recent influenza vaccines have consisted of highly purified, egg-grown, inactivated viruses in a trivalent preparation containing two type A strains and one type B strain. One dose intramuscularly in the deltoid muscle is required each year for residents.

Table 5.1   *Influenza Control Measures*

PREVENTION

- Resident vaccination
- Employee vaccination

MANAGEMENT OF OUTBREAKS

- Monitor residents for "influenza-like" illness
- Respiratory and secretion precautions for cases
- Monitor employees for illness
- Screen visitors and relatives for illness
- Vaccinate previously unvaccinated residents and staff
- Amantadine prophylaxis (if influenza A)

Acute local reactions, with mild to moderate soreness around the vaccination site, occur in approximately 33% of vaccines and last one to two days. Systemic reactions, including fever with or without an I-LI, occur in less than 1% of vaccinees, begin 6 to 12 hours postvaccination, persist for one to two days, and appear to be less severe in older persons.[2] Because influenza vaccine contains only noninfectious viruses, it cannot cause influenza. Contraindications to vaccination include an anaphylactic or documented hypersensitivity to eggs.[12] There are no studies to suggest an increased risk of exacerbations in persons with multiple sclerosis or other chronic neurologic demyelinating diseases, but persons with a previous history of Guillain-Barré syndrome may be at increased risk for a recurrence from influenza vaccines. Amantadine does not suppress the antibody responses to inactivated influenza vaccines.

The proportion of elderly vaccinees who develop protective serum HAI antibody titers of 1:40 or more postvaccination ranges from more than 85% for H3N2 antigens in healthy community-based older persons to 46% to 100% for H3N2 antigens and 20% to 69% for B antigens in ambulatory older persons in LTCFs.[13] Studies in skilled nursing facilities indicate that 39% to 64% and 17% to 63% of elderly vaccinees develop HAI antibody titers of 1:40 or more postvaccination to H3N2 and B antigens, respectively.[14] Although there is considerable heterogeneity among elderly residents, these responses overall are significantly lower than for healthy young and healthy older persons and suggest that older persons with chronic diseases, medications, or other conditions frequently associated with residence in LTCFs (or intensive home-based care) may be expected to respond less satisfactorily to inactivated influenza vaccines. Protective titers are not substantially improved by increasing the vaccine dose to two or three times the standard commercial dose nor providing booster vaccinations, and these measures are not recommended.[15,16]

When influenza vaccine antigens are closely matched with the epidemic strain and studied in placebo-controlled trials, the efficacy rate is 96% for reducing influenza infection in healthy older persons.[17] A retrospective study demonstrated that influenza vaccine reduced influenza-associated hospitalizations and deaths among community-residing older persons by 72% and 81%, respectively.[18] An uncontrolled prospective study of outbreaks in nursing homes indicated that, although the efficacy of influenza vaccine in uncomplicated illness was relatively low (28% to 37%), the efficacy in reducing complications, including hospitalization (47%), pneumonia (58%) and death (76%) was substantial.[1]

Annual influenza vaccination programs with the current standard trivalent inactivated influenza vaccine are recommended for all LTCFs by the Immunization Practices Advisory Committee (ACIP).[12] Only 55% to 60% of residents in LTCFs, however, receive annual influenza vaccination, with the lowest rates occurring in LTCFs that require annual written informed consent.[19] Efforts to improve influenza vaccination rates for residents in LTCFs have included (1) resident/guardian consent for annual influenza vaccination upon admission, (2) preprinted medication orders with renewals prior to the influenza season, and (3) careful review of late fall and winter admissions after vaccination programs and vaccination of those residents depending on immunization status.[20] The ACIP also recommends that vaccination should be routinely provided for all residents with the concurrence of attending physicians rather than obtaining individual vaccination orders for each resident. Consent for vaccination should be obtained from the resident or family member at the time of admission to the facility, and all residents should be vaccinated at one time. Because protective antibody titers rarely last more than a few months in elderly residents,[21] it is advisable to vaccinate this high-risk population as close to six weeks before the expected influenza season occurs.[12]

In addition to maximizing the protection of LTCF residents, the ACIP also recommends that all employees who have contact with these residents should be vaccinated.[12] Persons who live in the community where the influenza outbreak is occurring and who are clinically or subclinically infected can transmit the influenza virus to LTCF residents. Epidemiologic studies of several LTCF outbreaks have identified an employee as the index case; unfortunately, fewer than 30% of LTCF personnel receive influenza vaccine in any given year.[20] Nevertheless, several approaches have been utilized to achieve a vaccination rate for personnel approaching 80%, including (1) a mobile influenza vaccine cart that moves between nursing stations, (2) annual in-service "fairs" with immediate opportunities for vaccination, and (3) "thank you" notes to vaccinated staff.[20] Others have suggested that an approved immunization program in LTCFs for influenza vaccine for residents and personnel should be a requirement for state licensure.[22] A useful handbook on managing influenza vaccination programs in LTCFs is available from the Centers for Disease Control and Prevention (CDC).[23] The influenza vaccine for residents is also discussed in Chapter 17.

Amantadine is recommended as continuous chemoprophylaxis for LTCF residents during the interval when influenza A viruses are circulating in the community but prior to a LTCF influenza outbreak. Although this preoutbreak-initiated preventive program may have certain benefits versus an influenza vaccination program,[24] the most useful strategy for amantadine is to supplement the protection of residents already vaccinated. In this case, amantadine is intended as an additional margin of protection, especially for high-risk residents in LTCFs with cardiopulmonary disease. The duration of chemoprophylaxis is the duration of the community outbreak (i.e., 6 to 12 weeks). Occasionally amantadine is used as the only prophylactic measure for those few residents for whom influenza vaccine is contraindicated. In this case the duration of chemoprophylaxis is the duration of the influenza season (i.e., up to 12 weeks). Problems associated with these strategies are (1) the long duration of amantadine use with the increased likelihood of adverse reactions, (2) the development of amantadine-resistant influenza A strains (see below), (3) the uncertainty that influenza A virus will cause an outbreak, and (4) the expense (the cost of 100 mg per day per resident is approximately $15.00 or $20.00 for a 6- or 12-

week course, respectively), which is borne by the LTCF because of current limited reimbursement mechanisms.

Management of Outbreaks

The management of outbreaks begins with the knowledge that influenza A virus has been identified in the community and the recognition that there are several residents on the same LTCF unit with an I-LI. Retrospective studies have defined an outbreak as an overall attack rate of at least 10% within any 7-day period,[1] but concurrent management decisions require an alternative. A practical definition of a LTCF outbreak is the presence of more than one I-LI case occurring in the same unit within two consecutive days. Usually the identification of an outbreak is not difficult, however, because of the short incubation period (18 to 36 hours) and the rapid "explosive" spread of influenza viruses, primarily by small-particle aerosols. Surveillance measures should begin now with documentation by case–resident and case–employee line listings and by noting the sequence of cases on a diagram of the unit (see Chapter 11). Because other respiratory viruses can cause similar disease and LTCF outbreaks,[4] it is important to confirm that the current outbreak is due to influenza A virus. A practical approach is to obtain virus cultures within 24 to 36 hours of onset of I-LI from two or three of the first cases on each unit.

As soon as the outbreak is identified, control measures are instituted with the expectation that early intervention will limit its spread to the current unit.[20] Although there are no controlled studies, most restrictions for residents include placing all with an I-LI on respiratory and secretion precautions during the duration of their contagiousness (i.e., five days from the onset of the illness). Because roommates are at especially high risk for infection, well roommates are managed in the same way. All appointments that are not medically related are canceled. Most important, support services (i.e., occupational therapy, recreation therapy, social services, chaplains, volunteers, etc.) should establish programs and activities on the outbreak unit.

As noted, personnel play an important role in the introduction and spread of influenza in LTCFs. Ideally, a number of guidelines should be agreed to prior to the influenza season. When personnel with direct resident care call in sick, they should notify the department of the nature of the illness. Those with fever, cough, or other I-LI symptoms

should remain off work for three to five days from the onset of their clinical illness. Personnel with the onset of I-LI while at work should notify their supervisor and report to the employee health nurse before going home. "Floating" personnel on and off the outbreak unit should be strongly discouraged. Those temporarily assigned to the outbreak area should remain assigned to this area for the duration of this outbreak (i.e., four or five consecutive days with no new cases). Cohorting of nursing personnel (i.e., one nurse team cares for sick residents only and the other team cares for well residents only) should be attempted whenever feasible. In case of shortage of personnel, employees with mild I-LIs can work, especially with residents already ill, but must wear a mask with direct resident contact and practice vigorous handwashing techniques. Unfortunately, because of the shortage of LTCF personnel (especially nursing and administrative problems with sick leave) most of these guidelines can only be approximated.

Visitors with I-LI (or any signs or symptoms of a URI) should not visit residents at any time of the year, but especially not during the community's influenza outbreak. All visitors should be informed of the outbreak's progress before seeing the resident.

Other general measures include (1) closing the nursing unit to all new admissions after consultation with the infection control practitioner, the medical director, and the director of nursing and administration, (2) in-service training on respiratory secretion precautions by the infection control practitioner, handwashing techniques, and cohorting strategies, (3) restricting all but essential personnel from other areas of the LTCF from entering the unit, and (4) discharging asymptomatic residents, and transferring asymptomatic or symptomatic residents to other health care facilities provided the receiving persons are informed that the resident is from an outbreak area.

Vaccination programs should be reinstituted throughout the LTCF when an influenza outbreak is suspected. Because vaccination throughout the influenza season has potential benefit for the unimmunized,[25] vaccination should be offered again to residents and staff who previously refused. A 14-day course of amantadine chemoprophylaxis should be recommended as an adjunct to these "late vaccinees" during the interim period required to develop protective antibody levels postvaccination.

Chemoprophylaxis with amantadine is recommended by the ACIP and the CDC for all residents in LTCFs experiencing an influenza outbreak. Chemoprophylaxis is also recommended to all unvaccinated personnel who provide direct resident care.[12] Others are more selective in the use of amantadine prophylaxis in LTCFs because of concerns regarding amantadine efficacy and toxicity.[20] Renal function–adjusted amantadine chemoprophylaxis is initiated in residents without a seizure history when 10% of residents on the unit have an I-LI and influenza A has been documented in the community or LTCF. Chemoprophylaxis is also provided to consenting personnel on the outbreak unit, but it is not provided for residents and staff elsewhere in the LTCF. This more conservative use of amantadine chemoprophylaxis may help reduce the emergence and transmission of amantadine-resistant influenza viruses, which is most frequently noted in residents who are taking amantadine chemoprophylaxis during the onset of influenza.[26] The ACIP recommends that residents with influenza who are treated with amantadine should be separated from asymptomatic residents receiving amantadine chemoprophylaxis, but this is impractical in most LTCFs.

PNEUMONIA

Epidemiology

Nursing home (NH)–associated pneumonia is the second most common type of NH-associated infection and accounts for 15% to 50% of all NH-associated infections.[27] Prior to the pneumococcal vaccine era, the incidence of NH-acquired radiographically confirmed pneumonias ranged from 69 to 115 cases per 1000 residents, or 5.8 to 6.8 cases per 10,000 resident-care days.[28] During the pneumococcal vaccine era, the incidence of radiographically confirmed pneumonias ranged from 245 to 298 cases per 1000 resident-years in vaccinees and nonvaccinees.[29] More recent studies have noted an incidence of 11 to 12 cases per 1000 residents in two large chronic institutions[30] and 1.8 cases per 10,000 resident-care days in a Veterans Administration chronic care facility.[31]

Future development of methods to prevent pneumonia among LTCF residents requires identification of residents at increased risk for developing this infection. When compared to elderly patients with community-associated pneumonia admitted to a hospital, residents with LTCF-associated pneumonia have a significantly higher prevalence of dementia and cardiovascular disease.[32] When compared to elderly patients with hospital-acquired pneumonia, LTCF residents with pneumonia have more difficulty with oropharyngeal secretions, deteriorating health, and the occurrence of an unusual event—i.e., confusion, agitation, falls or wandering.[33] These studies identify the debilitated functionally disabled LTCF resident, especially those at risk for aspiration, as the resident most likely to develop pneumonia. Residents who have problems handling oropharyngeal secretions or with regurgitation of gastric contents are at especially high risk. Deteriorating health status may be a nonspecific "marker" for impaired host resistance. An "unusual event," such as a change in mental status or a fall, may relate more to its importance as an early manifestation of infection in this high-risk population. Although additional studies are needed to confirm these findings, they may be helpful in targeting specific prevention measures for these high-risk residents.

Pathogenesis

With few exceptions, most episodes of LTCF-associated pneumonia in the elderly are due to aspiration of oropharyngeal flora into the lung and failure of host defense mechanisms to eliminate the aspirated bacteria.[34] Residents in LTCFs have increased rates (approximately 40%) of oropharyngeal colonization with aerobic gram-negative bacilli.[35] Colonization is more frequent in residents with difficulty ambulating and performing activities of daily living or in those receiving treatment for cardiac or lung disease. This type of colonization can be transient.[36] or persist for many weeks.[37] The mechanism(s) whereby aerobic gram-negative bacilli colonize the oropharyngeal mucosa in LTCF residents are not well understood.

Another major component in the pathogenesis of pneumonia in LTCF residents is the aspiration of bacteria-laden oropharyngeal secretions. Although aspiration is generally thought of as regurgitation from the esophagogastric regions, this is seldom the cause of aspiration pneumonia in elderly residents in the absence of nasogastric intubation. Silent aspiration of oropharyngeal secretions can occur in up to 40% of healthy younger persons during their sleep and in up to 75% of persons with neurologic impairment.[38] In addition, aspiration in the older person may be associated with an ineffective cough mechanism, although this needs further study.

As a result of decrease in the mucociliary transport mechanisms in older persons,[39] there is retention of secr-

Table 5.2 *Presumed Etiology of Pneumonia in the Elderly*

	Setting		
	COMMUNITY ACQUIRED	INSTITUTION ACQUIRED	HOSPITAL ACQUIRED
Agent	Prevalence (%)		
Streptococcus pneumoniae	55	35	20
Hemophilus influenzae and other *Hemophilus species*	10	5	5
Staphylococcus aureus	1	1	5
Gram-negative bacilli	5	15	35
Mixed flora*	25	40	30
Other†	4	4	5

* Two or more respiratory pathogens, normal oropharyngeal commensals, or both
† Other = *Legionella, Chlamydia,* anaerobes, fungi, unknown

tions and consequent bacterial multiplication. Many different underlying diseases frequently occurring in older persons can also impair pulmonary host defenses.[40]

Etiology

The bacterial etiology of LTCF-associated pneumonia is poorly understood. Some of the reasons include the following: (1) The most frequently cultured specimen, expectorated sputum, is usually contaminated with respiratory pathogens; (2) more reliable specimens from the lower respiratory tract (e.g., transtracheal aspirates) require invasive procedures not appropriate in LTCFs; and (3) blood cultures seldom demonstrate the respiratory pathogen. In addition, aspiration of oropharyngeal secretions and poor clearance of bacteria-laden lower respiratory secretions lead to a substantial proportion of pneumonias with mixed flora (e.g., two or more respiratory pathogens, oropharyngeal commensals alone, or both). Despite these drawbacks, there is an emerging consensus that the etiology of LTCF-associated pneumonia is predominately due to *S. pneumoniae*, aerobic gram-negative bacilli, *Hemophilus species*, and mixed flora.[27,31,41] Table 5.2 illustrates these findings.

Clinical Features

Several authors have noted that the clinical presentation of pneumonia in the elderly in general and in the LTCF resident in particular, is different from younger patients.[32,42] The absence of fever and productive cough with purulent secretions

does not exclude the presence of pneumonia in LTCF residents. Frequently, the presentation is as an insidious and nonspecific deterioration. LTCF staff must pay close attention to subtle changes in residents that suggest the presence of pneumonia—i.e., anorexia, lethargy, and confusion (the latter may be difficult to assess with underlying dementia). An early but nonspecific clue to pneumonia is an increased respiratory rate (i.e., $\geq$ 26 breaths per minute), which may precede the clinical diagnosis by 24 hours.[43] On examination of the chest, signs of consolidation (i.e., bronchial breath sounds and egophony) are often absent, with dullness to percussion and decreased breath sounds being the only clues to pneumonia.

Diagnosis

The diagnosis of pneumonia in the LTCF resident is problematic because of several concerns, including (1) the frequent insidious and nonspecific presentation, (2) the absence of fever in 15% to 20% of residents, (3) the absent or ineffective cough and sputum production, (4) the contamination of secretions by bacteria colonizing the oropharynx, which severely limits the usefulness of nasopharyngeal aspirates, and (5) the frequent masquerading of other disorders as bacterial pneumonia on the chest radiograph.[42,44] The limited laboratory and radiologic services at LTCFs frequently result in residents being sent to hospitals for diagnosis and treatment. The problem is further compounded by the lack of on-site physician evaluation.[45]

Recommendations for diagnostic workup of suspected pneumonia in LTCF residents include (1) written documentation of relevant symptoms per the resident (if adequate communication is possible) and of relevant signs and symptoms per facility staff, (2) written documentation of relevant physical examination, including vital signs, and (3) vital signs, including temperature, pulse, respiratory rate, and blood pressure recorded every eight hours during the acute phase of the illness. Before treatment is begun, a sputum specimen should be obtained for culture and gram stain along with a chest radiograph and a peripheral white blood cell count and differential. If the temperature is greater than 103°F, shaking chills are noted, or hypotension is present, two blood cultures should be obtained.[46]

If laboratory results are available, criteria for the diagnosis of LTCF-associated bacterial pneumonia include (1) a new infiltrate on chest radiograph, plus [a] culture of the best available lower respiratory tract specimen demonstrating a respiratory pathogen(s) or normal throat flora, [b] temperature of 100°F or more, [c] peripheral white blood cell count greater than 10,000 per mm³, or [d] peripheral white blood cell count less than or equal to 10,000 per mm³ with a left shift, or (2) a blood culture demonstrating a respiratory pathogen with no other suspicious site of infection.[46]

If no laboratory results are available, diagnostic criteria for pneumonia include (1) a new cough and purulent respiratory secretions plus [a] temperature of 100°F or more, [b] tachypnea (26 respirations per minute or more), or [c] one physical sign of pneumonia (e.g., rales, dullness to percussion), (2) temperature greater than or equal to 100°F, plus [a] tachypnea (26 respirations per minute or more) or [b] one physical sign of pneumonia (e.g., rales, dullness to percussion), or (3) a new cough with increased purulent respiratory secretions (if the resident has chronic lung disease).[46]

Although these recommendations are appropriate, the availability and timeliness with which these studies can be obtained remains a significant concern. In order to improve the quality of care of LTCF residents with pneumonia there must be better access to routine diagnostic studies and more on-site evaluation of residents by physicians or other clinicians (nurse practitioners or physician assistants).

Treatment

As previously noted, the problem in treating residents with LTCF-associated pneumonia is the difficulty in iden-

tifying the etiologic agent for which a narrow-spectrum antibiotic regimen could be selected. Thus, empiric broad-spectrum antibiotic regimens with activity against *S. pneumoniae*, aerobic gram-negative bacilli, *Hemophilus species*, and mixed flora are often utilized in this high-risk population.[47]

There are no published studies comparing oral versus parenteral (intramuscular) antibiotic therapy for residents with LTCF-associated pneumonia when it is elected to treat the resident without hospitalization. Most often this decision is based on the clinical experience of the practitioner. Trimethoprim/ sulfamethoxazole or ciprofloxacin given orally are useful in this situation. Both of these agents offer twice-daily dosing; the major advantage of trimethoprim/sulfamethoxazole is that it is inexpensive and is more active against gram-positive organisms. Ciprofloxacin has better gram-negative activity but perhaps should be reserved for the penicillin- or cephalosporin-allergic resident. Ciprofloxacin appears to be as efficacious as the second-generation or third-generation cephalosporins, with the advantages of decreased drug cost and avoidance of intramuscular injections.[48] If the situation warrants parenteral therapy, ceftriaxone intramuscularly offers the convenience of once-a-day dosing. For the resident who develops pneumonia in the LTCF and is hospitalized, intravenous antibiotics are usually prescribed.[47] Further studies are needed to (1) assess the cost-effectiveness of treatment options (parenteral versus oral antibiotics) and treatment sites (hospital versus LTCF), (2) assess methods of improving availability of laboratory and other diagnostic studies, and (3) identify guidelines similar to those for persons with community-acquired pneumonia to assist LTCF staff in determining which residents with pneumonia should be hospitalized.[49]

Prevention

Methods to prevent LTCF-associated pneumonia include (1) vaccination of LTCF residents with pneumococcal and influenza vaccines, (2) identification of high-risk residents, and (3) elimination or reduction of known risk factors. The justification for pneumococcal vaccine for LTCF residents is the increased incidence of pneumococcal pneumonia in this setting: an estimated incidence of 13 to 16 cases per 100,000 per year[29] compared to an estimated incidence of 3 cases per 100,000 per year in the noninstitutionalized older person.[50] In a recent case-control study, the overall vaccine protective efficacy against invasive infection was 61%, with age-specific efficacy rates ranging from 93% in patients under 55 to 46% in patients age 85 or older and vaccinated within three years.[51] In the United States an observational nonrandomized trial in LTCFs demonstrated a vaccine efficacy of 30% to 40%.[29] In addition, pneumococcal vaccine is safe and inexpensive.

All elderly LTCF residents should be immunized with the 23-valent pneumococcal vaccine on admission to LTCFs unless there is written documentation of prior vaccination. Pneumococcal vaccine should be targeted for residents with cardiopulmonary conditions requiring active treatment and for all LTCF residents during an epidemic or high endemic rates of vaccine-type pneumococcal pneumonia. The reader is referred to Chapter 17 and to the latest recommendations from the CDC for complete details on the use of pneumococcal vaccine including recommendations for revaccination.[52]

As noted previously, residents who have difficulty with oropharyngeal secretions are more likely to develop pneumonia. This is probably associated with microaspiration of a few milliliters of bacteria-laden oropharyngeal secretions, which occurs frequently in the LTCF resident. Although efforts to prevent "silent microaspiration" may be impossible, other measures in preventing larger-volume aspiration (especially associated with eating) may be useful (i.e., maintaining the resident in the seated position or with the head elevated if in bed).

In residents requiring enteroalimentation by tube feeding, gastrostomy is frequently recommended because of the presumed higher risk of aspiration pneumonia with nasogastric tubes.[53] Moreover, the development of percutaneous endoscopic gastrostomy (PEG) has greatly simplified the procedure so that PEG placement for tube feeding has become commonplace in the United States. However, retrospective studies comparing complications of nasogastric and PEG tubes for enteral feeding have not demonstrated any advantage of PEG tubes in terms of reduced rates of aspiration pneumonia in hospitalized patients[54] or in LTCF residents.[55] In a recent randomized, prospective study in hospitalized patients with neurologic dysphagia, PEG tube feeding was associated with significantly fewer treatment failures, especially tube displacement. No complications occurred in the nasogastric group, but three complications (aspiration pneumonia—2, wound infection—1) were noted in the PEG group.[56] No prospective studies comparing the outcome of PEG and nasogastric tubes for

enteral feeding have been reported in LTCF residents; these studies are much needed.

Many LTCF residents are at increased risk for oropharyngeal colonization with gram-negative bacilli. Although there are no studies to date, strategies to eliminate or prevent oropharyngeal colonization by respiratory bacterial pathogens in LTCF residents may have a role in the prevention of subsequent pneumonia. Because many LTCF residents have poor oral hygiene,[57] some have suggested that this may be important in the development of pneumonia and other infections among LTCF residents.[58] Perhaps methods to improve oral hygiene may reduce pneumonia rates in LTCF residents by reducing the quantity of respiratory pathogens, including aerobic gram-negative bacilli associated with dental plaque, and other manifestations of poor oral hygiene. Further studies are needed to define more carefully the relationship between oropharyngeal colonization and pneumonia in LTCF residents and methods for prevention.

TUBERCULOSIS

Epidemiology

Tuberculosis infection is defined by a positive tuberculin skin test from a previous contact with *Mycobacterium tuberculosis* with no evidence of active disease. *Tuberculous disease* or TB is defined as tissue invasion by actively multiplying *M tuberculosis*. The tuberculin skin test may be positive or negative, and there is often evidence of a systemic response (fever, weight loss, anorexia, etc.) as well as specific localized signs (e.g., sputum production and shortness of breath) with pulmonary TB.

Persons age 65 and over constitute the largest reservoir of *M tuberculosis* infection in the United States today. Tuberculosis case rates in the United States are higher among the elderly (20.6 per 100,000) than among all other age groups (average 9.3 per 100,000).[59] Elderly nursing home residents are at greater risk for tuberculosis than older persons in the community: approximately 40 per 100,000 person-years versus approximately 20 per 100,000 person-years, respectively. The observed rate of tuberculosis among nursing home employees is approximately three times the rate expected in adults of similar age, race, and sex employed elsewhere.[60] The tuberculosis case rates for men and women residents in nursing homes in Arkansas (a state with one of the largest proportions of older persons) may be as high as 1014 per 100,000 and 376 per 100,000, respectively, or 5 to 30 times higher than the rates in older persons of comparable age and sex living in the community.[61]

In most circumstances TB is not a highly contagious infection. Transmission requires close, prolonged, household-like contact, or possible heavy contact of short duration (e.g., personnel who suction the oropharynx of residents with active pulmonary TB). The most dangerous transmitters of *M tuberculosis* are residents with large numbers of bacilli in their sputum, which can be correlated with a positive acid-fast stain of secretions from the lower respiratory tract. Transmission is decreased rapidly by 14 to 21 days (depending on the concentration of bacilli and the pulmonary lesions) of effective treatment.

However, as a nosocomial infection for nursing home residents and employees,[62–64] tuberculosis is a frequent occurrence in the LTCF setting. If residents with negative skin tests are retested after being in a LTCF for six months or more, the prevalence of positive skin tests increases twofold in all age groups.[61] The increase in the number of residents with tuberculous infection is due to several factors: exposure to an active case of pulmonary TB, improved nutrition, and a late booster phenomenon.[65] The most important factor, however, is exposure to a resident with an active case of pulmonary TB that is undetected.

Pathogenesis

Understanding the pathogenesis of tuberculous infection and disease is critical in developing methods of control and prevention in the LTCF setting. Infection with *M tuberculosis* occurs when one inhales air containing droplet nuclei contaminated with the organism. Organisms are released into the air when a person with untreated (or ineffectively treated) pulmonary TB coughs, speaks loudly, or sneezes. Transmission does not occur by fomites—e.g., clothes, books, food trays, personal articles, etc. The droplet nuclei traverse the upper airways and tracheobronchial tree and once in the lung (lower lobes) begin to multiply, usually inside macrophages. Spread occurs by lymphatics to regional lymph nodes and may disseminate hematogenously to other organs, especially the liver and kidney. If the normal cellular immune response is intact, most of the bacilli are killed in about two to four weeks. Most often, however, some bacilli remain dormant but viable in various organs including the lung. Sites with dormant bacilli have the

potential to reactivate at some later time. In areas of the body in which there is a rather exuberant immune response, fibrosis and calcification may occur. Most patients infected with M tuberculosis, however, have normal chest x-rays and are asymptomatic. The presence of a positive tuberculin skin test (see below) is an indication that a person is harboring viable tubercle bacilli and generally is the only evidence of infection.[66]

Approximately 80% of the cases of TB in the United States are due to reactivation of a dormant lesion.[67] Prior to careful studies of outbreaks of TB in LTCFs, it was also assumed that the development of TB in LTCF residents was due primarily to reactivation, with few cases of TB being due to recent exogenous infection. After all, elderly residents in LTCFs today were infected with *M tuberculosis* 50 years or more prior to admission. But in a series of studies in Arkansas LTCFs,[61,63,68] only 15% to 20% of residents on admission had a significant tuberculin skin test (10 mm or more of induration). Thus, although most of these residents were assumed to have been infected with the tubercle bacillus early in life, they apparently had outlived their infection and their tuberculin skin test had reverted to nonreactive (even after a booster skin test). Such residents are at risk for exogenous reinfection with this pathogen and a second primary infection.[63,69]

Clinical Features

The clinical diagnosis of TB in the elderly LTCF resident is a challenge for all clinicians. Cases are often missed because of the atypical presentation of TB in the elderly and the frequent inability of the elderly to communicate their complaints. This frequently leads to exposure and infection of susceptible residents and employees. It is therefore important for LTCF nursing staff, infection control practitioners, and physicians to have a high index of suspicion for the clinical presentation of TB. Some specific situations in which TB should be considered are illustrated here.

Reactivation of a dormant infection in the lung can occur at any time in a resident with a positive tuberculin skin test, if there has been no previous preventive therapy. Clinical features are frequently nonspecific: fatigue, anorexia, weight loss, and night sweats with or without low-grade fever. This is usually associated with a deterioration of clinical status without explanation. A productive cough with mucoid sputum may be a late sign and is often confused with chronic bronchitis. Chest radiographs usually demonstrate a fibronodular infiltrate in the upper lobe(s) of the lung with or without cavitation. These changes are often mistaken for cancer, however.[62]

Residents with recent exogenous reinfection may present with primary pulmonary tuberculosis with cough, weight loss, fever, and infiltrates in the lower lobes of the lung.[62,70] These features are often mistaken for bacterial pneumonia in the LTCF resident, and the diagnosis of TB is delayed or never made. Consequently, residents are often treated with antibiotics but do not respond, although occasionally the clinical syndrome may transiently improve when newer antibiotics with antituberculous activity (e.g., the quinolones) are prescribed. Thus, the diagnosis of TB should be strongly considered in LTCF residents with suspected pneumonia that is poorly responsive to antibiotic therapy.

Pleural effusion can also occur after a new tuberculous infection and can be confused with heart failure. Although less common, TB can develop in extrapulmonary sites in the elderly, including the kidney, pericardium, vertebrae, and meninges. Workup for these infections requires consultation and transfer to the hospital.

Diagnosis

From the preceding, it is evident that the diagnosis of TB in the LTCF resident is problematic. First, there is a need for a high index of suspicion clinically. Next, chest radiographs, both PA and lateral views (whenever possible), should be obtained whenever pulmonary TB is suspected. The radiologist should review these films and compare the findings with any previous films. Because LTCF residents frequently have abnormal chest films representing other more frequent pulmonary conditions, the x-ray requisition should ask the radiologist to comment as to whether "any abnormal findings are compatible with TB." Routine chest radiographs are not useful for detecting disease in the absence of symptoms.[71]

Due to the difficulty in obtaining appropriate specimens, the bacteriologic diagnosis of TB in the elderly LTCF resident is also problematic. If pulmonary TB is suspected, respiratory secretions should be obtained on three separate days for TB smear and culture. The optimal collection time is early in the morning prior to breakfast. Expectorated sputum is at best difficult to obtain from elderly disabled residents. Therefore, nasopharyngeal aspirates (which promote vigorous coughing) are frequently required. Often respira-

tory therapy services are necessary to assist in obtaining adequate lower respiratory secretions using preaspiration heated nebulization treatment.

If pulmonary TB is suspected and the laboratory workup is pursued, the resident should be placed in a private room appropriate for respiratory precautions (see "Infection Control Considerations" following). If these resources are not available, the resident will require transfer to a hospital setting.

The tuberculin skin test is not useful as a diagnostic test because it may be positive in residents who have only TB infection and may give false-negative reactions in up to 30% of residents with TB disease (tuberculosis).[60] Therefore, the diagnosis should be pursued, despite a negative skin test, especially if the clinical findings are compatible. The importance of the skin test is that it identifies people who are infected prior to the development of active TB. Thus, skin testing is one of the key components in the program for prevention of tuberculosis transmission in nursing homes.

Tuberculin Skin Testing

Infection with *M tuberculosis* usually results in a cell-mediated immune response within two to four weeks of the initial infection. This immune response can be detected by injecting intradermally 5 tuberculin units (TU) of purified protein derivative (PPD) and noting a positive reaction (10 mm or more of induration is considered a positive reaction in the nonexposure situation). The recommended method is to measure the extent of induration in two dimensions by the ballpoint pen technique with the results recorded in millimeters of induration.[72] Results of tuberculin skin testing should be recorded conspicuously and consistently in the resident's medical record. This should include the number of millimeters of induration, especially if it is less than 10 mm. Undetectable induration should be recorded as "nonreactive" rather than "negative". Accuracy and consistency in recording skin test results cannot be overemphasized because of its importance in interpretation of subsequent skin tests.

As previously noted, immunity to TB may wane with time in elderly residents, especially if there is no reexposure to the tubercle bacillus. This waning immunity may result in a negative skin test (<10 mm of induration) in some residents who, on repeat skin testing by the same method within 30 days of the first test, have a positive reaction. This phenomenon of an initially negative skin test (0 to 9 mm induration) that becomes positive after a repeat skin test is referred to as the *booster phenomenon*.[73] The technique of performing two skin tests in succession is referred to as the two-step PPD (tuberculin) test.[74] In the LTCF setting the *two-step PPD test* has identified an additional 3% of tuberculin reactors when the second skin test is given within 30 days of the initial test, which increases to 5% when the second test is given after 30 days.[63] If used routinely for both residents and employees, this technique will help distinguish true conversions in initial nonreactors in the event an exposure necessitates another test at a later date.[75] Residents whose skin tests are negative (0 to 9 mm of induration) should be retested after any exposure to a suspected or proven case of pulmonary TB.[60]

There is an important correlation between the size of the converted skin test reaction and the development of clinical tuberculosis in nursing home residents. In residents with two prior documented negative skin tests who become newly infected (converters), the skin test is usually greater than or equal to 15 mm of induration, and 90% will have an increment of greater than or equal to 12 mm of induration from the previous insignificant reaction.[61] In support of this, the tuberculosis rate is 3% for residents whose skin test converted with an increment of less than 12 mm induration; this is the same rate as for residents whose significant reaction was first noted on admission. This suggests that the positive skin test in this group of residents represents a "booster" of a previously waned positive reaction rather than a true conversion.

From the infection control viewpoint, identifying residents with tuberculin skin test reactivity or conversion is important because it is predictive of the resident's risk of developing active TB. Only 2% to 3% of residents who are tuberculin skin test positive or reactors on admission will develop active TB over several years of follow-up, primarily with reactivation of a dormant infection, but 8% of women and 12% of men residents who are initially skin test negative and convert their skin test (≥ 15 mm of induration with an increment of ≥ 12 mm) some time after admission will develop active TB within two years of the conversion.[61] This high rate of active disease among skin test converters in the LTCF argues strongly for an active surveillance program for tuberculous infection in

this setting and preventive treatment for all those who demonstrate conversion (see below).

Preventive Therapy

Until recently, it was always difficult to decide whether to use preventive therapy in the elderly LTCF resident with a positive tuberculin skin test. For years, it was standard practice to use established guidelines and a one-drug regimen (isoniazid) for preventive therapy for tuberculosis in children and younger adults.[71] In older persons, there was a great reluctance to accept these recommendations because of the risk of isoniazid-associated hepatitis which was said to increase with the age of the patient.[76] Stead and colleagues, however, in a series of studies in Arkansas LTCFs, have provided useful information with which to make decisions about isoniazid preventive therapy in this high-risk population. For the LTCF resident who is a tuberculin reactor, preventive therapy is not usually recommended because the risk of developing active TB is about 3% within five years, whereas the risk of isoniazid-associated hepatotoxicity is also about 3%.[77] There are exceptions to these recommendations, however: residents with diabetes mellitus or upper lobe changes on chest radiograph and those receiving corticosteroid therapy have an increased risk of developing active TB and should receive preventive therapy.[76]

The estimated number of cases of TB per 100,000 untreated converters ranges from approximately 175 per 100,000 (if no secondary cases occurred) to approximately 900 to 2,000 per 100,000 (if secondary cases occurred).[61] When no preventive therapy is offered, active tuberculosis occurs within two years of skin test conversion or approximately 45 to 80 times the rate (0.2%) in converters who receive preventive therapy.[61] Therefore, preventive therapy with isoniazid (300 mg orally per day) is recommended for 6 to 12 months for the resident who has converted to a positive skin test and whose chest radiographs do not reveal tuberculosis, unless there is a medical contraindication.[74]

Preventive treatment with isoniazid is surprisingly well tolerated in LTCF residents and is discontinued in less than 15% because of drug toxicity (4% to 5% hepatotoxicity) or intolerance.[77] However, debate about how closely residents should be followed for drug toxicity, especially hepatitis, continues. The most recent recommendation of Stead and colleagues is that residents should be closely monitored for early signs and symptoms of hepatitis (i.e., nausea, vomiting, or anorexia) rather than serially monitoring liver function tests. The latter should be obtained only when these signs or symptoms are noted; moreover, small rises in serum transaminases, observed in most patients taking isoniazid, may be difficult to interpret and confusing to the practitioner. On the other hand, others feel that periodic monitoring of liver function is important because the elderly resident may not demonstrate signs or symptoms of hepatitis.[78]

Treatment of Active Tuberculosis

The approach to the treatment of TB, using multidrug regimens, has evolved over the past 40 years with the development of effective tuberculocidal agents. These drugs have led to a marked reduction in the duration of treatment of TB from 18 to 24 months to as short as 4 to 6 months. Isoniazid and rifampin have become the cornerstones of therapy of TB in people of all ages, especially for older persons, when one wants to use as simple a regimen as possible.[79] Because drug resistance to these agents is infrequent at the present time among older persons in the United States, it is usually unnecessary to add a third drug to this regimen.

In most cases, the decisions regarding the choice of drugs and the need for respiratory precautions (until the 14 to 21-day period of effective treatment has been completed) will occur in the hospital setting. Several important treatment components in the LTCF (e.g., followup sputum smears and cultures, and monitoring for adverse reactions and complications) will require some outside consultation and assistance from state and local health departments.[80] LTCF medical and nursing personnel caring for residents under treatment for TB, however, should be aware of the side-effect profiles of the drugs being administered.

Infection Control Considerations

Guidelines for preventing the transmission of tuberculosis in hospitals have been available for many years[81] and were previously considered applicable to LTCFs.[82] Although specific guidelines for screening for tuberculosis in residents and employees in LTCFs had been published[83] and several state departments of health had developed similar guidelines,[84–86] until recently no comprehensive program targeted for the high-risk nursing home residents and employees was available. In 1990 the Advisory Committee for the Elimination of Tuberculosis established the first set of comprehensive guidelines and

---

Table 5.3 *Tuberculosis Control Measures*

SURVEILLANCE

- Identification of residents with pulmonary TB
- Identification of residents and staff with tuberculous infection (positive tuberculin skin test)

CONTAINMENT

- Prompt treatment of suspected or proven pulmonary TB
- Prevent further contacts for first 1–2 weeks of treatment
- Consult with local health department regarding need for specific isolation procedures (e.g., negative pressure ventilation room)
- Identification and evaluation of "exposed" residents and staff
- Preventive treatment for residents and staff with tuberculin skin test conversions

ASSESSMENT

- Monitor and evaluate surveillance and containment activities
- Staff education

---

recommendations for the control of TB in LTCFs.[60] The reader is urged to study and implement these recommendations. A recent review of this report by one of the consultants to the advisory committee will also be helpful in implementing these recommendations with current related policies and procedures despite current limited LTCF resources.[80] The Advisory Committee's recommended program contains three key elements (see Table 5.3), which are summarized here.

Surveillance

This includes identifying all cases of TB as well as infected residents and staff. For residents this will require the following:

1. Tuberculin skin testing (two-step PPD) programs of all newly admitted residents to define TB risk.

2. Conspicuous and accurate documentation of skin test results.

3. Those who are skin test reactors should have a chest radiograph to identify fibronodular, apical scarring, or active disease with special consideration for the radiologist as noted.

4. Skin test negative residents should be retested annually or at the time of a TB exposure to identify converters.

5. Residents who are skin test converters should have a chest radiograph performed; if the radiograph demonstrates no finding compatible with TB, preventive therapy is indicated. Residents who convert their tuberculin skin test provide evidence that an active case (of pulmonary TB) exists or existed in the facility. Efforts should be made to identify the index case(s) in order to identify others who have been exposed.

6. If residents refuse or are unable to complete recommended preventive treatment, they should be monitored for cough that persists for more than three weeks and/or a prolonged unexplained fever.

For employees this will require the following:

1. New employees should have a two-step PPD unless they can provide written evidence of a previously positive test.

2. Reactors less than age 35 (with no other risk factors) should receive preventive therapy with isoniazid for six to nine months.

3. Employees with a negative skin test should be retested yearly on the anniversary of their hiring and at the time of a suspected or confirmed TB exposure.

4. Skin test converters should be given preventive therapy regardless of age.

There are two major pitfalls in TB surveillance of LTCF employees, however. First, most LTCFs do not have formal employee health services, and maintenance of employee health records is less than optimal. As a result, employees are not always reevaluated at defined intervals (e.g., yearly). Second, it is often not well defined how those on preventive therapy will be followed up. This can create a liability issue for the facility. LTCFs should develop a specific TB policy that defines the mechanism whereby employees receiving preventive therapy are followed for compliance and adverse drug reactions. The prototype for

the TB Summary Record (Appendix II in reference 60) will be helpful here.

Containment

This program means ensuring that transmission of TB is stopped promptly after the diagnosis is made and consists of four elements: (1) appropriate isolation precautions (i.e., an isolation room under negative pressure for the first one to two weeks of treatment) are required unless [a] chemotherapy is promptly instituted at the time the diagnosis is suspected or confirmed, [b] recent and current contacts are evaluated and placed on appropriate therapy, and [c] new contacts can be prevented for a one- to two-week period. These recommendations may prove difficult to implement in LTCFs, however, because of the frequent delay in diagnosis, lack of private rooms for isolation, inadequate or limited engineering department resources and equipment to contain, exhaust, or disinfect the infectious particles in the air from the source case, and lack of expertise in initiating treatment for suspected tuberculosis. If it is determined after consultation with the local health department that resources for providing adequate precautions or the necessary workup are lacking, the residents should be transferred to the hospital.[80]

Appropriate ATS/CDC *treatment recommendations* should be followed for all residents with confirmed or suspected TB.[79] The recommendations also emphasize that nursing home staff must assure residents' compliance and monitor for drug toxicity, obtain follow-up sputum smears and cultures, and (with expert consultation) evaluate possible treatment complications.

General guidelines for conducting a contact investigation in a LTCF for "close contacts" are noted in Appendix III of the Advisory Committee's recommendations.[60] Health department personnel should be consulted to determine which contacts should be examined and by what methods.

Preventive therapy should be provided for all contacts who develop a skin test conversion. Other residents and staff with positive tuberculin reactions should be given preventive therapy and monitored according to previously published guidelines.[71]

Assessment

This means that the LTCF must monitor and evaluate the surveillance and containment activities. This will require a record-keeping system for tracking and assessing the status of persons with tuberculous infection including the overall effectiveness of tuberculosis control efforts. A record-keeping system, such as that shown in Appendix II of the Advisory Committee's Report[60] should prove helpful.

Although education is not included in the Advisory Committee's recommendations, it is an important complementary element. Education refers to imparting information and skills to residents, families, visitors, and employees so that they understand and participate in the implementation of surveillance, containment, and subsequent activities.[80] Yearly staff in-service training on TB should be mandatory to ensure that employees are aware of the reasons for using specific methods to control TB. Information sheets about TB should be developed and used to educate families and friends of residents with active TB about this infection so that they can cooperate with control efforts. Staff should be able to answer questions about TB posed by families. These educational efforts should emphasize that the disease, not the resident, is being isolated. The key resources for this effort will include the infection control practitioner and the education component of the nursing department, with the full support of the infection control committee and the administration.

To assure that these recommendations for tuberculosis prevention and control can be implemented, many LTCFs will require additional resources and support. LTCFs should designate an appropriately trained person as an infection control officer who is responsible for overseeing and operating a tuberculosis prevention and control program. In a multifacility system, there should be a qualified person or unit to oversee tuberculosis control activities throughout the facility. Smaller facilities will require substantial outside help from sources such as the state and local health departments. These resources, however, are already stretched beyond their limits. Therefore, assistance of others, especially local and regional professionals working in hospital-based infection control programs, such as members of the Association for Practitioners in Infection Control (APIC) and the Society for Hospital Epidemiology of America (SHEA), can play an important role during this difficult transition.

Acknowledgment

The authors wish to acknowledge several accomplished infection control practitioners—Lois Cheney, R.N.; Carolyn Hoden, R.N.; Ken Mamot, R.N.; Lorraine Moore, R.N.—from whom they have learned much, and the expert secretarial assistance of Amy Eglowstein.

REFERENCES

1. Patriarca PA, Weber JA, Parker RA, et al: Efficacy of influenza vaccine in nursing homes: reduction of illness and complications during an influenza A (H3N2) epidemic. *JAMA* 1985;253:1136–1139.
2. Betts RF, Douglas RG: Influenza virus. In Mandel GL, Douglas RG, Bennett JE (ed): *Principles and Practice of Infectious Diseases,* 3rd ed. New York, Churchill Livingstone, 1990, pp 1306–1325.
3. Gravenstein S, Miller BA, Ershler WB, et al: Low sensitivity of CDC case definition for H3N2 influenza in elderly nursing home subjects. *Clin Res* 1990;38:547A.
4. Falsey AR: Noninfluenza respiratory virus infection in long-term care facilities. *Infect Control Hosp Epidemiol* 1991;12:602–608.
5. Atkinson WL, Arden NH, Patriarca PA, et al: Amantadine prophylaxis during an institutional outbreak of type A (H1N1) influenza. *Arch Intern Med* 1986;46:1751–1756.
6. American Hospital Formulary Service: *AHFS Drug Information 1993.* Antivirals: amantadine hydrochloride. Bethesda,

MD, American Society of Hospital Pharmacists, 1993, pp 373–376.
7. Bryson YJ, Monahan C, Pollack M, et al: A prospective double-blind study of side effects associated with the administration of amantadine for influenza A virus prophylaxis. *J Infect Dis* 1980;141:543–547.
8. Arden NH, Patriarca PA, Fasano MB, et al: The roles of vaccination and amantadine prophylaxis in controlling an outbreak of influenza A (H3N2) in a nursing home. *Arch Intern Med* 1988;48:865–868.
9. Gravenstein S, Mast E, Drinka P, et al: Amantadine prophylaxis in 880 nursing home subjects: Strategies in toxicity reduction. *Gerontologist* 1989;29:252A.
10. Walters HE, Paulshock M. Therapeutic efficacy of amantadine HCl. *Mo Med* 1970;67:176–179.
11. Betts RE, Treanor JJ, Graman PS, et al: Antiviral agents to prevent or treat influenza in the elderly. *J Respir Dis* 1987;8(11A):S67–S72.
12. Centers for Disease Control: Prevention and control of

influenza. Recommendations of the Immunization Practices Advisory Committee (ACIP). *MMWR* 1992;41:1–17.

13. Bentley DW: Immunization for the elderly, in Fox RA (ed): *Medicine and Old Age: Immunology and Infection.* London, Churchill Livingstone, 1984, pp 333–370.

14. Arden NH, Patriarca PA, Kendal AP: Experiences in the use and efficacy of inactivated influenza vaccine in nursing homes, in Kendal AP, Patriarca PA (ed): *Options for the Control of Influenza.* New York, Alan R. Liss, 1986, pp 155–168.

15. Gross PA, Quinnan GV, Weksler ME, et al: Immunization of elderly people with high doses of influenza vaccine. *J Am Geriatr Soc* 1988;36:209–212.

16. Gross PA, Weksler ME, Quinnan GV, et al: Immunization of elderly people with two doses of influenza vaccine. *J Clin Microbiol* 1987;25:1763–1765.

17. Stuart WH, Dull HB, Newton LH, et al: Evaluation of monovalent influenza vaccine in a retirement community during the epidemic of 1965–1966. *JAMA* 1969;209:232–238.

18. Barker WH, Mullooly JP: Influenza vaccination of elderly persons: Reduction in pneumonia and influenza hospitalizations and deaths. *JAMA* 1980;244:2547–2549.

19. Patriarca PA, Weber JA, Meissner MA, et al: Use of influenza vaccine in nursing homes. *J Am Geriatr Soc* 1985;33:463–466.

20. Gravenstein S, Miller BA, Drinka P: Prevention and control of influenza A outbreaks in long-term care facilities. *Infect Control Hosp Epidemiol* 1992;13:49–55.

21. Levine M, Beattie BL, McLean DM, et al: Characterization of the immune response to trivalent influenza vaccine in elderly men. *J Am Geriatr Soc* 1987;35:609–615.

22. Bentley DW: Vaccinations. *Clin Geriatr Med* 1992;8(4):745–760.

23. *Managing an Influenza Vaccination Program in the Nursing Home.* Atlanta, GA, Influenza Branch, Center for Infectious Diseases, Centers for Disease Control, 1987, pp 1–32.

24. Patriarca PA, Arden NH, Koplan JP, et al: Prevention and control of type A influenza infections in nursing homes. *Ann Intern Med* 1987;107:732–740.

25. Gross PA, Rodstein M, LaMontagne JR, et al: Epidemiology of acute respiratory illness during an influenza outbreak in a nursing home. *Arch Intern Med* 1988;148:559–561.

26. Mast EE, Harmon MW, Gravenstein S, et al: Emergence and possible transmission of amantadine-resistant viruses during nursing home outbreaks of influenza A (H3N2). *Am J Epidemiol* 1991;134:988–997.

27. Crossley KB, Thurn KR: Nursing home–acquired pneumonia. *Semin Respir Infect* 1989;4:64–72.

28. Valenti WM, Jenzer M, Bentley DW: Type-specific pneumococcal respiratory disease in the elderly and chronically ill. *Am Rev Respir Dis* 1978;117:233–238.

29. Bentley DW, Ha K, Mamot K, et al: Pneumococcal vaccine in the institutionalized elderly: Design of a nonrandomized trial and preliminary results. *Rev Infect Dis* 1981;(Suppl.):S71–S81.

30. Vlahov D, Tenney JH, Cervino KW, et al: Routine surveillance for infections in nursing homes: experience at two facilities. *Am J Infect Control* 1987;15:47–53.

31. Farber BF, Brennen C, Puntereri AJ, et al: A prospective study of nosocomial infections in a chronic care facility. *J Am Geriatr Soc* 1984;32:499–502.

32. Marrie T, Durant H, Yates L: Community-acquired pneumonia requiring hospitalization: 5-year prospective study. *Rev Infect Dis* 1989;1:586–599.

33. Harkness GA, Bentley DW, Roghmann KJ: Risk factors for nosocomial pneumonia in the elderly. *Am J Med* 990;89:457–463.

34. Verghese A, Berk SL: Bacterial pneumonia in the elderly. *Medicine* 1983;62:271–285.

35. Valenti WM, Trudell RG, Bentley DW: Factors predisposing to oropharyngeal colonization with gram-negative bacilli in the aged. *N Engl J Med* 1978;298:1108–1111.

36. Irwin RS, Whitaker S, Pratter MR, et al. The transiency of oropharyngeal colonization of gram-negative bacilli in residents of a skilled nursing facility. *Chest* 1982;81:31–35.

37. Nicolle LE, McLeod J, McIntyre M, et al: Significance of pharyngeal colonization with aerobic gram-negative bacilli in elderly institutionalized men. *Age Aging* 1986;15:47–52.

38. Huxley EJ, Vroslav J, Gray WR, et al: Pharyngeal aspiration in normal adults and patients with depressed consciousness. *Am J Med* 1978;64:564–568.

39. Goodman RM, Yergin BM, Landa JF, et al: Relationship of smoking history and pulmonary function tests to tracheal mucous velocity in nonsmokers, young smokers, ex-smokers, and patients with chronic bronchitis. *Am Rev Respir Dis* 1978;117:205–213.

40. Esposito AL: Pulmonary host defenses in the elderly, in Niederman, MS (ed): *Respiratory Infections in the Elderly.* New York, Raven Press, 1991, pp 25–44.

41. Marrie T, Durant H, Kwan C: Nursing home–acquired pneumonia: A case-control study. *J Am Geriatr Soc* 1986;34:697–702.

42. Bentley DW: Bacterial pneumonia in the elderly. *Hosp Pract* 1988;23(12):99–116.

43. McFadden JP, Price RC, Eastwood HD, et al: Raised respiratory rate in the elderly patient; a valuable physical sign. *Br Med J* 1982;284:626.

44. Nunley D, Verghese A, Berk SL: Pneumonia in the nursing-home patient, in Verghese A, Berk SL (eds): *Infections in Nursing Homes and Long-Term Care Facilities.* Basel, Karger, 1990, pp 95–113.

45. Ouslander JG: Medical care in the nursing home. *JAMA* 1989;262:2582–2590.

46. Zimmer JG, Bentley DW, Valenti WM, et al: Systemic antibiotic use in nursing homes. A quality assessment. *J Am Geriatr Soc* 1986;34:703–710.

47. Mylotte JM, Ksiazek S, Bentley DW: Rationale approach to the antibiotic treatment of pneumonia in the elderly. *Drugs Aging* (in press).

48. Hirata-Dulas CA, Stein DJ, Guay DR, et al: A randomized study of ciprofloxacin versus ceftriaxone in the treatment of nursing home-acquired lower respiratory tract infections. *J Am Geriatr Soc* 1991;39:979–985.

49. Fine MJ, Smith DN, Singer DE: Hospitalization decision in patients with community-acquired pneumonia: A prospective

cohort study. *Am J Med* 1990;89:713–724.

50. Schwartz JS: Pneumococcal vaccine: Clinical efficacy and effectiveness. *Ann Intern Med* 1982;96:208–220.

51. Shapiro ED, Berg AT, Austrian R, et al: The protective efficacy of polyvalent pneumococcal polysaccharide vaccine. *N Engl J Med* 1991;325:1453–1460.

52. Centers for Disease Control: Recommendations of the Immunization Practices Advisory Committee (ACIP). Pneumococcal polysaccharide vaccine. *MMWR* 1989;38:64–67.

53. Jones JM: Enteral feeding: Techniques of administration. *Gut* 1986;27:47–50.

54. Fay DE, Poplausky M, Gurber M, et al: Long-term enteral feeding: A retrospective comparison of delivery via percutaneous endoscopic gastrostomy and nasoenteric tubes. *Am J Gastroenterol* 1991;86:1604–1609.

55. Ciocon, JO, Silverstone FA, Graver M, et al: Tube feedings in elderly patients: Indications, benefits, and complications. *Arch Intern Med* 1988;148:429–433.

56. Park RH, Allison MC, Lang J, et al: Randomised comparison of percutaneous endoscopic gastrostomy and nasogastric tube feeding in patients with persisting neurological dysphagia. *Br Med J* 1992;304:1406–1409.

57. Berkey DB, Berg RG, Ettinger DL, et al: Research review of oral health status and service use among institutionalized older adults in the United States and Canada. *Spec Care Dentist* 1991;11:131–136.

58. Limeback H: The relationship between oral health and systemic infections among elderly residents of chronic care facilities: A review. *Gerodontology* 1988;7:131–137.

59. Bloch AB, Rieder HL, Kelly BA, et al: The epidemiology of tuberculosis in the United States: Implications for diagnosis and treatment. *Clin Chest Med* 1989;297–313.

60. Prevention and control of tuberculosis in facilities providing long-term care to the elderly: Recommendations of the Advisory Committee for Elimination of Tuberculosis. *MMWR* 1990;39(No. RR-10):7–20.

61. Stead WW, To T: The significance of the tuberculin skin test in elderly patients. *Ann Intern Med* 1987;107:837–842.

62. Stead WW: Tuberculosis among elderly persons: an outbreak in a nursing home. *Ann Intern Med* 1981;94:606–610.

63. Stead WW, Lofgren JP, Warren E, et al: Tuberculosis as an endemic and nosocomial infection among the elderly in nursing homes. *N Engl J Med* 1985;312:1483–1487.

64. Brennen C, Muder RR, Muraca PW: Occult endemic tuberculosis in a chronic care facility. *Infect Control Hosp Epidemiol* 1988;9:548–552.

65. Welty C, Burstin S, Muspratt S, et al: Epidemiology of tuberculosis infection in a chronic care population. *Am Rev Respir Dis* 1985;132:133–136.

66. Stead WW: Pathogenesis of tuberculosis: Clinical and epidemiologic perspective. *Rev Infect Dis* 1989;11(Suppl 2):S366–S368.

67. Stead WW: Pathogenesis of a first episode of chronic pulmonary tuberculosis in man: Recrudescence of residuals of the primary infection or exogenous reinfection. *Am Rev Respir Dis* 1967;95:729–745.

68. Narain JP, Lofgren JP, Warren E, et al: Epidemic of tuberculosis in a nursing home: A retrospective study. *J Am Geriatr Soc* 1985;33:258–263.

69. Davidson PT: Tuberculosis. New ideas of an old disease. *N Engl J Med* 1985;312:1514–1515.

70. Alvarez S, Shell C, Berk SL: Pulmonary tuberculosis in elderly men. *Am J Med* 1987;82:602–606.

71. Centers for Disease Control: Screening for tuberculosis and tuberculous infection in high-risk populations, and the use of preventive therapy for tuberculous infection in the United States: Recommendations of the Advisory Committee for Elimination of Tuberculosis. *MMWR* 1990;39(RR-8):9–12.

72. Sokol JE: Measure of delayed skin test response. *N Engl J Med* 1975;293:501–502.

73. Thompson NJ, Glassroth JL, Snider DE, et al: The booster phenomenon in serial tuberculin testing. *Am Rev Respir Dis* 1979;119:587–597.

74. The American Geriatrics Society Statement on Two-step PPD testing for Nursing Home Patients on Admission. *J Am Geriatr Soc* 1988;36:77–78.

75. Dutt AK, Stead WW: Tuberculosis. *Clin Geriatr Med* 1992;8:761–775.

76. Kopanoff DE, Snider DE, Caras GJ: Isoniazid-related hepatitis: A US Public Health Service cooperative surveillance study. *Am Rev Respir Dis* 1978;117:991–1001.

77. Stead WW, To T, Harrison RW, et al: Benefit-risk consideration in preventive treatment for tuberculosis in elderly persons. *Ann Intern Med* 1987;107:837.

78. Yoshikawa TT: Tuberculosis in aging adults. *J Am Geriatr Soc* 1992;40:178–187.

79. American Thoracic Society, CDC: Treatment of tuberculosis and tuberculosis infection in adults and children. *Am Rev Respir Dis* 1986;134:356–363.

80. Bentley DW: Tuberculosis in long-term care facilities. *Infect Control Hospital Epidemiol* 1990;11:42–46.

81. *Guidelines for prevention of TB transmission in hospitals.* Atlanta, GA, Centers for Disease Control, June 1975.

82. Tuberculosis—North Dakota. *MMWR* 1979;27:523–525.

83. Kent DC, Atkinson ML, Eckmann BH, et al: Screening for pulmonary tuberculosis in institutions. *Am Rev Respir Dis* 1977;115:901–906.

84. Anderson, HR: Tuberculosis in nursing homes. *J Tenn Med Assoc* 1985;78:765–766.

85. Guidelines for prevention of tuberculosis transmission in nursing homes. *Texas Prevent Dis News* 1986;46:1–4.

86. State of New York Department of Health Memorandum: Recommendations for tuberculosis surveillance among residents of residential health care facilities 1986;86-117:1–3

CHAPTER

URINARY TRACT INFECTIONS

Lindsay E. Nicolle

GENERAL CONCEPTS OF URINARY TRACT INFECTION

Urinary tract infection is infection involving the bladder or kidneys (Fig. 6.1). Kidney or renal infection is also called *pyelonephritis*, and bladder infection is also known as *cystitis*.

URINARY TRACT

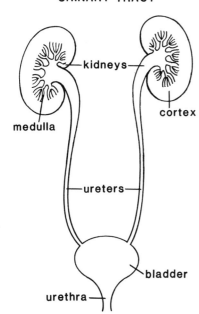

Figure 6.1 *The urinary tract*

Urinary infection usually results from bacteria present in the periurethral area or, in women, the vagina, ascending into the bladder and persisting in bladder urine. Subsequently, bacteria may ascend further to the kidney, leading to renal infection.

The urine and genitourinary tract are usually sterile proximal to the distal few centimeters of the urethra. The major host factor that maintains this sterility is intermittent, complete voiding of urine. Any abnormality that interferes with complete voiding, leading to an increase in "residual urine," is associated with a high likelihood of acquisition of urinary infection.

Urinary tract infection is classified as either complicated or uncomplicated. *Uncomplicated* urinary infection is bladder infection that occurs in young women with normal genitourinary tracts. *Complicated* urinary infection occurs in individuals with structural or functional abnormalities in their genitourinary tracts, including stones, tumors, strictures, and indwelling urinary catheters (Table 6.1). The appropriate management of urinary infection differs depending on whether the infection is complicated or uncomplicated.

Individuals who experience repeated urinary infection may have relapse or reinfection. *Relapse* is recurrent infection with the same organism, consistent with reemergence of the organism from a site within the urinary tract from which it has not been eradicated. *Reinfection* is recurrent infection with a new organism that has gained entry to the urinary tract.

Microbiology and Pathogenesis

Bacteria that cause urinary tract infection are primarily organisms of the normal gut flora.[1] For uncomplicated urinary

Table 6.1   *Abnormalities of the Genitourinary Tract Frequently Associated with Complicated Urinary Tract Infection*

ABNORMALITY	COMMON CAUSES

Intrinsic obstruction	Kidney, bladder stones
	Nephrocalcinosis
	Nephropathy: analgesics
	                      diabetic
	                      sickle cell disease
	
	Tumors

Extrinsic obstruction	Ureteral/urethral stenosis, valves, bands Benign prostatic hypertrophy Extrinsic ureteral compression
Functional obstruction	Neurogenic bladder Hydronephrosis Diverticuli Bladder prolapse
Nonobstructing calculi	Kidney, bladder stones
Foreign bodies	Indwelling catheter Ureteral stents Nephrostomy tubes

infection in women, *E. coli* is responsible for 85% of infections.[2] Other organisms that contribute include *Staphylococcus saprophyticus* (5%–10%), *Proteus mirabilis*, and *Klebsiella pneumoniae*. In diabetics and pregnant women, group B streptococci (*Streptococcus agalactiae*) may be isolated.

Individuals with complicated urinary tract infection frequently have repeated infections. *E. coli* is commonly isolated, particularly early in the course. However, due to frequent courses of antimicrobials for repeated infections, exposure to health care institutional environments, and frequent invasive procedures, organisms of increasing antimicrobial resistance occur more commonly. Thus, *Proteus mirabilis, Citrobacter freundii, Pseudomonas aeruginosa, Enterococcus faecalis*, and other organisms are frequently isolated from persons with complicated urinary infection.[3] In

institutional populations, *Providencia stuartii* may commonly be isolated.[4]

For acute uncomplicated urinary infection in women, the development of infection depends upon specific organism factors as well as host factors.[5] Women who are nonsecretors of the blood group substances are most likely to have recurrent urinary tract infections, and urinary infection is frequently precipitated by sexual intercourse.[6] For the development of acute nonobstructive pyelonephritis, organism factors appear to be paramount. In particular, *E. coli* isolated in acute, nonobstructive pyelonephritis invariably produce a specific bacterial surface component called a pilus.[1]

The picture is quite different for complicated urinary tract infection. In this instance, the most important factor appears to be obstruction with impaired voiding. With abnormalities in the genitourinary tract, organisms do not require specific virulence factors to allow them to ascend to the kidney and cause invasive infection. Thus the presence of anatomical or functional obstruction as a host factor is of paramount importance.

Diagnosis

Urinary tract infection may be symptomatic or asymptomatic. Clinical syndromes of symptomatic infection include acute pyelonephritis and cystitis. Acute pyelonephritis is diagnosed clinically by costovertebral angle pain and tenderness, usually accompanied by fever and leukocytosis. Symptoms of bladder infection may precede or accompany symptoms of pyelonephritis. Cystitis, or bladder infection, is characterized by irritative symptoms such as burning on voiding (dysuria), suprapubic pain, urgency, and frequency. Fever is not a manifestation of cystitis. The symptoms associated with these syndromes are nonspecific, however, and these symptoms by themselves are not diagnostic of urinary infection.

The diagnosis of urinary infection requires microbiological confirmation of the presence of bacteria in the urine[7–12] (Table 6.2). For a symptomatic individual, bacteria present in a quantitative count above 10^5 colony forming units (cfu)/ml in a properly collected voided specimen forwarded promptly to the laboratory is considered diagnostic of infection.[7] For asymptomatic subjects, two consecutive urine cultures with the same organism present in quantitative counts above 10^5 cfu/ml are required for a diagnosis of urinary infection.[7] Lower quantitative counts may represent contamination by bacteria colonizing the periurethral area in voided urine specimens. This is particularly a problem in specimens collected from women. For men, however, lower quantitative counts of potential uropathogens are frequently consistent with infection,[8] and for women with the syndrome of acute cystitis or acute uncomplicated infection, 25% to 50% will have quantitative counts below 10^5 cfu/ml.[9] Thus, although the use of the quantitative urine culture is an essential diagnostic technique for urinary tract infection, results of the urine culture must be interpreted within the clinical context.

Morbidity

Asymptomatic bacteriuria leads to significant morbidity only for pregnant women, where it is associated with a high risk of pyelonephritis and premature delivery,[13] and in individuals who undergo invasive procedures of the genitourinary tract, such as cystoscopy, which may be associated with bacteremia if urinary tract infection is present at the time of mucosal trauma.[14] For other individuals with asymptomatic bacteriuria, current evidence does not document significant short-term or long-term complications

Table 6.2 *Bacteriologic Diagnosis of Urinary Tract Infection by Quantitative Culture*

POPULATION	QUANTITATIVE URINE CULTURE (WITH REFERENCE)
Asymptomatic bacteriuria	
Female	$\geq 10^5$ cfu/ml on two consecutive specimens[7]
Male	$\geq 10^4$ cfu/ml of uropathogen[8]
Acute cystitis	$\geq 10^2$ cfu/ml of a gram negative or *S. saprophyticus*[9]
Clinical acute pyelonephritis	$\geq 10^4$ cfu/ml on one specimen[10]
Indwelling catheter	any quantitative count in aspirated specimen[11]
In and out catheter	any quantitative count
Male with external collecting device	$\geq 10^5$ cfu/ml[12]

from bacteriuria. Women with acute uncomplicated urinary infection may be frustrated and upset by the frequency of symptomatic episodes but will suffer no long-term adverse effects from these. However, these women are at increased risk of developing acute nonobstructive pyelonephritis.[15] Acute pyelonephritis is a serious illness that is associated with bacteremia in as many as one third of cases. Bacteremia is more common in diabetic women and women over age 65 years.[16] Rarely, it may lead to metastatic infection such as septic arthritis or endocarditis. Early diagnosis and treatment of pyelonephritis or other invasive urinary infection is essential.

For individuals with complicated urinary tract infection, the determinant of morbidity is more often the underlying abnormality that has led to the increased frequency of infections rather than the infections themselves. Thus it is essential in every case to identify the abnormality and correct it wherever possible. These patients often have repeated episodes of symptomatic and invasive urinary tract infection if the underlying abnormality is not corrected.

Management

Many antimicrobials are effective for the treatment of urinary tract infection.[2] The antimicrobial chosen should generally be one where there is substantial clinical experience and that is least costly. First-line oral agents include trimethoprim/sulfamethoxazole, trimethoprim alone, or nitrofurantoin. Second-line agents include amoxicillin, fluoroquinolone antimicrobials, amoxicillin/clavulanic acid, and cephalosporins such as cephalexin. Second-line agents should be selected where antimicrobial resistance or patient intolerance precludes using first-line agents. In selecting empiric therapy, where the infecting organism and susceptibilities have not yet been determined, it is helpful to know current antimicrobial susceptibilities in a population.

For invasive urinary infection, parenteral therapy with ampicillin plus an aminoglycoside remains the treatment of choice. For penicillin-allergic patients, the aminoglycoside by itself may be used, particularly if Gram stains of the urine exclude gram-positive organisms as the etiologic agent. Certain antimicrobials, including nitrofurantoin and nalidixic acid, must be avoided in individuals with significant renal impairment. Aminoglycoside therapy may be problematic in subjects with underlying renal failure, and other parenteral antimicrobials with a wide gram-negative spectrum may be considered in this case.

For young women with acute uncomplicated urinary infection, symptomatic episodes can be treated with short courses of selected antimicrobials of one or three days.[2] For women with frequent recurrent episodes, symptomatic cystitis is effectively prevented by prophylactic therapy with prolonged courses of low-dose antimicrobials.[17] Individuals with pyelonephritis or symptomatic episodes of complicated urinary infection should be treated with antimicrobials for 14 days. These individuals will usually continue to have recurrent infection if the underlying abnormality in the genitourinary tract that predisposed to urinary infection is not corrected. Rarely, individuals with recurrent episodes of symptomatic infection require "suppressive" therapy. This is therapy that is continued to prevent complications of urinary infection such as symptomatic episodes or bacteremia in individuals who have persistent urinary infection, usually with persistent underlying abnormalities, that cannot be cured.

URINARY TRACT INFECTION IN THE ELDERLY

Urinary infection is one of the most common bacterial infections occurring in elderly populations. For women there is a gradual increase in the prevalence of urinary infection from childhood through older age (Table 6.3).[18] At the age of 65, 5% to 6% of well elderly women in the community will have urinary infection.[19] This prevalence increases to about 15% for those over age 80.[20] For men,

Table 6.3 *Prevalence of Urinary Infection (Bacteriuria) in Different Populations by Age, Residence, and Sex (adapted from references 19-22).*

AGE	FEMALE	MALE
20–60 years	2%–5%	<1%
>60 years,		
community	5%–10%	2%–5%
geriatric apartment	10%–15%	5%–10%
nursing home	15%–50%	15%–35%

urinary infection is uncommon before 60 years, but increases markedly beyond this age. From 2% to 4% of men in the community at age 60 will have bacteriuria as will from 10% to 15% of those over 80 years.[21]

The reasons for this marked increase in urinary infection with age have not been fully characterized. It appears, however, that associated diseases that occur more commonly in older populations are the most important contributing factors. Diabetes is more common in older women, and diabetic women are three times more likely than nondiabetic women to have bacteriuria.[22] For men, development of prostatic hypertrophy is likely the most important factor promoting urinary infection. Neurologic diseases such as cerebrovascular disease, dementia, and Parkinson's disease, which are usually associated with a neurogenic bladder and impaired voiding, are also important contributors. Hormonal changes that accompany aging may contribute to the increased prevalence of bacteriuria, but their importance relative to other factors has not been defined.

Although urinary tract infection is one of the most common infections in the elderly, it is a relatively less important cause of morbidity or mortality in this population compared to pneumonia and certain noninfectious diseases. Estimates of morbidity of symptomatic urinary infection in noninstitutionalized elderly populations are not available. Although urinary tract infection is the most common cause of bacteremia in elderly noninstitutionalized populations, it accounted for only 0.5% of admissions to one acute care institution of all patients over 65 years.[23]

The association of asymptomatic bacteriuria and mortality in the elderly has been controversial.[21,24–26] Several early studies reported that relative to those with no bacteriuria, elderly individuals with asymptomatic bacteriuria had a decreased survival.[24,25] No explanation for this observed difference in survival was apparent. Subsequent studies in community-based populations have failed to confirm this difference.[21,26] It was felt that differences in comorbidities between bacteriuric and nonbacteriuric elderly, rather than a direct effect of bacteriuria itself, likely explained the earlier observations. Thus, there is at present no convincing evidence that asymptomatic bacteriuria contributes to decreased survival in the elderly community population.

Considerations with respect to the management of urinary infection are not different for older than for younger populations. There is currently no evidence to suggest a benefit for the routine treatment of asymptomatic bacteriuria.[27] Symptomatic infection, of course, warrants antimicrobial therapy. Antimicrobial treatment of urinary infection is less effective for older women than for younger women.[28–30] The reasons for this impaired efficacy in older women have not been clearly defined. In particular, the shorter courses of therapy that are highly successful in young women have much lower efficacy in older women. Thus, if treatment is necessary, an initial course of 7 days seems appropriate for presumed bladder infection, and 14 days for kidney infection.

Men with symptomatic urinary infection should be initially treated with a 14-day course of therapy. If infection relapses, prolonged courses of therapy of 6 or 12 weeks should be given.[31,32] Many elderly men have a focus of infection in the prostate. Once bacterial infection is established in the prostate, it is frequently impossible to eradicate due to several factors, including poor antimicrobial penetration into the prostate and the presence of prostatic stones. Thus relapsing infection is common. Antimicrobial pharmacokinetics in the elderly is discussed in Chapter 12.

URINARY TRACT INFECTIONS IN NURSING HOMES

Prevalence and Incidence

Urinary tract infection is extremely common in the nursing home population. Repeated studies have reported from 10% to 40% of men and 30% to 50% of women resident in nursing homes will have bacteriuria (urinary infection) at any given time (Table 6.3). The incidence of urinary tract infection in this population is also very high. In one group of highly functionally disabled elderly men, new infections occurred at a rate of 45 per 100 patient-years, with 10% of nonbacteriuric residents becoming bacteriuric in each three-month period.[33] An institutionalized population in Greece had an initial prevalence of bacteriuria of 19% for men and 27% for women, with a further 11% and 23%, respectively, having a positive urine culture at 6 or 12 months from admission.[34] Female nursing home residents in Philadelphia had an initial prevalence of bacteriuria of 25%, with an additional 8% identified with a positive urine culture each six-month period.[35]

Risk Factors

By themselves, age and duration of residence in the nursing home are not predictors of bacteriuria.[20,35–37]

However, urinary infection is most likely to occur in the most highly functionally disabled residents. For both men and women, urinary incontinence, bowel incontinence, and dementia are associated with an increased prevalence of bacteriuria. In some studies, impaired mobility has also been shown to be associated with bacteriuria, but this observation has not been consistent.[35,37]

Changes in resident status may be associated with a new onset of urinary infection. For instance, episodes of impaired mobility due to concurrent illness such as pneumonia may precipitate bacteriuria.[33] Many incontinent elderly men have voiding managed with external drainage devices such as condoms with leg bags. The use of condoms and leg bags is a risk factor for acquisition of urinary infection, particularly if the tubing becomes obstructed or twisted.[38]

The small proportion of elderly residents in nursing homes who have voiding managed with long-term indwelling bladder catheters have a 100% prevalence of bacteriuria.[39] The foley catheter allows ingress of organisms from the periurethral area into the bladder and then provides a focus on which the organisms can survive within the bladder.

Microbiology

Organisms isolated from urinary infection in elderly institutionalized individuals differ for men and women (Table 6.4). For women, *Escherichia coli* is the most common infecting organism with *Proteus mirabilis*, group B streptococci, and *Citrobacter freundii* occurring less frequently.[20,40] For men *P. mirabilis* appears to be the most frequent infecting organism, with *E. coli, P. aeruginosa* and *E. faecalis* also occurring frequently. Many of these organisms are relatively resistant to antimicrobials. One organism of particular interest to long-term care facilities is *Providencia stuartii*, an organism that is endemic in many facilities and may be highly antimicrobial-resistant. It is seldom isolated from urinary infection except in individuals who have acquired it in institutions. Urinary infection in a given individual may persist with the same organism for months or years, but other residents have serial modifications in their infecting organisms over time.[20,33,40]

Elderly subjects in nursing homes are frequently unable to cooperate to obtain voided urine specimens for culture. This may result in contamination of urine specimens and

Table 6.4 *Microbiology of Urinary Tract Infection in Nursing Home Populations*

	ORGANISMS	
	FEMALE	MALE
Common	E. coli P. mirabilis	P. mirabilis E. faecalis E. coli
Other		K. pneumoniae Citrobacter freundii Morganella morganii Providencia stuartii Pseudomonas aeruginosa Group B streptococcus

misidentification of urinary tract infection because of contaminated specimens. For men, a clean catch urine specimen is generally reliable and may frequently be obtained at the time of routine toileting. Several studies have validated the use of freshly applied clean condoms for the collection of urine specimens for culture.[12,41] If condoms are used, the quantitative cutoff of 10^5 cfu/ml for an infecting organism is appropriate for diagnosis of bacteriuria (Table 6.2). For women who are unable to cooperate to provide clean voided specimens, the collection of specimens may be problematic. A pedibag system has occasionally been employed, but the use of pedibags for specimen collection is associated with a high level of contamination and may not provide culture results that can be interpreted. This method has not yet been validated and cannot currently be recommended for specimen collection. If it is essential that a urine specimen be obtained for culture to assist in management decisions for a nursing home resident and that resident cannot cooperate to provide a satisfactory specimen, then in and out catheterization should be used for specimen collection. Catheterization, by itself, however, carries a risk of introduction of infection and should be used only when clinically appropriate.

Virtually all elderly residents of nursing homes with asymptomatic bacteriuria, over 90%, will have pyuria, or leukocytes in the urine.[40,42,43] Thus, the presence or absence of pyuria is not helpful in determining the clinical significance of a positive urine culture. In addition, as many as 30% of elderly residents who do not have urinary tract infection will also have pyuria.[43,44] The determinants of this pyuria in nonbacteriuric subjects are not known. The high frequency of pyuria without urinary tract infection indicates that the urinalysis by itself cannot be used to identify urinary infection in elderly residents of nursing homes.

Morbidity and Mortality

Urinary infection in nursing home residents is usually asymptomatic. Although discrete episodes of symptomatic infection do occur, they are infrequent relative to the extraordinarily high prevalence of bacteriuria.[37,40] Urinary infection is the most frequent source for bacteremia in the nursing home population.[45] Episodes of morbidity due to urinary infection may include bacteremia, fever with pyelonephritis, or symptomatic lower tract infection associated with irritative symptoms such as increased frequency, dysuria, and new or increased incontinence.

It is difficult to ascertain symptoms and their relevance to the urinary tract in many elderly nursing home residents because of associated functional disability and difficulties in communication. In addition, chronic genitourinary symptoms such as incontinence, frequency, and nocturia are frequent in elderly residents. Although a high proportion of individuals with these chronic symptoms may have bacteriuria, urinary infection is not the cause of chronic symptoms.[36,46] Acute onset of symptoms or changes in symptoms may be due to urinary infection, although other diagnostic possibilities must be considered. Another diagnostic challenge is the elderly nursing home resident with fever, a positive urine culture, and no apparent source for the fever. For residents without indwelling catheters, the source of fever is unlikely to be urinary infection unless other symptoms (e.g., hematuria) suggest genitourinary involvement. In the individual patient, however, it may be impossible to determine whether the source is urinary or nonurinary.

Elderly nursing home residents with chronic indwelling catheters are at particularly high risk for fever and, potentially, sepsis associated with urinary infection.[47] These residents have multiple organisms present at high quantitative counts in the urine. The indwelling catheter may traumatize the mucosa of the genitourinary tract, allowing ingress of organisms to the bloodstream.

Morbidity and mortality in elderly nursing home residents with chronic indwelling catheters is greater than in residents with bacteriuria but no indwelling catheters.[47,48]

As mentioned earlier, there has been controversy about the impact of asymptomatic urinary infection on mortality in the noninstitutionalized elderly. One study in a male institutionalized population found no association of bacteriuria with mortality.[37] Urinary infection is also an infrequent cause of mortality in autopsy series in the institutionalized elderly.[49,50] Thus there is no present evidence that asymptomatic bacteriuria is a determinant of survival in this population.

Management of Urinary Infection in Nursing Homes

Asymptomatic bacteriuria in the nursing home population does not require antimicrobial treatment unless the resident is to undergo an invasive genitourinary procedure. Attempts to treat elderly nursing home residents with asymptomatic bacteriuria with antibiotics are usually followed by early recurrence of infection, either relapse or reinfection, and limited decrease in prevalence in bacteriuria for the population.[33,40] In addition, elderly subjects may experience adverse effects secondary to the antimicrobials, and the antimicrobial pressure promotes the emergence of resistant organisms within the nursing home environment. Treatment of asymptomatic bacteriuria has not been shown to decrease the incidence of symptomatic episodes of urinary infection or influence long-term outcomes. Thus, asymptomatic bacteriuria in the nursing home population should not be treated with antimicrobials.

Episodes of symptomatic infection should be treated. For residents with lower tract symptoms suggesting bladder infection, a 7-day course of therapy is likely appropriate. If invasive infection occurs, usually characterized by the presence of fever, a 14-day course of therapy would be suggested. At present, no clinical studies document the optimal duration of therapy for treatment in the nursing home population.

One difficulty with the management of urinary infection in the nursing home population is the clinical uncertainty with respect to identification of symptomatic infection. With such a high prevalence of bacteriuria, over 50% in the most functionally impaired, a positive urine culture is not diagnostic of symptomatic urinary infection even in the presence of urinary tract symptoms or fever. However, a negative urine culture obtained prior to antimicrobial therapy may exclude urinary infection. In some cases, empiric treatment with antimicrobials and observing the clinical response is the only option. However, the goals to be achieved by such therapy should be determined beforehand and the situation reassessed if the desired response to antimicrobial therapy is not achieved.

Special Considerations with Respect to Indwelling Catheters

Short-term indwelling catheters are catheters that are maintained in an individual for less than 30 days. Generally, short-term catheterization is associated with a risk of acquisition of bacteriuria of approximately 5% per day. Women have a higher daily acquisition rate than men.

The larger issue in the nursing home population is the use of long-term indwelling catheters. Chronic indwelling catheters are used for a number of different reasons. For men, retention may require a chronic indwelling catheter. For women, incontinence is the most common indication leading to the use of a permanent indwelling catheter. As previously noted, residents with chronic indwelling catheters have persistent polymicrobial bacteriuria.[39] In the absence of antimicrobial therapy, organisms persist for variable durations. Some may be present only transiently; others persist for months.

Organisms that are present in the bladder in the patient with a chronic indwelling catheter are usually initially organisms that colonize the periurethral area.[51] These organisms gain access to the urinary system by ascending the urethra on the outside of the catheter. Infection occurs less commonly through the lumen of the catheter, when contaminated urine in the drainage bag refluxes or tubing is obstructed. Finally, any disruption of the closed drainage system may allow access of organisms to the urine column. Specimens for culture from chronic indwelling catheters should be collected aseptically from the sampling port. A number of studies[52–54] have suggested that specimens collected from "old catheters" differ quantitatively and qualitatively in microbiology from specimens isolated from freshly inserted catheters in the same patient. This has been interpreted to mean that the specimens from "old catheters" represent catheter colo-

nization rather than bladder infection. The clinical significance of this observation is not clear, nor have studies been performed in symptomatic patients to determine the validity of catheter specimen collection methods. At present, it seems premature to suggest routine catheter replacement prior to specimen collection.

Elderly residents of nursing homes with a chronic indwelling catheter clearly have excess morbidity and mortality compared to those without a chronic indwelling catheter.[48] They experience more febrile episodes of possible urinary source than noncatheterized bacteriuric individuals[47] and more frequently have pathologic evidence of kidney infection (manifested by abscess or inflammation at autopsy).[55] Thus, chronic indwelling catheters should only be used when there are no other options for patient voiding management.

The mechanisms through which chronic indwelling catheters lead to increased morbidity and mortality are not entirely clear. Catheters frequently may obstruct, leading to increased residual volume and reflux with sepsis. This allows organisms to gain access to the kidneys. The occurrence of catheter obstruction in nursing home residents with indwelling catheters is highly variable. Obstruction is due to struvite formation, the same substance present in stones formed by urease producing organisms, primarily *Proteus mirabilis*.[56] However, patient variables appear to be important to predict which residents with *P. mirabilis* catheter infections will obstruct.[57] The routine replacement of catheters to prevent obstruction is not recommended, however.

Trauma to the genitourinary mucosa when the catheter is manipulated is another important cause for invasive infection associated with indwelling urinary catheters. Patients with indwelling catheters have a large number of organisms present in their urine. Trauma to the mucosa with bleeding may be associated with direct access of these organisms or endotoxin to the blood stream, leading to fever and bacteremia. Thus, appropriate catheter care to limit trauma is important.

Bacteriuria in subjects with chronic indwelling catheters should only be treated if the patient is symptomatic. Treatment of asymptomatic subjects will not eradicate bacteriuria, but it will encourage the emergence of organisms with increased antimicrobial resistance. Symptomatic infection should be treated with as short a course of therapy as possible in hopes of minimizing bacterial resistance. There is no role for suppressive antimicrobial therapy in subjects with chronic indwelling catheters.

INFECTION CONTROL ASPECTS OF URINARY INFECTION IN NURSING HOMES

General Measures

It is not yet clear what measures, if any, can decrease the occurrence of urinary infection in noncatheterized nursing home populations. The prevalence of urinary infection is determined primarily by the concurrent chronic diseases associated with functional or structural abnormalities and impaired voiding. Measures to ensure optimal management of underlying diseases as well as optimal nutrition are, of course, desirable. Whether such general care interventions influence the prevalence of bacteriuria or incidence of symptomatic infection is not known. A decreased use of condom drainage catheters or indwelling foley catheters would certainly decrease the occurrence of infection. However, these devices are often necessary in incontinent or obstructed elderly subjects and cannot be avoided in some subjects even with optimal urologic and incontinence management.

There is an association between bacteriuria and the presence of urinary and fecal incontinence. Some authors have suggested that controlling incontinence may decrease the occurrence of urinary infection, speculating that periurethral contamination by feces, in particular, promotes bacteriuria. Although this may be true, it is equally true that subjects with incontinence are more likely to have neurologic abnormalities with associated impaired voiding and increased residua, which facilitate infection. Thus it is not clear that more careful management of incontinence would necessarily decrease urinary infection in the nursing home population.

As many elderly residents of nursing homes will be bacteriuric, urine of subjects with asymptomatic bacteriuria provides a large and ubiquitous reservoir for organisms, frequently of increased antimicrobial resistance. Careful handwashing following any contact with urine, contaminated bedding of an incontinent patient, or urinary devices such as condom and leg bags will decrease transmission of organisms among patients.

Rather than decreasing the prevalence of asymptomatic bacteriuria, the goal of management should be to prevent symptomatic infection. Episodes of invasive infection may be prevented by early identification of retention, avoiding indwelling catheters wherever possible, preventing mucosal trauma or kinking or obstruction of the catheter in individuals with indwelling catheters, and the use of preprocedure antimicrobials for individuals with infected urine prior to invasive procedures.

Epidemic Urinary Tract Infection

A number of outbreaks of urinary tract infection have been identified, primarily in acute care institutions.[58–61] These outbreaks have usually been identified because they are caused by unusual organisms or organisms of increased antimicrobial resistance. The actual frequency of "epidemic urinary tract infection" in nursing homes is not known. Factors associated with these outbreaks in acute and chronic care institutions include a high prevalence of asymptomatic bacteriuria in patients with chronic indwelling catheters, shared use of equipment such as urinometers, which facilitates cross-contamination among patients, and transmission on the hands of personnel caring for patients.

A systematic surveillance of organisms isolated from the urine to determine the usual infecting organisms and susceptibilities for a given institution and to identify crosstransmission should be developed. Where an outbreak of epidemic UTI is suspected, outbreak investigation including appropriate control measures should be initiated promptly (see Chapter 11).

Institutional policies should include appropriate management of catheters and condoms and cleaning of patient equipment, and should specifically preclude sharing of potentially contaminated equipment among patients. Appropriate handwashing by staff between patients must be facilitated.

Indwelling Catheters

A number of methods have been documented to delay the acquisition of bacteriuria in individuals with short term indwelling catheters (Table 6.5). The most important of these include maintenance of a closed sterile drainage system, use of aseptic technique at insertion, and ensuring that there is unimpaired drainage from the bladder to the drainage bag. Antimicrobial therapy during the first four

Table 6.5   *Methods Studied to Decrease Acquisition of Infection in Catheterized Patients*

PROVEN EFFICACIOUS:

Aseptic insertion
Closed drainage system
Individual drainage equipment
Unobstructed drainage
Antimicrobials first four days only

PROVEN NOT EFFICACIOUS:

Routine perineal care with soap or disinfectant
Antibiotic irrigation
Disinfectant in drainage tube
Silver-impregnated catheters

days an indwelling catheter is in situ decreases early acquisition of infection. Beyond that initial few days, however, there is no benefit in decreased infection, and infection that occurs will be with organisms of increased resistance. Thus, antimicrobial therapy is not recommended to prevent short-term catheter infection. Other interventions that have been well studied but have not been shown to decrease acquisition of infection include routine perineal care with either soap or a disinfectant, the addition of a disinfectant to the drainage bag,[62,63] and antibiotic irrigation of the catheter.[64] Irrigation, in fact, is associated with an increased risk of infection because of the need to open the drainage system to allow entry of the irrigating solution. The extent to which any of these observations made in subjects with short-term catheters are applicable to subjects with long-term indwelling catheters is not clear, but it seems reasonable to apply the information gained from these studies of short-term catheters to the care of long-term indwelling catheters.

The first approach to the prevention of urinary infection with indwelling catheters is, of course, to avoid the use of indwelling catheters. Alternate methods for control of incontinence should always be attempted, and obstruction causing retention should be corrected where possible. Indwelling catheters should be used only if essential for patient care, not for convenience of the staff. When short-term catheterization is necessary, the indwelling catheter should be discontinued as soon as possible.

Appropriate catheter care is necessary to decrease the complications of indwelling catheters secondary to catheter trauma and to decrease acquisition of organisms in the nursing home. Urine flow from the bladder to the drainage bag should be unimpeded, so twisting or kinking of the catheter should be avoided and the drainage bag should always be maintained below the level of the bladder. Catheters and tubing must be well secured so there will not be tension on them. The catheter and drainage tubing and bag should be replaced when obstructed or leaking, but replacement on a routine schedule is not necessary if the system is functioning well. Staff members should be aware that when providing catheter care or manipulating the tubing or drainage bag they are likely to become contaminated with organisms, and they should use gloves if contamination with urine is likely, with careful handwashing after any manipulations of catheters in patients whether or not gloves are worn.

Antimicrobial Use

Elderly residents of nursing homes have a high prevalence of bacteriuria, and asymptomatic bacteriuria is a large reservoir for gram negative organisms, which may become resistant. One problem that undoubtedly contributes to the development of resistance is the widespread use of antimicrobials in nursing home patients.[65] This intense antimicrobial use for nonurinary infections may lead to the emergence of resistant organisms, with the asymptomatic bacteriuric subject then serving as a reservoir for such resistant organisms. Thus, programs for the appropriate use of antimicrobials including restrictions in use and duration and avoidance of broad-spectrum agents where possible are an integral part of the infection control program (see Chapter 12).

REFERENCES

1. Svanborg Edén C, De Man P: Bacterial virulence in urinary tract infection. *Infect Dis Clin North Am* 1987;1:731–750.

2. Johnson JR, Stamm WE: Diagnosis and treatment of acute urinary tract infections. *Infect Dis Clin North Am* 1987;1:773–791.

3. Preheim LC: Complicated urinary tract infections. *Am J Med* 1985;79(suppl 2A):62–66.

4. Gaynes RP, Weinstein R, Chamberlin W, et al: Antibiotic resistant flora in nursing home patients admitted to the hospital. *Arch Intern Med* 1985;145:1804–1807.

5. Sobel JD: Pathogenesis of urinary tract infections: Host defences. *Infect Dis Clin North Am* 1987;1:751–772.

6. Nicolle LE, Harding GKM, Preiksartas J, et al: The association of urinary tract infection with sexual intercourse. *J Infect Dis* 1982;146:579–583.

7. Kass EH: Asymptomatic infections of the urinary tract. *Trans Assoc Amer Physicians* 1956;69:56–64.

8. Lipsky BA, Ireton FC, Fihn SD, et al: Diagnosis of bacteriuria in men: Specimen collection and culture intervention. *J Infect Dis* 1987;155:847–854.

9. Stamm WE, Counts GW, Running KR, et al: Diagnosis of coliform infection in acutely dysuric women. *N Engl J Med* 1982;307:463–468.

10. Robert FJ: Quantitative urine cultures in patients with urinary tract infection and bacteriuria. *Am J Clin Path* 1986;85:616–618.

11. Stark RP, Maki DG: Bacteriuria in the catheterized patient. What quantitative level of bacteriuria is relevant? *N Engl J Med* 1984;311:560–564.

12. Nicolle LE, Harding GKM, Kennedy J, et al: Urine specimen collection with external devices for diagnosis of bacteriuria in elderly incontinent men. *J Clin Microbiol* 1988;26:1115–1119.

13. Patterson TF, Andrade VT: Bacteriuria in pregnancy. *Infect Dis Clin North Am* 1987;1:807–822.

14. Cafferkey MT, Falkiner FR, Gillespie WA, et al: Antibiotics for the prevention of septicemia in urology. *J Antimicrob Chemother* 1982;9:471–477.

15. Stamm WE, McKevitt M, Roberts PL, et al: Natural history of recurrent urinary tract infections in women. *Rev Infect Dis* 1991;13:77–84.

16. Gleckman RA, Bradley PJ, Roth RM, et al: Bacteremic urosepsis: A phenomenon unique to elderly women. *J Urol* 1985; 133:174–175.

17. Nicolle LE, Ronald AR: Recurrent urinary tract infection in adult women: Diagnosis and treatment. *Infect Dis Clin North Am* 1987;1:793–806.

18. Kaye D: Urinary tract infection in the elderly. *Bull N Y Acad Med* 1980;56:209–220.

19. Evans DA, Williams DN, Laughlin LW: Bacteriuria in a population-based cohort of women. *J Infect Dis* 1978;138:768–773.

20. Boscia JA, Kobasa WD, Knight RA, et al: Epidemiology of

bacteriuria in an elderly ambulatory population. *Am J Med* 1986;80:208–214.

21. Nordenstam GR, Brandberg CA, Oden AS, et al: Bacteriuria and mortality in an elderly population. *N Engl J Med* 1986;314:1152–1156.

22. Zhanel G, Harding GKM, Nicolle LE: Asymptomatic bacteriuria in diabetes. *Rev Infect Dis* 1991;13:150–154.

23. Gleckman R, Blagg N, Hibert D, et al: Community-acquired bactermic urosepsis in elderly patients: A prospective study of 34 consecutive episodes. *J Urol* 1983;128:79–81.

24. Sourander LB, Kasanen A: A five-year follow-up of bacteriuria in the aged. *Gerontol Clin* 1972;14:274–281.

25. Dontas AS, Kasviki-Charvati P, Papanayiotou PC, et al: Bacteriuria and survival in old age. *N Engl J Med* 1981;304:939–943.

26. Heinamaki P, Haavisto M, Hakulimen T, et al: Mortality in relation to urinary characteristics in the very aged. *Gerontology* 1986;32:167–171.

27. Boscia JA, Kobusa WD, Knight RA, et al: Therapy vs. no therapy for bacteriuria in elderly ambulatory non-hospitalized women. *JAMA* 1987;257:1067–1071.

28. Cardenas J, Quinn EL, Booker G, et al: Single dose cephalexin therapy for acute bacterial urinary tract infections and acute urethral syndrome with bladder bacteriuria. *Antimicrob Agents Chemother* 1986;29:383–385.

29. Harding GKM, Nicolle LE, Ronald AR, et al: Management of catheter acquired urinary tract infection in women: Therapy following catheter removal. *Ann Intern Med* 1991;114:713–719.

30. Saguinar R, Nicolle LE: Canadian Infectious Diseases Society Clinical Trials Group. Single dose or three days norfloxacin for acute uncomplicated urinary infection in women. *Arch Intern Med* 1992;152:1233–1237.

31. Gleckman R, Crowley M, Natsios GA: Therapy for recurrent invasive urinary tract infections in men. *N Engl J Med* 1979;301:878–880.

32. Smith JW, Jones SR, Reed WP, et al: Recurrent urinary tract infections in men: Characteristics and response to therapy. *Ann Intern Med* 1979;91:544–548.

33. Nicolle LE, Bjornson J, Harding GKM, et al: Bacteriuria in elderly institutionalized men. *N Engl J Med* 1983;309:1420–1426.

34. Kasviki-Charvati P, Drolette-Kefakis B, Papanyiotou PC, et al: Turnover of bacteriuria in old age. *Age Ageing* 1982;11:169–174.

35. Abrutyn E, Mossey J, Levison M, et al: Epidemiology of asymptomatic bacteriuria in elderly women. *J Am Geriatr Soc* 1991;39:388–393.

36. Brocklehurst JC, Dillance JB, Griffiths L, et al: The prevalance and symptomatology of urinary infection in an aged population. *Gerontol Clin* 1968;10:242–243.

37. Nicolle LE, Hendersen E, Bjornson J, et al: The association of bacteriuria with resident characteristics and survival in elderly

institutionalized men. *Ann Intern Med* 1987;106:682–686.

38. Hirsh DD, Fainstein V,. Musher DM: Do condom catheter collecting systems cause urinary tract infections? *JAMA* 1979;242:340–341.

39. Warren JW, Tenney JH, Hooper JM, et al: A prospective microbiologic study of bacteriuria in patients with chronic indwelling urethral catheters. *J Infect Dis* 1982;146:719–723.

40. Nicolle LE, Mayhew WJ, Bryan L: Prospective, randomized comparison of therapy and no therapy for asymptomatic bacteriuria in institutionalized elderly women. *Am J Med* 1987;83:27–33.

41. Ouslander JG, Greengold BA, Silverblatt FJ, et al: An accurate method to obtain urine for culture in men with external catheters. *Arch Intern Med* 1987;147:286–288.

42. Nicolle LE, Muir P, Harding GKM, et al: Localization of site of urinary infection in elderly institutionalized women with asymptomatic bacteriuria. *J Infect Dis* 1988;157:65–70.

43. Boscia JA, Abrutyn E, Levison ME, et al: Pyuria and asymptomatic bacteriuria in elderly ambulatory women. *Ann Intern Med* 1989;110:404–405.

44. Rodgers K, Nicolle LE, McIntyre M, et al: Pyuria in institutionalized elderly subjects. *Can J Infect Dis* 1991;2:142–146.

45. Senay H, Goetz MB: Epidemiology of bacteremic urinary tract infections in chronically hospitalized elderly men. *J Urol* 1991;145:1201–1204.

46. Boscia JA, Kobasa WD, Abrutyn E, et al: Lack of association between bacteriuria and symptoms in the elderly. *Am J Med* 1986;81:979–982.

47. Warren JW, Damron D, Tenney JH, et al: Fever, bacteremia, and death as complications of bacteriuria in women with long-term urethral catheters. *J Infect Dis* 1982;155:1151–1158.

48. Kunin CM, Dorthitt S, Danung J, et al: The association between the use of urinary catheters and morbidity and mortality among elderly patients in nursing homes. *Am J Epidemiol* 1992;135:291–301.

49. Kohn RR: Cause of death in very old people. *JAMA* 1982;247:2793–2797.

50. Puxty JAH, Horan MA, Fox RA: Necropsies in the elderly. *Lancet* 1983;i:1262–1264.

51. Warren JW: Catheter-associated urinary tract infections. *Infect Dis Clin North Am* 1987;1:823–854.

52. Grahn D, Norman DC, White ML, et al: Validity of urinary catheter specimens for diagnosis of urinary tract infec-

tion in the elderly. *Arch Intern Med* 1985;145:1858–1860.

53. Berggvist D, Bronnestam R, Hedilin H, et al: The relevance of urinary sampling methods in patients with indwelling Foley catheters. *Br J Urol* 1980;52:92–95.

54. Tenney JH, Warren JW: Long-term catheter-associated bacteriuria. Species at low concentration. *Urology* 1987;30:444–446.

55. Warren JW, Muncie HL, Hall-Craggs M: Acute pyelonephritis associated with bacteriuria during long-term catheterization. A prospective clinico-pathologic study. *J Infect Dis* 1988;158:1341–1346.

56. Hedelin H, Eddeland A, Larsson L, et al: The composition of catheter encrustations, including the effects of allopurinol treatment. *Br J Urol* 1984;56:250–254.

57. Kunin CM: Blockage of urinary catheters. Role of microorganisms and constituents of the urine on formation of encrustations. *J Clin Epidemiol* 1989;42:835–842.

58. Schaberg DR, Weinstein RA, Stamm WE: Epidemics of nosocomial urinary tract infection caused by multiply resistant gram-negative bacilli: Epidemiology and control. *J Infect Dis* 1976;133:363–366.

59. Rutala WA, Kennedy VA, Loflin HB, et al: *Serratia marcescens* nosocomial infections of the urinary tract associated with urine measuring containers and urinometers. *Am J Med* 1981;70:659–663.

60. Kocka FE, Roemusch E, Carsey WA et al: The urometer as a reservoir of infectious organisms. *Am J Clin Path* 1977;67:106–107.

61. Fierer J, Ekstrom M: An outbreak of Providentia stuartii urinary tract infections: Patients with condom catheters are a reservoir of the bacteria. *JAMA* 1981;245:1553–1555.

62. Gillespie WA, Jones JE, Teasdale C, et al: Does the addition of disinfectant to urine drainage bags prevent infection in catheterized patients? *Lancet* 1983;i:1037–1039.

63. Thompson RL, Haley CE, Searcy MA, et al: Catheter-associated bacteriuria: Failure to reduce attack rates during periodic installations of a disinfectant into urinary drainage systems. *JAMA* 1984;251:747–751.

64. Warren JW, Platt R, Thomas RJ, et al: Antibiotic irrigation and catheter-associated urinary-tract infections. *N Eng J Med* 1978;299:570-573.

65. Warren JW, Palumbo FB, Fitterman L, et al: Incidence and characteristics of antibiotic use in aged nursing home patients. *J Am Geriatr Soc* 1991;39:963–972.

CHAPTER 7

PRESSURE ULCERS

Joyce M. Black and Steven B. Black

BACKGROUND

Definition

Pressure ulcers have plagued human beings since the time of Hippocrates. The term *decubitus* derived from a Latin word meaning "to lay down," has also been used to describe these ulcers. For many years the terms *decubitus* and *bedsores* were popular and appropriate terms, because these ulcers are common in the bedridden. Today, the term *pressure ulcers* is preferred, as it more clearly describes the condition and the fact that more than bedridden patients develop pressure ulcers. In contrast to the long history of pressure ulcers, scientifically proven techniques for their treatment are relatively recent. This chapter reviews causes of pressure ulcers and medical, surgical, and nursing management of them.

Pressure ulcers are graded to help in treatment plans (see Fig. 7.1) The stages are as follows:

Stage 1: Nonblanchable erythema of intact skin. This stage is present when an area remains red after pressure is removed. It is important to recognize that Stage 1 ulcers are not areas of reactive hyperemia. Compensatory reactive hyperemia is the flow of additional blood upon the release of pressure in an area of tissue hypoxia. Reactive hyperemia also appears as red areas but normally persists only for one half to three fourths as long as pressure was applied.

Stage 2: Partial thickness loss of epidermis and/or dermis. The ulcer is superficial and presents clinically as an abrasion, blister, or shallow crater.

Stage 3: Full thickness skin loss involving damage or necrosis of subcutaneous tissue that may extend to, but not through, underlying fascia. The ulcer presents as a deep crater.

Stage 4: Full thickness skin loss with extensive destruction, tissue necrosis or damage to muscle, bone, or other supporting structures. Undermining and sinus tracts may also be associated with ulcers in this stage.

Significance of the Problem

Pressure ulcers continue to be a significant problem. An estimated 1.5 to 3 million persons in the United States have pressure ulcers.[1] Among residents of skilled care facilities and nursing homes, the prevalence of pressure ulcers ranged

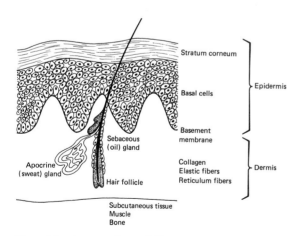

Figure 7.1 *Anatomy of normal skin*

from 2.4 percent[2] to 23 percent.[3] This wide range in prevalence of pressure ulcers is probably due to the wide variation in cases and staffing. The prevalence of more than one ulcer was 9.2% in a 1990 study. The sacrum and heel were the most common sites. The greater trochanter had the most stage 4 ulcers.[4]

Not only are the incidence and prevalence of pressure ulcers a concern, the ulcers are costly. Approximately 60,000 deaths per year from bacteremia are associated with the complications of pressure ulcers.[5] The cost of repair for ulcers depends upon the stage of the ulcer. A stage 2 left heel ulcer was healed for $4,255. Care of multisite ulcers of the ischial tuberosity, trochanter, and gluteal fold cost $23,301.[5]

EXTRINSIC AND INTRINSIC RISK FACTORS

Several causes of pressure ulcers exist. They are divided into extrinsic and intrinsic factors. Extrinsic factors exist outside of the patient and are pressure, friction, shear, and moisture. Intrinsic factors are within the patient and include limited mobility, advanced age, malnutrition, incontinence, and other specific clinical disorders.

Extrinsic Factors

Pressure is the key element in pressure ulcer development. Pressure ulcers develop when the external pressure applied to the skin exceeds the capillary pressure to perfuse the skin. Normally the capillary pressure ranges from 12 to 32 mm Hg, depending upon the body part. Pressure that exceeds 70 mm Hg for over two hours will result in tissue damage from hypoxia. The skin can tolerate more pressure than can fat and muscle tissue without developing hypoxia. However, if pressure is relieved every one to two hours, compensatory reactive hyperemia occurs and restores blood supply to the hypoxic tissues.

The compression of soft tissue between a bony prominence and the skin surface results in a cone-shaped pressure area. A cone of tissue destruction occurs from the skin through fat and muscle tissue to the bone. The tip of the cone, like the tip of an iceberg, is visible at the skin surface, whereas the majority of tissue damage occurs below the visible surface of the skin.

Friction occurs when two surfaces are moved across each other, such as skin across bedsheets. Friction removes the outer surface of the skin. Although friction most commonly results in blisters and abrasions, it can contribute to more serious injury. Friction has been shown to reduce the amount of external pressure needed to produce a pressure ulcer.[6]

Tissue injury from *shear* occurs when the skin remains stationary and the underlying tissue shifts. Shear injury can occur when patients are pulled up toward the head of the bed by their shoulders or slide down toward the foot of the bed. As a result of shear, blood vessels in the sacral area are likely to become twisted and distorted. Underlying tissue can become ischemic and necrotic. Shear forces have likely contributed to the undermining seen with sacral ulcers.

The presence of *moisture* created by perspiration or urinary or fecal drainage increases the risk of pressure ulcers fivefold. As tissues become damp, there is an increase in static friction between the surface and the skin. Moisture also macerates the skin, which makes it more susceptible to infection.

Intrinsic Factors

The protective mechanism of spontaneous *movement* occurs during waking and sleeping hours. When tissue tolerance of pressure and ischemia has been reached, the body automatically moves to reduce pressure and restore blood flow. Several intrinsic factors may exist within a patient that impair this mechanism. Paraplegia and hemiplegia impair sensation. Sedation from narcotics or anesthesia and decreased levels of consciousness reduce the central nervous system's perception. Movement may also be restricted due to pain or devices. Diabetic neuropathy may prevent sensory information from reaching the brain, inhibiting awareness of the need to move.

The *aged* patient is more susceptible to skin ulceration because there is less subcutaneous fat. Other changes in the skin due to age also increase risk. These changes include increased fragility of skin, decreased turnover rate of epidermal cells, stiffening of dermal collagen, decreased number of oil glands, and a decrease in dermal blood vessels.

Several studies have clearly associated *malnutrition* with ulcers.[7] In one study, pressure ulcers were found only in severely malnourished patients.[8] Further, the stage of the ulcer correlated with the degree of low albumin levels. Malnutrition plays a greater role in the development of pressure ulcers in the elderly, whereas pressure alone plays a more significant role in the neurologically impaired patient.

The serious nature of malnutrition in pressure ulcer development is seen at the cellular level. Inadequate protein allows plasma in the capillary to move into the interstitial spaces around the cells. This shift in fluid creates edema and mechanically impairs tissue oxygenation and nutrition. Once a pressure ulcer is present, proteins can also be lost through the wound drainage. Low protein levels also prolong inflammation and delay wound healing. In addition, low and high levels of glucose impair the function of leukocytes, which remove debris from the wound. The usual patient with ulcers has low levels of serum albumin, serum protein, and hemoglobin, and low total lymphocyte counts. In addition, the patient's weight is often below ideal body weight for height. Without adequate levels of protein and hemoglobin the tissues become hypoxic.

Several minerals are also important components of wound healing and delay healing when they are inadequate. Copper, calcium, zinc, and vitamins A , B, and C are needed for collagen synthesis, generating new cells, and giving the wound strength.

The elderly patient should have a dietary history completed that examines several factors. Present weight should be compared to ideal weight for height. A recent unintentional weight loss or a weight that is less than 85% of the ideal for height is considered malnutrition. Factors that increase metabolic needs such as fever, infection, tremor, and tissue injury should be noted. Factors that increase protein losses (including draining or open wounds, effusions, and chronic blood loss) should be identified. Chronic respiratory, endocrine, cardiac, or gastrointestinal diseases deter the ability to eat, digest food, or excrete waste. Several social factors (such as the inability to procure or cook food, the need to eat alone, and lack of money) are common in the elderly. The elderly patient may also have changes in the condition of the mouth, poorly fitting dentures, or a lack of taste/smell, all of which impair adequate eating. A nutritional assessment guide has been published.[8] Malnutrition is also discussed in Chapter 2.

Incontinence has been associated with pressure ulcer development for many years. Incontinence causes maceration of the skin, increasing the risk of ulceration. Once the tissue has macerated, the skin barrier is lost and the fluid from the incontinence is absorbed by the skin, increasing the risk of bacterial growth and shear.

Clinical disorders increase the risk of pressure ulcers by impairing circulation to the extremities. Uncontrolled diabetes with hyperglycemia, especially blood glucose levels over 200 mg, impairs the ability of leukocytes (white blood cells) to function. In addition, diabetes leads to peripheral vessel occlusion and decreased circulation, which increases further the risk of ulceration and gangrene.

Fractures, contractures, or arthritic disorders impair mobility and thereby increase pressure ulcer risk. Confused, demented, or depressed patients are also at higher risk because they do not understand and/or fail to cooperate with treatment plans. Spasms place the patient at increased risk of shear forces and often limit the number of options for position changes.

Steroids decrease the rate of new cell growth, new vessel formation, and wound contraction. They also decrease the natural inflammatory response, which assists with wound healing. Vitamin A has been shown to counteract the anti-inflammatory properties of steroids and should be considered for patients who have delayed healing while taking steroids. Caution is necessary to prevent overdosage of vitamin A over time. Prolonged stress can stimulate the body's natural steroids (cortisol) to be released and delay healing.

Infection and contamination of a wound will delay its healing. Contamination delays healing when more than 10^5 (100,000) organisms per gram of tissue are found.

Data from 5,000 nursing home residents revealed several similarities in the residents who had ulcers on admission: older age, male, nonwhite, dismissed from a hospital, unable to perform own bath or transfer, being bedridden or chair-ridden, requiring catheterization, experiencing fecal incontinence, and having no rehabilitation potential.[9]

Identification of the High-Risk Patient

Prevention of pressure ulcers is a goal of all health care providers. Patients at high risk of developing pressure ulcers should be identified so that preventive actions can be taken. The primary risk factor for pressure ulcer development is immobility. Therefore, patients who cannot turn or move themselves should be systematically assessed frequently, at least once a day, for pressure ulcer development. Stage 1 and 2 ulcers can develop quickly. Other risk factors for pressure ulcers can be assessed by using an assessment tool, several of which exist. Braden's tool has been extensively tested, and appears to be the best tool for prediction of risk (see Fig. 7.2). Using this tool, scores totaling more than 16 indicate high risk for pressure ulcer development. Systematic skin assessment should be performed once a day.

INTERVENTIONS FOR THE HIGH-RISK PATIENT

Reducing Pressure

Pressure is the primary cause of pressure ulcers. Preventive measures to reduce the risk of pressure ulcers cannot be emphasized enough. Lifting and turning of immobile patients is the simplest and most common method to relieve pressure, and an every-two-hour turning schedule

BRADEN SCALE
FOR PREDICTING PRESSURE SORE RISK

Patient's Name _____   Evaluator's Name _____   Date of Assessment [   ]

SENSORY PERCEPTION ability to respond meaningfully to pressure-related discomfort	1. Completely limited: Unresponsive (does not moan, flinch, or grasp) to painful stimuli, due to diminished level of consciousness or sedation. OR limited ability to feel pain over most of body surface.	2. Very Limited: Responds only to painful stimuli. Cannot communicate discomfort except by moaning or restlessness. OR has a sensory impairment which limits the ability to feel pain or discomfort over 1/2 of body.	3. Slightly Limited: Responds to verbal commands, but cannot always communicate discomfort or need to be turned. OR has some sensory impairment which limits ability to feel pain or discomfort in 1 or 2 extremities.	4. No Impairment: Responds to verbal commands. Has no sensory deficit which would limit ability to feel or voice pain or discomfort.	
MOISTURE degree to which skin is exposed to moisture	1. Constantly Moist: Skin is kept moist almost constantly by perspiration, urine, etc. Dampness is detected every time patient is moved or turned.	2. Very Moist: Skin is often, but not always moist. Linen must be changed at least once a shift.	3. Occasionally Moist: Skin is occasionally moist, requiring an extra linen change approximately once a day.	4. Rarely Moist: Skin is usually dry, linen only requires changing at routine intervals.	
ACTIVITY degree of physical activity	1. Bedfast: Confined to bed	2. Chairfast: Ability to walk severely limited or non-existent. Cannot bear own weight and/or must be assisted into chair or wheelchair.	3. Walks Occasionally: Walks occasionally during day, but for very short distances, with or without assistance. Spends majority of each shift in bed or chair.	4. Walks Frequently: walks outside the room at least twice a day and inside room at least once every 2 hours during waking hours.	
MOBILITY ability to change and control body position	1. Completely Immobile: Does not make even slight changes in body or extremity position without assistance.	2. Very Limited: Makes occasional slight changes in body or extremity position but unable to make frequent or significant changes independently.	3. Slightly Limited: Makes frequent though slight changes in body or extremity position independently.	4. No Limitations: Makes major and frequent changes in position without assistance.	
NUTRITION usual food intake pattern	1. Very Poor: Never eats a complete meal. Rarely eats more than 1/3 of any food offered. Eats 2 servings or less of protein (meat or dairy products) per day. Takes fluids poorly. Does not take a liquid dietary supplement. OR is NPO and/or maintained on clear liquids or IV's for more than 5 days.	2. Probably Inadequate: Rarely eats a complete meal and generally eats only about 1/2 of any food offered. Protein intake includes only 3 servings of meat or dairy products per day. Occasionally will take a dietary supplement. OR receives less than optimum amount of liquid diet or tube feeding.	3. Adequate: Eats over half of most meals. Eats a total of 4 servings of protein (meat, dairy products) each day. Occasionally will refuse a meal, but will usually take a supplement if offered. OR is on a tube feeding or TPN regimen which probably meets most of nutritional needs.	4. Excellent: Eats most of every meal. Never refuses a meal. Usually eats a total of 4 or more servings of meat and dairy products. Occasionally eats between meals. Does not require supplementation.	
FRICTION AND SHEAR	1. Problem: Requires moderate to maximum assistance in moving. Complete lifting without sliding against sheets is impossible. Frequently slides down in bed or chair, requiring frequent repositioning with maximum assistance. Spasticity, contractures or agitation leads to almost constant friction.	2. Potential Problem: Moves feebly or requires minimum assistance. During a move skin probably slides to some extent against sheets, chair, restraints, or other devices. Maintains relatively good position in chair or bed most of the time but occasionally slides down.	3. No Apparent Problem: Moves in bed and in chair independently and has sufficient muscle strength to lift up completely during move. Maintains good position in bed or chair at all times.		

© Copyright Barbara Braden and Nancy Bergstrom, 1988

CON-63 (12/88)

Total Score [   ]

Figure 7.2 *Braden Scale for predicting pressure sore risk (copyright B. Braden and N. Bergstrom, used with permission).*

has become a common part of nursing care. For many patients a position change every two hours is adequate, but the time frame is not absolute. Each patient's tolerance for lying in one position for two hours must be assessed, and a turning schedule developed for that patient. If the patient is found to have reddened areas after two hours, more frequent turning or additional protection is needed. The problem, of course, is maintaining a frequent turning schedule around the clock.

There are several devices on the market for pressure relief that should not be used as adjuncts to frequent turning. The ideal mattress is one that relieves pressure and provides comfort. Eggcrate mattresses are not pressure-reduction devices and should never be used for this reason. Eggcrates can provide some comfort. The device used for any given patient must be chosen based upon its ability to reduce capillary pressure below 32 mm Hg. A 1992 study[10] found that several pressure-reducing devices produce significantly lower heel and trochanter pressures than a standard mattress. The researchers caution, though, that the patient's height and weight must be considered before choosing a pressure-relief device. Prior to changing to another pressure-relief device for the high-risk residents of nursing homes, the ease of using the device and evidence that the device can reduce pressure in the debilitated elderly (some devices have been studied on well, ambulatory people) need to be determined.[11]

The heel is especially prone to pressure because of the small surface area and lack of padding. The heels should be suspended from the mattress by placing small pillows under the entire calf of the leg. The knee should not be flexed with a pillow. Sponge rings (donuts) should not be used to elevate the heel. These devices are known to cause venous congestion and edema, and they are more likely to cause pressure ulcers than prevent them.

Chair-bound patients are at risk of pressure ulcers on the ischial tuberosities. The patient should be taught to shift weight by doing chair push-ups every 15 minutes or should be moved slightly in the chair every hour by the staff. Pressure-reducing devices should be used for chair-ridden patients; examples are foam, gel, air, or a combination. Donuts should again be avoided. Postural alignment, weight distribution, balance, stability, and ability to perform self-care should also be considered when choosing a pressure-relief device for a wheelchair-bound patient.

Bedfast patients should be positioned with pillows or foam wedges to keep the bony prominences from direct contact. When the patient is turned on the side, avoid a position directly on the trochanter. A detailed plan of care including the turning schedule should be developed on these high-risk patients and followed around the clock.

Range of motion (ROM) exercises should be performed every eight hours on all extremities. Active ROM is preferred because it maintains some muscle strength. If the patient cannot perform active ROM, passive ROM assists in maintaining muscle stretch and joint motion.

Massage over bony prominences has been used for decades to stimulate circulation to the skin. Scientific evidence that massage could stimulate blood and lymph flow has never been established. More important, preliminary new evidence reveals that massage may be harmful to deep tissues, tearing them apart from nearby layers.[12,13]

Reducing Shear and Friction

To reduce shear, the head of the bed should be maintained at the lowest degree of elevation allowed by the patient's medical condition. To reduce friction, the patient should be lifted with a turning or lifting sheet rather than dragged by the shoulders toward the head of the bed. In addition, friction can be reduced by the use of lubricants, such as creams, protective films, protective dressings, and protective padding.

Improving Nutrition

Because of prospective payment systems, the federal government is most concerned about prevention and treatment of malnutrition in nursing home residents. Unfortunately, the ability of caregivers to feed patients against their will is severely limited. Even when patients are known to be malnourished, third-party payment systems seldom pay for feeding pumps to correct malnutrition. Sadly, under federal regulations nursing home residents with ulcers cannot be transferred to a hospital unless they are septic. This is interpreted as having a fever and a white blood cell count over 15,000. Sepsis is often compounded by malnutrition and failure to initiate and maintain an adequate immune response. At this stage of progression, the ulcers and malnutrition are so far advanced that healing is nearly impossible. The ideal is probably not possible with tightening health care dollars, so health care providers are being called on to be creative, identify patients at risk early, and promote nutrition on an ongoing basis for all patients.[14,15]

High-calorie diets are not enough. Protein must be restored. The average diet should contain 0.8 gm of protein per kg of body weight. When patients are stressed from surgery, illnesses or attempting to heal a wound they need 1.0 gm of protein per kg. Patients should also eat 1500 to 3500 Cal per day, depending upon level of activity. In one study healing began three to four days after a positive protein balance (anabolism) was reached.[7]

MANAGEMENT OF PATIENTS WITH ULCERS

Team Evaluation

The most logical first step when initiating management is to assess the patient as an individual based on a thorough history and comprehensive physical examination. The wound is not just a wound but a wound in the context of a unique patient. The etiology and complicating factors should be defined. The intrinsic and extrinsic factors should be assessed, and thought should be given to using these factors as a guide to maximize healing potential. There has been a tendency to try to distill wound healing into a "cookbook" or algorithm to cover all patients. Algorithms may be food for thought, but they are not a substitute for problem solving in the individual patient.

Difficult or complicated patients are best dealt with using a team approach. Using the initial evaluation and healing factors as a guide, appropriate members of the team are called to see the patient. A conference among team members results in a wound healing plan or options that can be discussed with the patient and primary physician. Once agreement is reached, the plan is instituted. Depending on progress (or lack of progress), the team may need to reassess the situation and plan. The important point is to get the experts involved in the beginning so that valuable time and resources are not wasted in the scenario of calling in a new expert every three or four days when progress stalls.

Members of the team are a plastic surgeon, a wound nurse specialist, an infectious disease specialist, a vascular and general surgeon, an endocrinologist (including a diabetes nurse specialist/educator), a hyperbaric oxygen specialist/pulmonologist, an orthopedic surgeon, a nurse for education and reinforcement, a dietician, a physical therapist, an occupational therapist, orthotics, social service, and a home health care nurse. Not all members of the team are necessary for most cases. There is no significance to the order of the members mentioned.

Medical Management

Systemic antibiotics are not usually advised for colonized ulcers unless the patient has sepsis, osteomyelitis, or cellulitis. However, antibiotics may be indicated when organisms (quantitative cultures) are in numbers greater than 10^5 per gram of tissue. Antibiotics do not reach the organisms because the organisms exist in the eschar, which is avascular. *Eschar* is nonviable tissue that increases the risk of infection. Topical antibiotics can be used in wound packing. The goal is to correct the causative factors and maximize the intrinsic and extrinsic healing factors. The choice of wound dressing is important. Ideally, the dressing is chosen to facilitate fibroblasts and epithelium. However, dressings must also control infection, as bacteria will also destroy not only healing tissue but the ulcer bed as well.

Operative Management

When the surgeon assesses a pressure ulcer (or any other defect for that matter) the assessment follows a very logical pattern. The pertinent questions are:

What tissue is missing (skin, skin + subcutaneous fatty tissue, etc.)?

What tissue is needed for satisfactory reconstruction (function and appearance)?

What tissue is available?

What factors can be changed to optimize chances for healing?

What is the risk for the patient (including the risk of no surgical treatment)?

To determine what tissue is missing, the wound must be clean and debrided of devitalized tissue. There is no way to determine the extent of tissue missing in a wound with eschar. Sinus tracts and undermined areas also have to be investigated and sometimes unroofed.

Depending on the situation, all missing tissue may not need to be replaced. A pressure ulcer eroding into an underlying bony prominence may destroy some bone. The bone does not need to be replaced; in fact, it may be advisable to excise more of the bony prominence. When planning reconstruction, plastic surgeons mentally use a "reconstructive ladder" that progresses from simple to more complex solutions:

1. Primary suture closure
2. Skin graft
3. Adjacent (pedicle) flap
4. Muscle or musculocutaneous flap
5. Free flap

Primary Suture Closure

A very small ulcer can sometimes be successfully dealt with by simply excising it and closing it primarily with sutures.

Skin Graft

The next most simple method of achieving a healed wound is skin graft. The outer layer of skin is "shaved off," leaving the donor site to heal from the deeper remaining layer of skin. This split thickness skin graft is placed over the ulcer and heals as blood vessels grow from the bed into the graft. A skin graft requires less blood supply to heal than any other method. It is usually a very satisfactory way to deal with lower leg and foot ulcers. However, it is difficult for skin grafts to heal when placed directly on open bone. They will not provide adequate padding for sitting or lying for sacral or ischial or trochanter ulcers if subcutaneous tissue is missing. Skin grafts require a period of four to seven days or longer of immobilizing the recipient site area, so strict bed rest is usually ordered when grafts are placed on the pelvis or lower extremities.

Adjacent (Pedicle) Flap

Ulcers in the pelvic weight-bearing regions usually require a flap closure. In the past pedicle flaps of skin and subcutaneous tissue were shifted or rotated from nearby nonulcerated skin to close these ulcers. However, the survival of these flaps depended on the random blood supply in the flap's pedicle. With the random pattern, there frequently was not enough blood flowing into the flap to heal the skin at the edge of the flap farthest away from the pedi-

cle; unfortunately, this is usually the area of the flap used to close the ulcer.

Muscle or Musculocutaneous Flap

A technique for flaps that provided a more reliable blood supply was essential. Muscle and musculocutaneous flaps were then discovered. The blood supply for these flaps is based on the larger arteries that supply the muscle. Blood vessels in many muscles have branches that perforate the muscle and supply overlying skin. The skin and subcutaneous tissue over these muscles will survive nicely if moved

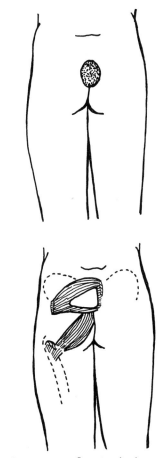

Figure 7.3 *A myocutaneous flap using the gluteus maximus muscle to surgically repair a sacral ulcer.*

with the underlying muscle (musculo- or myocutaneous flap, see Fig. 7.3). The advantage of this type of flap in pressure ulcers in the pelvic area is that bulky subcutaneous tissue (and muscle) with overlying skin can be moved with a known arterial blood supply rather than a random subdermal plexus. Muscles have abundant blood vessels (for energy), which help bring red blood cells, white blood cells, antibodies, and antibiotics to the wound to speed healing. This is especially helpful if there is relatively avascular bone in the base of the wound. However, the surgeon must chose muscles carefully so that functions performed by the muscle are taken over by other muscles. Pressure, stretching, and shearing forces must be kept to a minimum during the healing phase to avoid damage to the flap before it has healed firmly in its bed.

Free Flap

Free flaps are essentially muscle-type flaps that have had their artery and vein "disconnected" at the donor site and then "reconnected" under the microscope to vessels at the recipient site. They have the same advantages as muscle flaps but are more complicated surgically, require more operative time, and introduce another element of uncertainty into healing (the blood vessel anastomoses).

Musculocutaneous flaps are usually the surgical procedures of choice for pressure ulcers in the pelvic area, and usually it is advisable to remove or "shave down" any underlying bony prominence that focused the pressure in the first place (e.g., ischial tuberosity, trochanter). As one can imagine, rotating muscles is rather a significant operation, frequently requiring blood transfusion and always requiring immobilization in special reduced-pressure beds postoperatively for two weeks or longer. Therefore, the surgeon carefully assesses the risks of the procedure for each particular patient. In many debilitated or elderly patients the risks of this major procedure are unacceptably high compared to the risk of the ulcer slowly healing in without surgery. Leaving an ulcer to heal in without surgery is not risk-free, however, as many people die yearly from infections starting in pressure ulcers, so decisions have to be carefully weighed for each individual patient.

Skin grafts are usually the procedures of choice for ulcers distal to the mid-calf, as blood vessels to muscles are more unreliable in this area. Skin grafts require immobilization of the recipient area, which usually means strict bed rest. If

venous stasis or edema is associated with the ulcer, it may be a week or two before the skin graft will tolerate swelling associated with having the leg or foot down (sitting, standing, walking).

If reconstructive surgery is decided upon, wound care tactics frequently need to be changed. Dressings need to be modified from those designed to facilitate epithelium to ones designed to debride the surface and promote granulation tissue. Granulation tissue is composed of capillary buds, increasing blood supply and resistance to infection. The ulcer is usually completely excised surgically, as epithelium just gets in the way. Therefore, the dressing regime is frequently changed from moist dressings to wet-to-dry debriding dressings preoperatively. Patient mobility is encouraged preoperatively, recognizing the period of forced immobility postoperatively. Bowel preparations, minimum residue diets, and stool softeners are instituted to minimize postoperative fecal contamination. Nutrition must be assessed and maintained for healing after these large operations. Intrinsic and extrinsic factors have to be reassessed and maximized for healing. Hyperbaric oxygen is often helpful, depending on the degree of tissue hypoxia measured in the area of the ulcer and the extent to which hyperbaric oxygen treatment can increase measured tissue oxygen.

There are several important factors to remember when surgical treatment is undertaken:

1. Surgical procedures for pressure ulcers are frequently significant undertakings involving risks in debilitated patients, including the risks associated with bed rest and postoperative immobility.
2. Surgical procedures seldom correct the underlying problem(s) that led to the ulcer, and further rehabilitation directed to the problem(s) will be necessary or the ulcer will recur.
3. There is the risk of "winning the battle" with the ulcer and "losing the war" with the total patient, especially in debilitated patients.
4. The most successful results are obtained when members of the Wound Care Team coordinate efforts to optimize intrinsic and extrinsic factors for healing.

In the properly selected patient and circumstance, surgical reconstruction will result in superior healing with superior tissue in much shorter time than allowing the wound to heal in secondarily. Tissue integrity and barrier to infection will be restored much more quickly. However, it is important that the relative risks are appropriate. After healing is complete, special attention must be paid to correcting the factors that resulted in the ulcer forming in the first place.

Nursing Management of Patients with Ulcers

Nursing management of the patient with an ulcer begins with the realization that areas that do not blanch when pressure is removed are stage 1 ulcers. These red areas indicate that tissue damage is present in the dermis and epidermis.

Assessment

Assessment of a wound includes an accurate description of the wound's size and depth. The presence of sinus tracts (channels off of the sides of the wound) should be noted. Photographs may provide some of the best descriptors of wound size and extent. The color of the wound indicates its degree of healing or extent of infection. A red wound is usually filled with granulation tissue and fragile capillaries. A yellow wound is one that is covered with a soft yellow or ivory eschar. A black wound is also covered with eschar that is black or brown. The type of drainage and presence of infection should be documented.

Management

One of the simplest methods for wound care is based upon the color of the wound.[16]

A *red* wound is healing and needs protection. It needs to be kept moist and should never be treated with heat lamps, alcohol, or Maalox. These treatments should be abandoned completely, as they do more harm than good. Red wounds should not be treated with lotions, ointments, salves, or soaps because these materials may irritate the wound and delay healing.

If the wound is red and shallow, it can be covered with occlusive dressings or a thin layer of antibiotic ointment and a nonadhesive dressing. If the wound is deep, it should be kept moist with saline-soaked gauze. This type of dressing is called a moist-to-damp dressing, as it is not allowed to dry. It is important to use only gauze and avoid dressings made with cotton filling on open wounds. The cotton in these dressings sticks to the open wound. Dressings should be cut to the approximate size of the wound. Avoid putting

wet dressings on the skin surrounding the wound because it will macerate. Moisture barrier creams or sprays should be applied to the surrounding skin before using the wet-to-damp dressings. The dressing should be changed every three, four, or six hours depending upon the moisture in the wound.

A *yellow* wound needs cleaning (debridement). Debridement can be accomplished with whirlpool baths to soften the eschar, wet-to-dry dressings, or enzymatic agents. Surgery may also be required to remove eschar.

Damp gauze dressings are applied to the wound bed (not the surrounding skin) and allowed to dry and adhere to the eschar, using a wet-to-dry dressing technique. Dry dressings are removed and take with them pieces of the eschar that have adhered to the dressings. Dressing removal can be painful, and the patient should be given analgesics as needed.

Various solutions are often applied to a wound for debridement. Solutions such as bacitracin, neomycin, and

Table 7.1   *Use of Dressings for Various Ulcers*

ULCER DRAINAGE	PREFERRED DRESSING
Superficial, little drainage	Transparent
	These dressings should not be used on infected wounds and have no absorptive capacity.
Low drainage	Hydrogel
	Dressings are not transparent; they provide soothing coolness.
Moderate drainage	Hydrocolloid
	Dressings are not transparent and can melt down onto normal tissues.
Large drainage	Alginates
	These require a secondary dressing for cover; normal skin needs to be protected from maceration.

COMMENTS:

Date __/__/__

Vitals: B/P:____ Temp:____ R:____ P:____

Wound #/Location:_____
Measurement: L___c.m. W___c.m. D____c.m.
Drainage: Y N Color:_____
Amount: SM MO LG   Odor:Y N_____

Wound Bed
Moist: Y N
Color: Pale Pink Red Bluish Black Yellow
Areas of necrosis present: Y N
Is wound painful? Y N   Sharp Dull Burning Other_____
Photographs done: Y N Focus distance:_____inches

Treatment Plan:_____
_____
_____
_____

COMMENTS:

Wound #/Location:_____
Measurement: L___c.m. W____c.m. D____c.m.
Drainage: Y N   Color:____
Amount SM MO LG Odor: Y N_____

Wound Bed
Moist: Y N
Color: Pale Pink Red Bluish Black Yellow
Areas of necrosis present: Y N
Is wound painful? Y N Sharp Dull Burning Other_____

Photographs done: Y N Focus distance:_____inches

Treatment Plan:_____
_____
_____
_____

Date __/__/__

Vitals: B/P:____ Temp:____ R:____ P:____

Wound #/Location:_____
Measurement: L___c.m. W___c.m. D____c.m.
Drainage: Y N Color:_____
Amount: SM MO LG   Odor:Y N_____

Wound Bed
Moist: Y N
Color: Pale Pink Red Bluish Black Yellow
Areas of necrosis present: Y N
Is wound painful? Y N   Sharp Dull Burning Other_____
Photographs done: Y N Focus distance:_____inches

Treatment Plan:_____
_____
_____
_____

COMMENTS:

Wound #/Location:_____
Measurement: L___c.m. W____c.m. D____c.m.
Drainage: Y N   Color:____
Amount SM MO LG Odor:Y N_____

Wound Bed
Moist: Y N
Color: Pale Pink Red Bluish Black Yellow
Areas of necrosis present: Y N
Is wound painful? Y N Sharp Dull Burning Other_____
Photographs done: Y N Focus distance:_____inches

Treatment Plan:_____
_____
_____
_____

Date__/__/__

Vitals: B/P:____ Temp:____ R:____ P:____

Wound #/Location:_____
Measurement: L___c.m. W___c.m. D____c.m.
Drainage: Y N Color:_____
Amount: SM MO LG   Odor:Y N_____

Wound Bed
Moist: Y N
Color: Pale Pink Red Bluish Black Yellow
Areas of necrosis present: Y N
Is wound painful? Y N   Sharp Dull Burning Other_____
Photographs done: Y N Focus distance:_____inches

Treatment Plan:_____
_____
_____
_____

COMMENTS:

Wound #/Location:_____
Measurement: L___c.m. W____c.m. D____c.m.
Drainage: Y N   Color:____
Amount SM MO LG Odor:Y N_____

Wound Bed
Moist: Y N
Color: Pale Pink Red Bluish Black Yellow
Areas of necrosis present: Y N
Is wound painful? Y N Sharp Dull Burning Other_____
Photographs done: Y N Focus distance:_____inches

Treatment Plan:_____
_____
_____
_____

Figure 7.4   *Pressure ulcer flow sheet*

kanamycin are not toxic to fibroblasts, even when used full strength. In sharp contrast are solutions such as povidone-iodine, acetic acid, hydrogen peroxide, and chlorhexidine, which are damaging to healing tissues. These solutions are often used to control infection, but they are indiscriminately damaging to tissues, increasing the extent of the wound, killing normal cells, and delaying healing. Rarely is their use warranted.

A *black* wound is filled with leathery eschar and needs debridement because the risk of infection increases in proportion to the amount of eschar present. Surgical debridement is the method of choice. For the patient who cannot withstand surgery, enzymatic debriding agents can be used. These agents burn and should only be used to debride a two-inch-square area of tissue at one time. They will remove the black eschar and leave a yellow one, so the remaining wound still needs further work. Antibiotics alone will not control infection in these ulcers. Neither systemic nor topical antibiotics reach the wound, as they cannot penetrate the avascular eschar.

Dressings

The use of dressings in management of pressure ulcers is a continuing controversy. More and more products appear on the market; it is hard to tell them apart and difficult to know how to use them correctly.

Before applying a dressing, make sure that the wound is clean and dry. Use a skin protectant around the wound to protect the normal, intact skin. Adherent dressings can only be used when there is intact skin to apply them to. When applying hydrocolloids or hydrogels, place your hand over the dressing for one minute after applying. The heat significantly increases the adhesion of the dressing.

To remove dressings, gently push the skin away from the dressing instead of pulling the dressing off of the skin. The dressing may need to be soaked off. Table 7.1 describes the types of wounds commonly seen and the preferred dressings for their treatment.

Documentation

Documentation about the patient's risk for pressure ulcers should be done by using a pressure ulcer flow sheet (see Fig. 7.4). The staff assessing the patient must be consistent and trained in the interpretation of the sections of the form. Once a plan of care is developed, it must be recorded clearly and provide methods for consistent care and ongoing evaluation of the treatment plan based upon the patient's response.

Trends in Research

The future of pressure ulcer assessment, risk reduction, and management is bright. With the increasing age of the American public, more and more research dollars are being funded into study of pressure ulcers. Great advances in the care of these ulcers have been made over the past decade and continue to be made today.

Research is being conducted on the role of electrical stimulation, hyperbaric oxygen, growth factors, and the use of epithelium grown in the laboratory. Other advances are being made in the development of products to reduce risk and treat existing ulcers. These advances will certainly change the management of patients in the future.

REFERENCES

1. Parish LC, Witkowski JS, Crissey JT: *The Decubitus Ulcer.* New York, Masson, 1983.

2. Petersen NC, Bittmann S: The epidemiology of pressure ulcers. *Scand J Plastic Surg* 1971;5:65–66.

3. Young L: Pressure ulcer prevalence and associated patient characteristics in one long-term care facility. *Decubitus* 1989;2:52.

4. Meehan M: Multisite pressure ulcer prevalence survey. *Decubitus* 1990;3:14–17.

5. Bryan CS, Dew CE, Reynolds KL: Bacteremia associated with decubitus ulcers. *Arch Intern Med* 1983;143:2093–2095.

6. Dinsdale SM: Decubitus ulcers: Role of pressure and friction in causation. *Arch Phys Med Rehab* 1974;55:147–152.

7. Breslow R: Nutritional status and dietary intake of patients with pressure ulcers: Review of research literature 1943 to 1989. *Decubitus* 1991;4:16–21.

8. Pinchcofsky GD, Kaminski MV: Increasing malnutrition

during hospitalization: Documentation by a nutritional screening program. *J Am Coll Nutr* 1985;4:471–479.

9. Spector WD, Kapp MC, Tucker RJ: Factors associated with the presence of decubitus ulcers at admission to nursing homes. *Gerontologist* 1988;28:830–834.

10. Thompson-Bishop JY, Mottola CM: Tissue interface pressure and estimated subcutaneous pressure of 11 different pressure-reducing support surfaces. *Decubitus* 1992;5:42–48.

11. Lazzara DL, Buschmann MT: Prevention of pressure ulcers in elderly nursing home residents: Are special support surfaces the answer? *Decubitus* 1991;4:42–48.

12. Dyson R: Bed sores—The injuries hospital staff inflict on patients. *Nurs Mirror* 1978;146:30–32.

13. Olson B: Effects of massage for prevention of pressure ulcers. *Decubitus* 1989;2:3237.

14. Kaminski MV, Pinchcofsky-Devin G: Nutritional management of decubitus ulcers in the elderly. *Decubitus* 1989;2:20–30.

15. Bobel LM: Nutritional implications in the patient with pressure sores. *Nurs Clin North Am* 1987;22:379–390.

16. Cuzzell J: The RYB color code. *Am J Nurs* 1988;88:1342–1346.

CHAPTER

GASTROINTESTINAL INFECTIONS

Jane S. Roccaforte

OVERVIEW

Gastroenteritis is an important but relatively uncommon cause of nosocomial infection in the long-term care facility (LTCF).[1] In prevalence studies conducted in Wisconsin, Utah, and Maryland, gastroenteritis ranks well behind better known entities such as infected pressure ulcers, urinary tract infections, and respiratory tract infections.[2–4] Better recognition of the problem of gastroenteritis in the elderly is exemplified by a large national database study that quantified age specific indicators of hospitalization and death involving gastroenteritis. Of all age groups hospitalized with gastroenteritis, the elderly were at greatest risk for death.[5] The authors estimated the annual mortality rate in the United States for elderly with fatal gastroenteritis to be four to six times that of children.

Increasing attention has been focused on gastroenteritis in LTCFs in recent years, and more information regarding the epidemiology, diagnosis, and treatment of diarrhea and gastroenteritis in the elderly is published.[6–8] Gastroenteritis outbreaks in the LTCF are a major concern because of the high frequency of fecal incontinence in that setting.

Gastrointestinal Immunity

Large numbers of organisms enter the gastrointestinal tract by way of the mouth, but most are killed by gastric acid. The normal bacterial flora of the intestine is protective: It competes with potential invaders for space and nutrients. Once an infection develops, diarrhea serves as a protective mechanism by increasing clearance of pathogens or toxins. Achlorhydria, gastric surgery, H2 antagonists, and antacids lower gastric acidity and thereby predispose to bacterial and parasitic infections of the gut. Disturbance of normal gut flora by antibiotics lowers the dose of *Salmonella* needed to cause infection. Opiates and anticholinergics decrease intestinal motility and may increase the severity of infectious gastroenteritis.

Classification

The agents causing infectious diarrhea in the LTCF may be classified epidemiologically or pathologically. Epidemiologically, infectious agents causing diarrhea have a *reservoir* that is either humans or food/water. Organisms in the latter category are often pathogens of animals spread to humans by ingestion of contaminated food, whereas organisms carried by people are spread from person to person by the fecal-oral route (see Table 8.1). *Staphylococcus aureus* resides in humans but is spread by contaminated food.

Outbreaks of food poisoning (epidemic *common-vehicle* gastroenteritis related to food or water contamination) are quite common in the LTCF setting. Alternatively, epidemics of gastroenteritis in the LTCF may be spread

Table 8.1   *Epidemiologic Classification of Gastrointestinal Pathogens*

RESERVOIR = MAN	RESERVOIR = FOOD/WATER
Salmonella typhi	Nontyphoid *Salmonella**
Viral gastroenteritis*	*Clostridium perfringens**
*Shigella**	*Clostridium botulinum*
*Staphylococcus aureus**	*Yersinia enterocolitica*
Amoebae	*Campylobacter*
*Escherichia coli**	*Bacillus cereus*
Giardia	

*Common pathogen in the LTCF

from *person to person* by the fecal-oral route (see Chapter 11). In a survey conducted by the Centers for Disease Control and Prevention (CDC), 115 outbreaks of foodborne disease were reported in LTCFs throughout the United States, representing 2% of all foodborne outbreaks and 19% of outbreak-associated deaths from 1975 to 1987.[9] Of note, a pathogen was found in fewer than half of these outbreaks. *Salmonella* was the leading cause of confirmed foodborne outbreaks in the United States, accounting for about 50% of such outbreaks and 80% of deaths. Other common causes of foodborne outbreaks are *Staphylococcus aureus*, *Clostridium perfringens*, *C. botulinum*, and *Shigella*.

Table 8.2   *Pathologic Classification of Gastrointestinal Pathogens*

INVASIVE ORGANISMS	TOXIN-PRODUCING ORGANISMS
Shigella	*Clostridium perfringens*
Salmonella	*Staphylococcus aureus*
Amoebae	*Escherichia coli* 0157:H7
Giardia	*Vibrio cholerae*
Yersinia enterocolitica	*Bacillus cereus*
Campylobacter jejuni	*Clostridium botulinum*

Outbreaks may be traced to a variety of foods that serve as the common source. Factors that contribute to outbreaks include improper holding temperatures for food, inadequate cooking of food, contaminated equipment, and poor personal hygiene of food preparers.

Pathologic organisms can be conveniently classified into two groups: those that produce disease by *invasion* of the intestine and those that produce disease by means of a *toxin* (see Table 8.2). In general, invasive pathogens cause fever and frequent small stools containing mucus and blood. The incubation period is 12 to 72 hours. Toxin-mediated diseases have shorter incubation periods; nausea, vomiting, and diarrhea develop 1 to 36 hours after ingestion. For the most part, stool cultures are of no value in the diagnosis of toxin-related diarrhea. Diagnosis depends on history and culture of the suspected food.

SPECIFIC AGENTS OF GASTROENTERITIS

Toxin-Mediated Gastroenteritis

Staphylococcus aureus and *Clostridium perfringens* are the leading causes of toxin-mediated foodborne outbreaks. Precooked foods, particularly baked goods, may become contaminated with *S. aureus*. A food handler colonized or infected with *S. aureus* in the nares or in skin lesions may contaminate these food items. Staphylococcal enterotoxin is acid-stable. Nausea and vomiting begin one to six hours after ingestion. *C. perfringens* has an incubation period of 10 to 24 hours and is often associated with ingestion of gravy or beef products; 3% of *C. perfringens* outbreaks occur in LTCFs.[10]

C. perfringens and *S. aureus* cause outbreaks of toxin-mediated gastroenteritis in the LTCF or hospital setting.[11] In institutional outbreaks, most episodes were traced to preheated meat and poultry dishes that had been cooked one day earlier and inadequately cooked or stored before serving the following day. The incriminated foods were stews, pies, meats, and chicken dishes. Toxin-mediated gastroenteritis due to *S. aureus* and *C. perfringens* is self-limited, and antibiotic therapy is not helpful.

Bacillus cereus can also cause toxin-mediated gastroenteritis. It has two enterotoxins, each of which causes a distinct symptom complex. "Early incubation" *B. cereus* has an incubation period of one to six hours, and vomiting is prominent. Fried rice has been implicated as a commonsource vehicle in outbreak situations.[12] The second syndrome caused by this organism occurs 10 to 12 hours following ingestion of contaminated meats, sauces, and soups. Diarrhea is the foremost symptom.

Invasive Organisms

Salmonella Infections

Typhoid fever, the best-known type of *Salmonella* infection, is rare in the United States compared to other strains of nontyphoid *Salmonella*. Even a single case of typhoid fever in a LTCF should be viewed with great concern and prompt a search for a human carrier.

Nontyphoid salmonellosis may occur with a variety of different strains and is known to be a very important problem in LTCFs. The leading serotypes of nontyphoid *Salmonella* isolated from humans in the United States are *Salmonella typhimurium*, *S. enteritidis*, *S. newport*, and *S. heidelberg*. Salmonellosis tends to be unusually severe in LTCFs, where the mortality for outbreaks can be as high as 11%.[9] Most outbreaks in LTCFs are common-source outbreaks associated with contaminated food, where an explosive cluster of cases is seen 12 to 48 hours after exposure. Epidemics may be continued or propagated by a secondary person-to-person or hand-to-mouth contact. The most common vehicles are poultry and egg products.

Residents with salmonellosis manifest fever, abdominal pain, and diarrhea. Bacteremia, common with *Salmonella typhi*, is an unusual complication in nontyphoid salmonellosis. The diagnosis is made by stool culture. Antibiotic therapy is generally not necessary for nontyphoid *Salmonella*, and antibiotics may actually prolong fecal excretion of the organism. Enteric precautions should be employed for all infected individuals. This means a private room if the resident is incontinent or a regular room if the resident is continent of stool, with good handwashing and wearing of gloves by persons having direct contact with the resident or articles contaminated with fecal material. In large outbreaks, it

may be necessary to cohort infected residents. Good food-handling practices should be followed, with periodic review of principles of hygiene for dietary employees. Outbreaks may involve both residents and staff; an example of a *Salmonella* outbreak is presented in Chapter 11.

Shigella Infections

Like salmonellosis, shigellosis presents with fever, cramping, abdominal pain, and diarrhea. This invasive organism is the cause of bacillary dysentery, and stools contain blood, mucus, and white blood cells. The incubation period is 36 to 72 hours. Occasionally, severe and bloody diarrhea may be seen. Infection can occur after ingestion of as few as ten organisms, and the severity of illness correlates with the underlying condition of the host. The diagnosis is made by stool culture or rectal swab.

Although *Shigella* generally causes outbreaks by person-to-person transmission, occasional common-source outbreaks of foodborne illness may be seen. When these outbreaks occur, they can almost always be traced to contamination of food by an infected food handler. Antibiotics are indicated for residents with *Shigella* infection, and enteric precautions must be enforced to prevent further spread of the organism.

Yersinia Infections

Yersiniosis is usually caused by *Y. enterocolitica*. This organism causes a wide variety of manifestations, including fever, headache, vomiting, watery diarrhea, and enterocolitis. It has animal reservoirs, and many cases are related to ingestion of undercooked pork. Epidemics have occurred because of contaminated chocolate milk and tofu.[13] The fecal-oral route is the usual mode of transmission, and the incubation period is four to eight days. Diagnosis is made by stool culture. Antibiotic therapy is required for the septicemic form of this disease.

Campylobacter Infections

C. jejuni causes diarrhea in the community, with cattle and poultry serving as reservoirs. Contact with animals or ingestion of contaminated food, water, or unpasteurized milk are the most common modes of transmission. After an incubation period of three to five days, a diarrheal illness of variable severity occurs. Diagnosis is made by stool culture or dark field microscopy. The need for antimicrobial treatment is unclear, but fluid and electrolyte replacement is indicated for severe disease.

Parasitic Gastroenteritis

Amebiasis

Amebiasis is caused by the intestinal protozoan, *Entamoeba histolytica*, which exists in the trophozoite and cyst forms. Ingestion of contaminated food and water as well as person-to-person spread occur, and asymptomatic cyst carriers serve as reservoirs. Manifestations of infection range from mild diarrhea with abdominal pain to bloody diarrhea with toxicity (amebic dysentery). The diagnosis is made by finding *Entamoeba histolytica* trophozoites or cysts in the stool. Institutional outbreaks of amebiasis have been reported in the United States.[14]

Giardiasis

Giardia lamblia is a parasite principally of the upper small intestine. It causes mild diarrhea, abdominal cramps, and bloating. Malabsorption, fatigue, and weight loss may occur. The asymptomatic carrier is important in the spread of this organism. This disease is also diagnosed by stool examination, although examination of duodenal fluid may be necessary in situations of strong clinical suspicion and negative stool studies.

G. lamblia has caused community-wide waterborne and foodborne outbreaks.[15] Person-to-person transmission occurs, especially in institutions. The first reported outbreak in an LTCF had multiple modes of transmission.[16] Children in an affiliated day care center were implicated in the spread of this disease to their "adopted grandparents" in the LTCF.

Both *E. histolytica* and *G. lamblia* require antibiotic therapy of infected residents, and both require enteric precautions to prevent spread of the infection, especially to those who have direct contact with feces.

Viral Gastroenteritis

Viral gastroenteritis is a very common, usually self-limited infectious disease that causes diarrhea and occasionally low-grade fever. Norwalk virus, rotavirus, and enteroviruses are the usual causes of viral gastroenteritis.

Norwalk virus has been implicated in about one third of nonbacterial gastroenteritis outbreaks in the community and has also caused a number of LTCF outbreaks.[17–20] The incubation period is one to two days, and transmission is most likely via the fecal-oral route. In one severe outbreak in a LTCF in Los Angeles County, the attack rate was 55% among residents and 25% among employees.[20]

Rotavirus causes gastroenteritis in children as well as adults. It can be a major seasonal nosocomial pathogen, occurring in the cooler months. The incubation period is approximately 48 hours, and the mode of transmission is fecal-oral. Symptoms include fever and vomiting as well as watery diarrhea. Rotavirus infections are also generally mild, although they may be more severe in the elderly population.[21,22] In LTCFs, outbreaks have been reported with mortality rates ranging from zero to 10%.[21,23,24] Astroviruses and the Snow Mountain agent virus have also caused outbreaks of gastroenteritis in LTCFs.[22,25]

The agents of viral gastroenteritis are identified in stool or rectal swabs by a variety of immunologic techniques not available in most laboratories. Serologic testing with acute and convalescent titers can also be useful.

Antibiotic therapy is of no benefit in the treatment of viral gastroenteritis. Fluid and electrolyte support is indicated. Enteric precautions are advisable for residents with viral gastroenteritis because these infections spread by the fecal-oral route; this involves careful handwashing and proper disposal of feces.

E. coli 0157:H7

Enterohemorrhagic *E. coli* can cause diarrhea in the LTCF setting. *E. coli* 0157:H7 is a newly identified *E. coli* of this type and is responsible for both sporadic and outbreak cases.[26,27] This organism is associated with hemorrhagic colitis and the hemolytic uremic syndrome (HUS). Undercooked meats, particularly hamburger, are implicated as vehicles of transmission. Person-to-person spread has also been suggested in several outbreaks, and LTCFs have been involved in outbreaks.[28–30] The very young and the very old appear to be particularly susceptible to *E. coli* 0157:H7, and the mortality rate can be high for both groups.

The incubation period for illness caused by *E. coli* 0157:H7 ranges from three to eight days, which is longer than that for most enteric pathogens. Often, mild diarrhea is followed quickly by grossly bloody stools. Fever is unusual. HUS—a syndrome of microangiopathic hemolytic anemia, thrombocytopenia, and acute renal failure—is a complication of *E. coli* 0157:H7 infection. Eleven of twelve patients with this complication in one LTCF outbreak died.[30]

The diagnosis of this entity is based on stool culture. Because all stool specimens have *E. coli* in them, testing for *E. coli* 0157:H7 requires special techniques and must be specifically requested. Serotyping and the use of DNA probes can aid an outbreak investigation. Proper attention to food preparation, particularly correct cooking temperatures, can help prevent the morbidity and mortality associated with this organism.

PSEUDOMEMBRANOUS COLITIS

In 1978, Bartlett et al. published a report associating toxin-producing *Clostridia* with the entity known as pseudomembranous colitis (PMC).[31] *C. difficile*–associated diarrhea following antibiotic administration occurs in the elderly, both in sporadic cases and in epidemics.[32–35] This organism causes 20% to 25% of postantibiotic diarrhea.

C. difficile colonizes the intestinal tract of 3% of adults. Alteration of the normal protective colonic flora by antibiotic administration allows overgrowth of *C. difficile* with subsequent toxin production. Almost every antibiotic, given by any route, can lead to pseudomembranous colitis. Significantly, some cases of PMC do not occur until after the antibiotic course is completed, before the colon is recolonized with its usual flora.

Manifestations of PMC vary widely. Mild cases consist of diarrhea alone. However, the typical resident will have profuse diarrhea with some degree of abdominal cramping and perhaps a low-grade fever. High fever, abdominal pain, and bloody diarrhea occur in severe cases. Fecal white blood cells are found in 50%.

The diagnosis of PMC can be made by several methods. Flexible sigmoidoscopy confirms the presence of acute colitis, as well as plaques and nodules. *C. difficile* can be grown from the stool if special media are used. However, because some adults are merely colonized with this organism, growth from the stool does not necessarily correlate with pathogenicity.

Tissue culture is used to detect toxin activity, but this test can be expensive and labor intensive. Recently, commercial latex agglutination tests have been developed to aid in the diagnosis of *Clostridium difficile*–associated diarrhea. These rapidly performed tests are the usual means of diagnosis of LTCF cases.

Mild cases of PMC are treated by stopping the offending antibiotic and administering fluid and electrolyte support. More severe cases require antibiotic therapy aimed at reducing toxin production in the colon. Vancomycin, given orally in a dose of 125 mg to 500 mg every six hours is the drug of choice. Alternate therapy consists of metronidazole in a dose of 250 mg by mouth every six hours. Although metronidazole is less expensive than vancomycin, it may not be as effective in severe disease. Care should be taken to avoid antimotility agents when treating PMC, lest toxic megacolon occur.

Although symptomatic relief usually occurs in seven to ten days, relapses of PMC are not uncommon. These require retreatment. The resident with PMC should practice good hygiene, and isolation for enteric pathogens may be indicated. Nosocomial transmission of *C. difficile* does occur, and outbreaks of PMC in LTCFs are not uncommon.[33,35] Health care workers should wear gloves and use good handwashing techniques.

VIRAL HEPATITIS

Hepatitis A

Hepatitis A, or infectious hepatitis, has an incubation period of two to six weeks and tends to occur in epidemics. Spread is from person to person by the fecal-oral route. Many patients with hepatitis are asymptomatic, but fever, anorexia, nausea, and right upper quadrant abdominal pain may occur. Laboratory tests demonstrate liver injury with elevation of serum transaminases and bilirubin. Hepatitis A has a very good prognosis. Symptoms usually resolve within several weeks, and chronic liver disease does not develop.

The spread of hepatitis A is from person to person by the fecal-oral route. Shellfish, contaminated water, and infected food handlers have been responsible for outbreaks. The virus is found in the stool two weeks prior to the onset of symptoms and remains until liver function tests begin to return to normal; 20 to 60% of the population in the United States have hepatitis A antibodies, implying past infection.

Institutional outbreaks of hepatitis A are not uncommon. A resident with hepatitis A, particularly one with vomiting, diarrhea, and fecal incontinence, poses a hazard to other residents and LTCF personnel. In one outbreak, 10% of susceptible exposed employees acquired hepatitis A from an incontinent resident with hepatitis A.[36] Enteric precautions are appropriate measures for hepatitis A or hepatitis of unknown type.

There is no specific therapy for hepatitis A, although a number of preventive measures are available. Pooled immune serum globulin (ISG) confers significant protection against hepatitis A when given within two weeks of exposure. It is 80% to 90% effective and is indicated for household contacts of hepatitis A cases at a dose of 0.02 ml/kg by the intramuscular route. There currrenly is no vaccine for hepatitis A.

Hepatitis B

Hepatitis B is less common than hepatitis A. It has a much longer incubation period, from one to six months. The virus can be found in blood and body secretions. Transmission of the virus is usually by the parenteral route. Blood transfusion, hemodialysis, and injectable drug use are significant risk factors. Health care workers, especially those who have close contact with blood or blood products, are at increased risk. Hepatitis B leads to chronic active hepatitis in as many as 10% of cases. Cirrhosis, or scarring of the liver, may eventually result.

A variety of particles relating to the hepatitis B virus have been identified, including hepatitis B surface antigen (HBsAg), hepatitis B core antigen, and e antigen. These particles or the antibodies produced against them have been used to diagnose hepatitis B. The hepatitis B surface antigen and the e antigen correlate well with infectivity. Most patients eliminate hepatitis B surface antigen from their blood in several months and develop protective anti-HBsAg antibody, although 5% to 10% become chronic HBsAg carriers.

Hepatitis B vaccine consists of surface antigen of the virus (HBsAg). The vaccine is recommended for health care workers who have the potential for exposure to blood and body fluids. Three injections are recommended—the primary inoculation and two subsequent doses at one and six months. Universal precautions are appropriate for the resident with hepatitis B and for HBsAg carriers. Employee vaccination for hepatitis B is discussed in Chapters 15 and 16.

Although standard ISG does not reliably protect against hepatitis B, special high-titer hepatitis B immune globulin (HBIG) may offer some protection, especially following accidental needlestick of an unvaccinated employee. The recommended dose of HBIG is 0.06 ml/kg intramuscularly within one week of exposure, followed by a second dose one month later.

Other Hepatitis

Hepatitis C causes most cases of "non-A, non-B" hepatitis. It is similar to hepatitis B in its route of spread (parenteral) and its tendency to cause chronic liver injury. Diagnosis is by serum antibody. Hepatitis E resembles hepatitis A; this infection is spread by the enteric route and rarely causes cirrhosis.

ENTERAL FEEDINGS

Many residents of LTCFs are given enteral feedings for nutritional support. For this purpose, nasoenteral, gastrostomy, and jejunostomy tubes can be used. Diarrhea is a common side effect of these feedings. Causes of diarrhea in this setting include osmolarity of the formula, the delivery rate, and the concomitant use of medications including antibiotics and antacids.[37]

Inadequate hygiene or infection control techniques increase the risk of infection from contamination of the feeding solution. However, infectious diarrhea can result from contamination of the enteral feedings despite strict attention to handwashing, use of clean equipment in preparation, and appropriate "hang times."[38] The bacteria involved often come from the resident's own flora; gram-negative bacilli as well as staphylococci and streptococci can cause diarrhea and, occasionally, bacteremia.

Other infectious complications of enteral nutrition include otitis media and sinusitis (nasogastric tubes), local wound infection and peritonitis (gastrostomy tubes), and aspiration pneumonia.[37] Aspiration pneumonia can occur in greater than 50% of residents, even in the presence of gastrostomy tubes.[37,39–42] Preventive measures include elevation of the head of the resident's bed, making sure the tube is correctly positioned, and monitoring residual volumes. Policies and procedures should be developed for prevention of infections associated with enteral feedings.[43]

Enteral feedings are available commercially in liquid and powder forms, or they can be prepared in the LTCF kitchen. Liquid feedings that are purchased as sterile can probably be hung for 24 hours before changing.[38,44] Reconstituted (i.e., powder) or homemade feedings should be changed more frequently, however, due to the risk of bacterial contamination and overgrowth. Any materials used for the preparation of these feedings should be washed thoroughly between uses. This includes the blender, which should be disassembled for cleaning.[45] Flushing the bag and tubing between uses and before new feedings are added is prudent.

CONCLUSION

Although gastroenteritis in the LTCF is not as common as other entities discussed in this book, it can cause significant morbidity and even mortality. Several steps can be taken in order to prevent gastroenteritis in the facility (Table 8.3). Among these are measures to prevent cross-infection (handwashing, outbreak recognition, isolation) and measures to control the reservoir of infection (diagnosis and treatment of diarrhea cases, proper techniques

Table 8.3 *Prevention of Gastroenteritis in the LTCF*

Handwashing

Appropriate isolation of residents with diarrhea

Prompt outbreak recognition

Recognition and treatment of gastroenteritis cases

Judicious use of antibiotics

Proper enteral feeding preparation and administration

Kitchen personnel hygiene

Kitchen sanitation and cleaning

Appropriate cooking and refrigeration temperatures

for preparing and storing both food and enteral feeding solutions). The infection control aspects of the LTCF kitchen are discussed further in Chapter 18. Finally, judicious use of antibiotics preserves the resident's intestinal flora, an important defense mechanism against infectious gastroenteritis.

REFERENCES

1. Duma RJ: Approach to the patient with infectious diarrhea and gastrointestinal illness, in *Recognition and Management of Nursing Home Infections*. Bethesda, MD, National Foundation for Infectious Diseases, 1992, pp 51–60.
2. Garibaldi RA, Brodine S, Matsumiya S: Infections among patients in nursing homes: Policies, prevalence, and problems. *N Engl J Med* 1981;305:731–735.
3. Hoffman N, Jenkins R, Putney K: Nosocomial infection rates during a one-year period in a nursing home care unit of a Veterans Administration hospital. *Am J Infect Control* 1990;18:55–63.
4. Magaziner J, Tenney JH, DeForge B, et al: Prevalence and characteristics of nursing home-acquired infections in the aged. *J Am Geriatr Soc* 1991;39:1071–1078.
5. Gangarosa RE, Glass RI, Lew JF, et al: Hospitalizations involving gastroenteritis in the United States, 1985: The special burden of the disease among the elderly. *Am J Epidemiol* 1992;135:281–290.
6. Maasdam CF, Anuras S: Are you overlooking gastrointestinal infections in your elderly patients? *Geriatrics* 1981;36:127–134.
7. Smith IM: Infections in the elderly. *Hosp Pract* 1982:69–85.

8. Leu LF, Glass RI, Gangarosa RE, et al: Diarrheal deaths in the United States, 1979 through 1987. *JAMA* 1991;265:3280–3284.
9. Levine WC, Smart JF, Archer DL, et al: Foodborne disease outbreaks in nursing homes, 1975 through 1987. *JAMA* 1991;266:2105–2109.
10. Shandera WX, Tacket CO, Blake PA: Food poisoning due to *Clostridium perfringens* in the United States. *J Infect Dis* 1983;147:167–170.
11. Sharp JCM, Collier PW: Food poisoning in hospitals in Scotland. *J Hyg Camb* 1979;83:231–236.
12. Gilber RJ, Stringer MF, Peace TC: The survival and growth of Bacillus cereus in boiled and fried rice in relation to outbreaks of food poisoning. *J Hyg Camb* 1974;73:433.
13. Black RE, Jackson RJ, Tsai T, et al: Epidemic *Yersinia enterocolitica* infection due to contaminated chocolate milk. *N Engl J Med* 1978;298:76–79.
14. Petri WA, Ravdin JI: Amebiasis in institutionalized populations, in Ravdin JI (ed.): *Amebiasis: Human Infections by Entamoeba histolytica*. New York, Churchill Livingstone 1988, pp 576–581.
15. Craun GF: Waterborne giardiasis in the United States,

1965–1984. *Lancet* 1986;ii:513–514.

16. White KE, Hedberg CW, Edmundson LM, et al: An outbreak of giardiasis in a nursing home with evidence for multiple modes of transmission. *J Infect Dis* 1989;160:298–304.

17. Kaplan JE, Gary GW, Baron RC, et al: Epidemiology of Norwalk gastroenteritis and the role of Norwalk virus in outbreaks of acute nonbacterial gastroenteritis. *Ann Intern Med* 1982;96:765–771.

18. Kaplan JE, Schonberger LB, Varano G, et al: An outbreak of acute nonbacterial gastroenteritis in a nursing home. *Am J Epidemiol* 1982;116:940–948.

19. Pegues DA, Woernle CH: An outbreak of acute nonbacterial gastroenteritis in a nursing home. *Infect Control Hosp Epidemiol* 1993;14:87–94.

20. Gelbert GA, Waterman SH, Ewert D, et al: An outbreak of acute gastroenteritis caused by a small round structured virus in a geriatric convalescent facility. *Infect Control Hosp Epidemiol* 1990;11:459–464.

21. Cubitt WD, Holzel H: An outbreak of rotavirus infection in a long-stay ward of a geriatric hospital. *J Clin Pathol* 1980;33:306–308.

22. Lewis DC, Lightfoot NF, Cubitt WD, et al: Outbreaks of astrovirus type I and rotavirus gastroenteritis in a geriatric inpatient population. *J Hosp Infect* 1989;14:9–14.

23. Marie TJ, Lee SHS, Faulkner RS, et al: Rotavirus infection in a geriatric population. *Arch Intern Med* 1982;142:313–316.

24. Halvorsrud J, Orstavik I: An epidemic of rotavirus-associated gastroenteritis in a nursing home for the elderly. *Scand J Infect Dis* 1980;12:161–164.

25. Gordon SM, Oshiro LS, Jarvis WR, et al: Foodborne Snow Mountain agent gastroenteritis with secondary person-to-person spread in a retirement community. *Am J Epidemiol* 1990;131:702–710.

26. Karmali MA, Petric M, Lim C, et al: The association between idiopathic hemolytic uremic syndrome and infection by verotoxin-producing *Escherichia coli*. *J Infect Dis* 1985;151:775–782.

27. Riley LW, Remis RS, Helgerson SD, et al: Hemorrhagic colitis associated with a rare *Escherichia coli* serotype. *N Engl J Med* 1983;308:681–685.

28. Ryan CA, Tauxe RV, Hosek GW, et al: *Escherichia coli* 0157:H7 diarrhea in a nursing home: Clinical, epidemiological and pathological findings. *J Infect Dis* 1986;154:631–638.

29. Spike JS, Parsons JE, Nordenberg D, et al: Hemolytic uremic syndrome and diarrhea associated with *Escherichia coli* 0157:H7 in a day care center. *J Pediatr* 1986;109:287–291.

30. Carter AO, Borczyk AA, Carlson JAK, et al: A severe outbreak of *Escherichia coli* 0157:H7-associated hemorrhagic colitis in a nursing home. *N Engl J Med* 1987;317;1496–1500.

31. Bartlett JG, Chang TW, Gurwith M, et al: Antibiotic associated pseudomembranous colitis due to toxin-producing Clostridia. *N Engl J Med* 1978;298:531–534.

32. Bender BS, Laughon BE, Gaydos C, et al: Is *Clostridium difficile* endemic in chronic-care facilities? *Lancet* 1986;ii:11–13.

33. Bentley DW. *Clostridium difficile*–associated disease in long-term care facilities. *Infect Control Hosp Epidemiol* 1990;11:434–438.

34. Thomas DR, Bennett RG, Laughon BE, et al: Post-antibiotic colonization with *Clostridium difficile* in nursing home patients. *J Am Geriatr Soc* 1990;38:415–420.

35. Brooks SE, Veal RO, Kramer M, et al: Reduction in the incidence of *Clostridium difficile*–associated diarrhea in an acute care hospital and a skilled nursing facility following replacement of electronic thermometers with single-use disposables. *Infect Control Hosp Epidemiol* 1992;13:98–103.

36. Goodman RA, Carder CC, Allen JR, et al: Nosocomial hepatitis A transmission by an adult patient with diarrhea. *Am J Med* 1982;73:220–226.

37. Fisher RL: Indications and complications of enteral and parenteral therapy. *Contemp Intern Med* 1992;39–52.

38. FDA Drug Bulletin. Bacterial contamination of enteral formula products. US Department of Health and Human Services, Rockville, MD, November, 1988, p 34.

39. Boscoe MJ, Rosin MD: Finebore enteral feeding and pulmonary aspiration. *Br Med J* 1984;289:1421–1422.

40. Miller SK, Tomlinson JR, Sahn SA: Pleuropulmonary complications of enteral tube feedings. *Chest* 1985;88:230–233.

41. Metheny NA, Eisenber P, Spies M: Aspiration pneumonia in patients fed through enteral tubes. *Heart Lung* 1986;15:256–261.

42. Ciocon JO, Silverstone FA, Graver L, et al: Tube feedings in elderly patients. *Arch Intern Med* 1988;148:429–433.

43. Smith PW, Rusnak PG: APIC guideline for infection prevention and control in the long-term care facility. *Am J Infect Control* 1991;19:198–215.

44. Levy J. Enteral nutrition: an increasing recognized cause of nosocomial bloodstream infections. *Infect Control Hosp Epidemiol* 1989;10:395–397.

45. Simmons B, Trusler M, Roccaforte J, et al. Infection control for home health. *Infect Control Hosp Epidemiol* 1990;11:362–370.

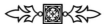

SECTION THREE

THE INFECTION CONTROL PROGRAM

CHAPTER
9

INFECTION CONTROL
PROGRAM ORGANIZATION

Philip W. Smith

REASONS TO HAVE AN INFECTION CONTROL PROGRAM

The reasons for developing an infection control program are listed in Table 9.1. The importance of infection control programs will probably increase in the future; nursing home infections are likely to increase because of the expanding elderly population and the vulnerability of nursing home residents to infections. There is an increasing number of patients requiring nursing home care;[1] it is projected that for persons who turned 65 in 1990, 43% will enter a nursing home at some point.[2] The hospital perspective payment system resulted in a shift of sick and terminally ill patients from hospitals to nursing homes,[3] with a subsequent increase in nursing home deaths.[4] In addition,

more AIDS patients are likely to receive terminal care in LTCFs. The increased patient acuity will magnify the risks of LTCF-acquired infections.

Protection of Residents and Employees

In Chapter 4, the risk of infection for nursing home residents was delineated. The nosocomial infection rate for nursing homes appears to be as high as that for hospitals, with significant morbidity, mortality, and financial cost for treatment. Infections in the nursing home are responsible for a large percentage of acute medically attended problems, transfers to acute care hospitals and deaths.[5,6] Certain nursing home infections pose a threat to the health of employees (see Chapter 16). In view of the frequency of infection and the fact that an important proportion of nosocomial infections may be prevented by an effective infection control program, it is incumbent upon the nursing home to develop such a program for the safety of residents and employees. Infection control is the prototype quality assurance program.

Requirements

An infection control program for nursing homes is mandated by the Standards for Certification and Participation in Medicare and Medicaid Programs, the Occupational Safety and Health Administration, and the Joint Commission on Accreditation of Health Care Organizations as

---

Table 9.1 *Reasons to Have a Nursing Home Infection Control Program*

1. Protection of residents from infectious complications
2. Protection of employees from infectious complications
3. Maximization of quality of care
4. Compliance with state and federal regulations
5. Avoidance of legal liability
6. Avoidance of adverse publicity

---

reviewed in Chapter 13. In addition, many states have statutory infection control requirements for licensure of nursing homes.[7] The guidelines require an infection control program providing all services necessary to maintain a sanitary and comfortable environment and to prevent infection in the nursing home.[8–10]

Legal Aspects

Several lawsuits have been decided in the area of hospital infections; this has stimulated interest in preventing legal liability by an effective infection control program. The same general principles should be applicable to nursing homes. Malpractice cases are based on the legal theory of negligence. In order to hold the defendant guilty of negligence, the plaintiff must prove that the defendant had a duty to care for the plaintiff, that this duty was breached, that the breach of duty was the proximate cause of the plaintiff's injury, and that the plaintiff suffered damages.[11] The health care institution is expected to deliver a standard of care appropriate to the community.

Lawsuits can be successfully avoided by having rules and regulations that are up-to-date and observed. Good record keeping to document compliance with accepted standards is also crucial to effective defense against malpractice in the area of infection control. A strong infection control program demonstrates that the nursing home is interested in providing the resident reasonable protection against the hazards of nursing home–acquired infection. An infection control program can also minimize the risk of another adverse event—publicity stemming from an infectious disease epidemic.

COMPONENTS OF AN INFECTION CONTROL PROGRAM

There are a number of approaches to infection control in the nursing home setting, depending on the interest and resources of the nursing home. A program needs to assign responsibility for infection control to a person, the infection control practitioner (ICP), who is usually a nurse. This person probably will not perform infection control activities on a full-time basis. This person may receive direction from a multidisciplinary body, the infection control committee (ICC).

Infection Control Program

Hospitals are required to have an active ICC. This committee must have the support of the hospital administration and must also have the written authority to intervene when a dangerous situation (such as an outbreak of *Staphylococcus aureus* infections) arises in the hospital.[12]

Past Medicare regulations also mandated an ICC in nursing homes, and such a committee is still required by the JCAHO and many state regulations.[7] The makeup of this committee is similar to that recommended for hospitals, including medical and nursing staffs, administration, and representatives from dietetics, pharmacy, housekeeping, maintenance, and laundry services. The chairman should have knowledge of or special interest or experience in infection control. The ICC carries out most infection control activities through the infection control practitioner and provides medical direction to this person.

Medicare now requires an infection control program rather than a specific committee. The facility must have a program for detecting, preventing, controlling, and reporting infections. The program must address food handling, laundry, waste disposal, employee health, pest control, traffic, visitation, asepsis, quality control, and safety.[8] Other aspects of the program include developing isolation procedures and enforcing employee handwashing.

Infection Control Practitioner

The infection control practitioner (ICP) is the key person who effects the infection control program. A background in clinical medicine, usually nursing, is helpful in carrying out the duties of the ICP. Knowledge of basic microbiology is beneficial. The person who performs the duties of infection control should be familiar with resident care problems in the nursing home; often the director of nursing is chosen.

The ICP must have well-defined authority and support from the administration, the medical director, and the infection control committee. The ICP should have written authority to institute infection control measures (such as isolation or visitor restrictions) in emergency situations.[13]

It is also very important that this person be extremely tactful in dealing with nursing home personnel, physicians, residents, and families. A number of potential problems unique to nursing home ICPs have been identified, including role confusion (because the ICP frequently has many other responsibilities), lack of authority to initiate isolation or to perform cultures, high turnover rate, lack of visibility of the ICP in the institution, and lack of time to fulfill infection control duties.

The ICP can play a very exciting and important role in the nursing home. Although residents tend to have a number of underlying chronic and degenerative diseases that are not reversible, infectious diseases are frequently preventable or treatable. Infections are an important problem in nursing homes (see Chapter 4). Finally, because of decreased physician availability in nursing homes compared to acute care hospitals, the ICP may well have a greater responsibility for the diagnosis and prevention of infections.

INFECTION CONTROL PROGRAM ACTIVITIES

A number of elements of an infection control program can be defined (see Table 9.2).

Surveillance: Data Collection and Evaluation

One of the most important elements of an infection control program is surveillance. An effective infection control program cannot be conducted without knowledge of the specific and unique problems of each nursing home. Infection rates must be determined and compared to the usual (baseline) infection rate so that epidemics can be detected early. In addition, surveillance provides an excellent opportunity for on-the-spot education of personnel in infection control techniques. Surveillance by itself may serve to decrease infections in the nursing home by reminding personnel of the importance of adhering to good infection control practices and by demonstrating that the administration of the institution is committed to the infection control program.

There are several techniques for data collection, including continuous surveillance and periodic prevalence surveys of the entire nursing home population. Surveillance information should be used in the control activities of the ICP. For example, an increase in the rate of urinary tract infection may lead to discovery of an epidemic that can be terminated by appropriate measures. Infection control problems in the nursing home may be used in educational programs for personnel. Surveillance is discussed in depth in Chapter 10.

Epidemic Investigation

One of the major purposes for having a surveillance program in a nursing home is early detection of epidemics. It is

Table 9.2   *Elements of a Nursing Home Infection Control Program*

ELEMENT	EXAMPLE
Surveillance	Calculate monthly infection rates
Epidemic control	Investigate a cluster of skin infections
Education	Develop in-service program for handwashing
Policy formation	Develop isolation policies
Procedure formation	Write catheter insertion procedure
Employee health program	Monitor employee TB screening results
Resident health program	Provide resident influenza vaccinations
Environmental control	Inspect laundry and kitchen
Antibiotic monitoring	Review standing antibiotic orders
Quality improvement	Monitor compliance with universal precautions
Public health impact	Report diseases to health department

the responsibility of the infection control program to detect, document, evaluate, and try to control outbreaks of infections in the nursing home. Chapter 11 provides a detailed discussion of the approach to an epidemic.

Education

Education of the nursing home staff is a major ongoing responsibility of the ICP. Because of high turnover rate in many nursing homes, it is imperative to instruct new employees about infections in the nursing home and the role that personnel play in transmission and prevention of these infections.

In the course of the daily routine, employees may become careless about certain infection prevention techniques. The ICP needs to periodically remind personnel about the importance of policies and procedures relating to careful handwashing, universal precautions, aseptic bladder catheter insertion, adherence to isolation procedures, maintenance of good personal hygiene, and the susceptibility of the elderly to infection. This may be accomplished by periodic in-service education on basic infection control practices, including a review of policies and procedures. Educational techniques and resources are discussed in depth in Chapter 14.

Policies and Procedures

The ICP plays a vital role in developing and updating policies and procedures in the nursing home. An example is isolation policies. General guidelines are available for isolation (see Chapter 19), but the ICP can play an important role in adapting these general guidelines to the specific needs of the nursing home and serving as a resource person for answering questions about these procedures.

Many aspects of the nursing home environment that affect resident care will be covered by infection control policies or procedures, including employee health, visitor regulations, isolation, disinfection/sterilization, housekeeping, engineering, food preparation, laundry, waste disposal, handwashing procedures, and policies relating to admission and transfer of residents with infection. Some policies, such as universal precautions, are designed primarily to protect the employee (see Chapter 15).

Policies and procedures need to be clearly written, widely distributed throughout the nursing home, and periodically updated; they should contain a provision for monitoring of compliance. Policies and procedures are discussed in more detail in Chapter 13.

Employee Health Program

Employees may serve as a source for spread of infections to nursing home residents or may acquire an infection in the line of duty. An active employee health program will minimize both of these risks.

The majority of employee health problems relate to infectious diseases; hence, the ICP is a logical person to oversee an employee health program in the nursing home. Elements of a nursing home employee health program include screening of new employees for infectious diseases, education of employees about their role in transmission of nosocomial infections, updating employee immunizations, periodic screening for infectious diseases (such as tuberculosis), assuring employee safety from bloodborne pathogens (universal precautions), and investigation of employees as potential agents for the spread of infectious diseases during epidemics. Employee health programs are reviewed in Chapter 16.

Resident Health Program

The infection control program should address various aspects of resident health, including resident hygiene, skin care, urinary catheter care, aspiration prevention, TB screening and immunizations (see Chapter 17).

Environmental Control

The ICP is frequently involved in monitoring the inanimate environment in the nursing home and overseeing the maintenance of an appropriately clean environment. Sanitation or disinfection of various parts of the environment are appropriate; specific procedures and policies for these methods should be delineated and monitored. Almost any part of the nursing home environment that comes in contact with the resident may occasionally serve as a vehicle for spread of infection. As a result, the ICP needs to be somewhat familiar with a number of housekeeping and maintenance areas, including ventilation and air conditioning, water distribution and plumbing, cleaning of environmental surfaces, laundry, waste disposal, kitchen and food operations, insect and rodent control, and safety programs.

Routine microbiologic sampling of the environment is

costly and not indicated. Selected environmental cultures may play an important role in epidemic investigations, however. Environmental control is discussed in Chapter 18.

Antibiotic Monitoring

The problems of antibiotic overuse and antibiotic-resistant bacteria are not confined to hospitals but are also of major importance in the nursing home. Antibiotic misuse results in wasted resources, side effects, and selection of resistant bacteria. Antibiotic-resistant bacteria such as MRSA cause serious epidemics in the nursing home. The ICP should work in cooperation with the pharmacist to monitor antibiotic resistance and usage in the nursing home. This issue is covered in depth in Chapter 12.

Quality Improvement/Assurance

The nursing home is required to have a quality assurance program.[14] The infection control program was actually one of the first "quality assurance" programs and now overlaps with formal quality improvement methods.[15,16]

Quality improvement (QI) programs, also known as quality assurance or quality management programs, emphasize continuous improvement in health care by analyzing and improving the process. Process analysis identifies areas of improvement; after changes are implemented, it is important to measure results to see if improvement actually occurred.

There are many similarities between QI programs and infection control programs:

* Both use data collection and analysis tools
* Both search for process improvements (or adverse events that can be prevented)
* Both rely on education to modify behavior
* Both do follow-up studies to assess the impact of the planned interventions

Because of the similarities, LTCFs may find that combining QI and infection control is efficient.

Community Health Impact—Disease Reporting

Infection control programs at individual nursing homes have public health responsibilities and interact with health agencies in several ways.

A number of diseases that may be seen in the nursing home are reportable on national or state levels, including hepatitis A, hepatitis B, tuberculosis, salmonellosis, shigellosis, amebiasis, and Legionnaires' disease. Diseases that are first diagnosed in the nursing home may have been communicable prior to hospitalization; hence, persons in the community would be at risk. State health departments are in a position to take measures to protect public health. In addition, epidemics may involve more than one nursing home or hospital.

Health departments in turn help infection control programs by facilitating various diagnostic tests, coordinating investigations of epidemics, providing literature, serving as liaison with the Centers for Disease Control and Prevention (CDC), and providing information on infectious diseases in the community.

Ideally, nursing home, hospital, and public health officials should work together to solve problems of mutual interest and public health importance. Statewide infection control organizations exist in a number of states. In Nebraska, for instance, the Nebraska Infection Control Network (NICN) is an organization cosponsored by the State Health Department, state nursing home association, state hospital association, and local chapter of the Association for Professionals in Infection Control and Epidemiology (APIC). The network organizes educational seminars and publishes a newsletter.[17]

Nursing Home–Hospital Interaction

As was mentioned in Chapter 4, the LTCF ICP needs to have some knowledge of nosocomial infections in hospitals; there is a dynamic microbiologic equilibrium between hospitals and nursing homes because of patient transfers. This impacts the infection control program at several levels.

Infection is one of the most common medical problems necessitating transfer of the LTCF resident to an acute care hospital.[5,18] Most nursing home residents transferred to an acute care hospital are treated and return to the same location and level of care afterwards.[18] One aspect of community health impact, in addition to disease reporting, is communication from the LTCF ICP to the hospital ICP when infection control matters of note are involved (e.g., isolation for MRSA). Conversely, hospitalized patients have long been known to have the potential for introducing resistant bacteria from hospitals to the LTCF.[19,20] As part of the surveillance function, the ICP needs to develop a program for screening incoming hospital transfers for possible communicable infections, and will, it is hoped, receive open communication from the hospital ICP prior to transfer of the patient.

CURRENT STATUS OF INFECTION CONTROL PROGRAMS

Several surveys during the last decade have provided insight into the status of infection control programs in the LTCF[21–27]; all noted that the vast majority of LTCFs have an ICP and an infection control committee. From these studies, one can develop a composite picture of the LTCF ICP as an individual who spends from 8 to 57 hours per month on infection control activities, depending on facility size, nursing intensity, and facility commitment to infection control (see Table 9.3). The ICP frequently has other duties such as general duty nursing, nursing supervision, inservice education, employee health, and quality assurance.[24] The ICP usually does not have specific training in infection control, and the turnover rate for nursing home ICPs is quite high.[21]

Most infection control programs include surveillance, which accounts for 26% to 38% of the time devoted to infection control by the ICP.[23,25] Surveillance activities are frequently hampered by the absence of written definitions of infections and excessive focus on chart review, and nosocomial infection rates are usually not calculated.[25] A prospective surveillance system with calculation of appropriate incidence rates is the basis for planning effective infection control efforts.[13]

Most LTCFs in the United States do have an employee health program, although only 49% to 74% require preemployment screening for relevant contagious diseases.[23,24] Most do not require a preemployment physical examination, and nearly half do not record contagious diseases occurring during employment.[23] An employee health program should also include baseline and periodic TB skin testing, an immunization history, appropriate immunizations, and periodic education in infectious diseases (see Chapter 16).

Few LTCFs provide a comprehensive resident health program[24] including preadmission screening for relevant contagious diseases (history, physical examination), pread-mission and periodic TB skin testing, an immunization history, and vaccination for tetanus/diphtheria, influenza, and pneumococcal pneumonia.[23,25] Commonly recommended immunizations such as influenza are often not offered to residents.

Some aspects of infection control are cost inefficient. For instance, a Maryland survey found that one third of nursing homes still performed routine environmental cultures.[24] Deficiencies in policy and procedure development in areas such as isolation and catheter care are common.[23,24] Price found deficiencies in isolation facilities such as inadequate number of sinks, and recirculated, inadequately filtered air.[22] Crossley did find, however, that most Minnesota nursing homes performed antibiotic utilization studies.[23]

Infection control programs have advanced greatly in the last decade, but ICPs have variable background training, have variable time available to devote to infection control duties, and perform surveillance with variable intensity. Educational programs designed for the ICP may help address these deficiencies.[28,29]

COST CONTAINMENT—IDEAS FOR INSTITUTIONS WITH LIMITED RESOURCES

In spite of the complex job description of an infection control practitioner and the important role such a person plays in preventing infections, many nursing homes lack the resources to employ a full-time ICP. A number of shortcuts are available for these institutions.

Perhaps the most time-consuming duty of an infection control practitioner is data collection and evaluation. There is no doubt that surveillance of infections is very important in order to provide accurate data for decisions concerning infection prevention. However, surveillance systems vary in complexity and time requirements. Walking rounds with chart review and discussions with nursing personnel on a frequent basis are ideal, but alternatives such as periodic prevalence surveys or screening of high-risk residents (e.g., those with indwelling bladder catheters) may be suitable. Any system that is used must be consistent. A system that removes the ICP from contact with nursing home personnel may dilute the effect of spontaneous teaching and encouragement (see Chapter 10).

Ideally education should be relevant to the institution's

own experience. Prepackaged educational programs, such as self-learning modules or audiovisual instructional programs are available. Time may be saved by borrowing ideas on policies, procedures, and isolation manuals from nursing homes or hospitals that have already developed them (see Chapter 14).

Finally, it may be most practical to combine the role of ICP with a number of other roles of importance in the nursing home. For instance, the ICP may be responsible for quality assurance or may oversee the institutional safety program, two functions required by accrediting agencies.[8] The ICP in a nursing home is frequently also a staff nurse. In view of the predominant concern with infectious diseases of employee health issues, the ICP may also be in charge of the employee health program. Another function is to work with the pharmacists on antibiotic audits, antibiotic appropriateness reviews, or antibiotic resistance surveillance.

HOW TO START A PROGRAM

The development of an effective infection control program usually follows these steps:

1. Appoint a responsible individual to be the infection control practitioner (ICP). This person needs to have support from administration and a clearly defined responsibility and time allotment for managing the infection control program.
2. The ICP will require training and resource materials. Brief introductory courses in infection control are available in many locations, and in-depth courses are offered by the Association for Professionals in Infection Control and Epidemiology (APIC), the Nebraska Infection Control Network, and others. Basic reference materials of great assistance in development of a program are available; several are given in this chapter's appendix. Local nurse epidemiologists, hospital epidemiologists, and health departments are often valuable resources.

3. Generally, the first duty of the new ICP is the development of some sort of surveillance system. Initially, definitions of infection can be obtained from reference sources or other institutions, and a simple recording form may be developed. Knowledge of the infection control problems of the particular nursing home is essential in order to make intelligent decisions about appropriate control measures. Surveillance also facilitates early detection and prevention of epidemics.
4. Policy and procedure development and review should be the next goal. Every facility should have written policies for isolation/precautions, visitation, disinfection/sterilization, aseptic insertion of bladder catheters, decubitus care, food sanitation and universal precautions.
5. Educational programs for nursing home personnel should begin quickly, because this is one of the most effective control measures. The institution's surveillance data should be used in educational programs.
6. As time goes on, the infection control practitioner may well evolve additional roles. The ICP serves as a resource person for many employees in the nursing home, including nursing, housekeeping, maintenance, administration, and other personnel.

Table 9.3 *LTCF Infection Control Practices*

Author	Ref.	Infection Control (total hrs/month)	Perform Surveillance (%)	ICP-Prior Training (%)
Price	22	8	83%	0
Crossley	23	7% > 40	74% < 20	60%
Khabbaz	24	14	64%	16%
Daly	25	10	74%	28%
Pearson	26	57	100%	>90%

The nursing home resources and commitment to infection control determine how quickly the preceding steps take place and how far the infection control program develops. An ICP who is willing to learn and seek advice can overcome deficiencies in training or background.

AN OVERVIEW OF CONTROL MEASURES

The development of nosocomial infection involves (see Fig. 4.1)

1. A reservoir of the infectious agent
2. A means of transmission of the infectious agent to the resident
3. Actual invasion of the host to produce an infectious disease

The development of a nursing home–acquired (nosocomial) infection can be blocked at any one of the three stages.

Both animate and inanimate *reservoirs* are important in the nursing home. The control methods address residents, visitors, and employees, all part of the animate reservoir (see Fig. 9.1). Other control measures necessary to maintain an appropriately clean inanimate environment in the nursing home are elaborated in Chapter 18.

The second step that may be interrupted is the *transmission* of agents. The single most important step in preventing transmission of infectious diseases in the nursing home is good handwashing; this measure also acts at the first step by decreasing the cutaneous reservoir. The other methods (see Fig. 9.2) address spread by airborne or direct-contact methods. Surveillance and education impact transmission by

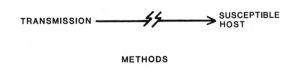

METHODS

Handwashing
Isolation
Closed urinary catheter systems
Air filtration/ventilation
Surveillance
Epidemic investigation
Education

Figure 9.2   *Infection control measures—transmission*

detecting epidemics and reminding personnel of correct infection control practices, respectively. Various aspects of control of transmission of infection are discussed in Chapter 19.

The final step is the transition from colonization to infection. *Host resistance* may be improved in a number of ways. General resistance may be improved by treating the residents' underlying medical illnesses to the greatest extent possible, providing good nutrition, and minimizing antibiotics (see Fig. 9.3). Other options include improving local defenses (e.g., good respiratory toilet) and enhancing specific immunity (e.g., influenza vaccine). Host measures are reviewed in Chapter 17.

Last, it should be remembered that nosocomial infections cannot be completely eliminated, but they can be minimized by a good infection control program. The realities of resident care do not permit the prevention of *all* infections, a situation analagous to infections in the hospital. When nosocomial infections do occur in the nursing

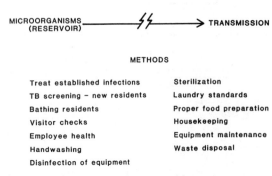

Figure 9.1   *Infection control measures—the reservoir*

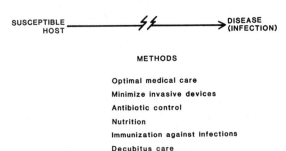

Figure 9.3   *Infection control measures—the host*

home, they pose a threat to the health of residents, and an infection control program must be prepared to detect the problem promptly and apply appropriate control measures. An integrated program will address all major areas in Table 9.2 that interface with infection control.

The 1980s saw the birth and development of LTCF infection control programs. The descriptive epidemiology of nursing home infections and epidemics were defined, the elements of an infection control program were described, and the unique problems of LTCF infection control programs were recognized.[30] Additional research is necessary to define risk factors for infection, ideal definitions of infection, effectiveness of specific control measures, and cost effectiveness of LTCF infection control programs.

REFERENCES

1. Shaughnessy PW, Kramer AM: The increased needs of patients in nursing homes and patients receiving home health care. *N Engl J Med* 1990;322:21–27.

2. Kemper P, Murtaugh CM: Lifetime use of nursing home care. *N Engl J Med* 1991;324:595–600.

3. Sager MA, Easterling DV, Kindig DA, et al: Changes in the location of death after passage of Medicare's prospective payment system—a national study. *N Engl J Med* 1989;320:433–439.

4. Lyles YM: Impact of Medicare diagnosis-related groups (DRGs) on nursing homes in the Portland, Oregon metropolitan area. *J Am Geriatr Soc* 1986;34:573–578.

5. Tresch DD, Simpson WM Jr, Burton JR: Relationship of long-term and acute-care facilities: The problem of patient transfer and continuity of care. *J Am Geriatr Soc* 1985;33:819–826.

6. Mott PD, Barker WH: Treatment decisions for infections occurring in nursing home residents. *J Am Geriatr Soc* 1988;36:820–824.

7. Crossley K, Nelson L, Irvine P: State regulations governing infection control issues in long-term care. *J Am Geriatr Soc* 1992;40:251–254.

8. US Department of Health and Human Services, Health Care Financing Administration. Medicare and Medicaid requirements for long term care facilities. *Federal Register* 1991;56:48826–48880.

9. Occupational Safety and Health Administration. Occupational exposure to bloodborne pathogens. *Federal Register* 1991;56:64175–64182.

10. The Joint Commission on Accreditation of Healthcare Organizations: *Long-Term Care Standards Manual.* Chicago IL, 1990.

11. Hesson WW, Thu CW: Legal commentary, Part I: Basics of liability law. *Infect Control Hosp Epidemiol* 1988;9:127–129.

12. *Accreditation Manual for Hospitals.* Joint Commission on Accreditation of Health Care Organizations, Chicago, IL, 1993.

13. Smith PW, Rusnak PG: APIC guideline for infection prevention and control in the long-term care facility. *Am J Infect Control* 1991;19:198–215.

14. *Omnibus Budget Reconciliation Act of 1987—Subtitle C—Nursing Home Reform.* 101 Stat 1330: 160 ff.

15. Crede W, Hierholzer WJ Jr: Linking hospital epidemiology and quality assurance: Seasoned concepts in a new role. *Infect Control Hosp Epidemiol* 1988;9:42–44.

16. APIC position paper 1985. *Am J Infect Control* 1989;17:66–68.

17. Smith PW: The Nebraska Infection Control Network. *Neb Med J* 1983;68:394–395.

18. Stark AJ, Gutman GM, McCashin B: Acute care hospitalizations and long term care: An examination of transfers. *J Am Geriatr Soc* 1982;30:509–515.

19. Hsu CCS, Macaluso CP, Special L, et al: High rate of methicillin-resistance of *Staphylococcus aureus* isolated from hospitalized nursing home patients. *Arch Intern Med* 1988;140:569–570.

20. Gaynes RP, Weinstein RA, Chamberlin W, et al: Antibiotic-resistant flora in nursing home patients admitted to the hospital. *Arch Intern Med* 1985;145:1804–1807.

21. Garibaldi RA, Brodine S, Matsumiya S: Infections among patients in nursing homes: Policies, prevalence and problems. *N Engl J Med* 1981;305:731–735.

22. Price LE, Sarubbi FA Jr, Rutala WA: Infection control programs in twelve North Carolina extended care facilities. *Infect Control* 1985;6:437–441.

23. Crossley KB, Irvine P, Kaszar DJ, et al: Infection control practices in Minnesota nursing homes. *JAMA* 1985;254:2918–2921.

24. Khabbaz RF, Tenney JH: Infection control in Maryland nursing homes. *Infect Control Hosp Epidemiol* 1988;9:159–162.

25. Daly PB, Smith PW, Rusnak P: Effectiveness of an infection control course for long-term care facility nurses (abstract). Atlanta, GA, Third International Conference on Nosocomial Infections, 1990.

26. Pearson DA, Checko PJ, Hierholzer WJ Jr, et al: Infection control practitioners and committees in skilled nursing facilities in Connecticut. *Am J Infect Control* 1990;18:167–175.

27. Pearson DA, Checko PJ, Hierholzer WJ Jr, et al: Infection control practices in Connecticut's skilled nursing facilities. *Am J Infect Control* 1990;18:269–276.

28. Smith PW, Daly PB, Rusnak PG, et al: The design and dissemination of a multiregional long-term care infection control training program. *Am J Infect Control* 1992;20:275–277.

29. Daly PB, Smith PW, Rusnak PG, et al: Impact on knowledge and practice of a multiregional long-term care facility infection control training program. *Am J Infect Control* 1992;20:225–233.

30. Smith PW, Daly PB, Roccaforte JS: Current status of nosocomial infection control in extended care facilities. *Am J Med* 1991;91(suppl):281–285.

APPENDIX

Reference Library for the Beginning Infection Control Practitioner

Guidelines for the Prevention and Control of Nosocomial Infections, 1981–1983. US Department of Health and Human Services, Public Health Service, Centers for Disease Control, Atlanta, GA 30333. Price (1983) = $55.00. Can be ordered by phone (703-487-4650). (Covers isolation, employee health, environmental control, prevention of urinary tract infections, etc.)

Benenson AS (ed): *Control of Communicable Diseases in Man*, 15th ed. 1990. American Public Health Association, 1015 Fifteenth Street NW, Washington, DC 20005. Price (1993) = $15.00. (Lists infectious diseases with signs, symptoms, epidemiology, contagious periods, and treatment).

Association for Practitioners in Infection Control. "Long term care curriculum," in Berg R: *The APIC Curriculum for Infection Control Practice*, Vol 3. Kendall Hunt, Dubuque IA, 1988:1329–1389.

Smith PW, Rusnak PG: APIC guideline for infection prevention and control in the long-term care facility. *Am J Infect Control* 1991;19:198–215. May be ordered from APIC by phone (708-949-6052). Price (1993) = $10.00.

Duma RJ (ed): *Recognition and Management of Nursing Home Infections*, 1992, National Foundation for Infectious Diseases, Bethesda, MD.

Secondary Reference Materials

Sanford JP: Guide to antimicrobial therapy. Can be ordered by phone 214-750-5783. Price (1993) = $5.50.

Wenzel RP, ed: *Prevention and Control of Nosocomial Infections*, 2nd ed, 1993. Williams & Wilkins. Baltimore, MD, Price (1993) = $87.00. (discusses basics of nosocomial infections in hospitals).

Mayhall CG, ed: *Hospital Epidemiology and Infection Control* (in press), Williams & Wilkins. Baltimore, MD, (discusses basics of nosocomial infections in hospitals).

Davis BD, Dulbecco R, Eisen HN, Ginsberg HS (eds): *Microbiology*, 4th ed, 1990. JB Lippincott, Philadephia, PA, Price (1993) = $79.50, (discusses basic microbiology in depth).

CHAPTER

SURVEILLANCE IN THE LONG-TERM CARE FACILITY

Patricia G. Rusnak and Linda A. Horning

APPROACH TO SURVEILLANCE

The Importance of Surveillance—The Why

As discussed in Chapter 9, surveillance is a critical component of any infection control program. It provides the foundation for the entire program. Surveillance has been defined as the collection, collation, and analysis of data and the dissemination of that data to those who need to know so that an action can result.[1] When applied to infection control, *surveillance* identifies the activity that the long-term care facility (LTCF) employs in order to find and analyze *nosocomial infections* (infections that develop in the LTCF).

Time and energy spent in surveillance activity become an indirect investment in prevention and control of infections. Surveillance data provide a LTCF with valid information for establishing a baseline and determining which control measures are needed. Surveillance data are used primarily to plan control activities and educational programs and to prevent epidemics, but surveillance may also detect infections that require therapeutic actions.[2] This data base is often used in formal educational programs as well (see Chapter 14). Infection control policies and procedures may be modified to address problems detected by surveillance. Finally, surveillance activities may even decrease nosocomial infections through informal educational efforts on rounds by reminding personnel of the factors involved in nursing home infections

Table 10.1 *Surveillance Components*

1. The infection control practicioner
2. Definitions of infections
3. Surveillance procedure
4. Forms
5. Infection rate calculations
6. Data analysis
7. Communication

and the importance of good infection control techniques.

In establishing a surveillance program for a LTCF, consideration must be given to the size of the facility, the level of care provided by the facility, and the type and extent of information the program needs. Requirements by state and other regulatory agencies also affect the development of an effective surveillance program (see Chapter 13). Committment from the administration of a LTCF to a comprehensive surveillance program is essential. Most administrators appreciate the impact of nosocomial infections on residents; nosocomial infections in LTCFs occur with a frequency that approximates that of hospital nosocomial infections annually in the United States (see Chapter 4). The availability of resources and personnel to conduct surveillance must also be considered. The components of a surveillance program are listed in Table 10.1.

INFECTION CONTROL PRACTITIONERS—THE WHO

It is essential that one employee have defined responsibility for surveillance. This person, the infection control practitioner (ICP), must detect and record nosocomial infections. The person responsible for surveillance in a LTCF should ideally be a registered nurse with clinical experience. In addition, well-defined administrative support and the ability to interact tactfully with personnel, physicians, residents, and families are critical to the success of the ICP. Knowledge of infectious diseases and of their transmission and epidemiology are important qualifications. Background knowledge in basic microbiology and statistics is helpful. Data collection will most likely consume the majority of the ICP's time. The designated ICP is said to be the eyes, ears, and feet of the infection control program.

In hospitals, the amount of time and personnel devoted to surveillance is customarily determined by the acuity of the patients and the number of beds. Most LTCFs can conduct surveillance with more conservative resources. The population of a LTCF is generally more stable and made up of less critically ill individuals, which eliminates some of the high-risk areas of the hospital setting such as intensive care, surgery, and the emergency department. Resources, requirements by regulatory agencies, the number of beds in the facility, occupancy, and the level of care the facility provides determine the number of personnel-hours dedicated to infection surveillance.

SURVEILLANCE—THE WHEN

Surveillance activities vary among LTCFs depending on the extent of the surveillance program. Collection of data by retrospective review of charts is regarded as being of limited use due to the lack of descriptive information in the clinical records of most LTCF residents. Concurrent prospective collection of *incidence* data performed at least once a week is recommended to provide timely data.[2]

Periodic or targeted designated time frames for focused surveillance on specific types of nosocomial infections may be most efficient and cost effective. However, before this type of surveillance is implemented, it is recommended that at least one year of baseline data be collected. As discussed in Chapter 4, some surveys of LTCF infections have been done by review of all charts on a given day, yielding *prevalence* data. Prevalence data provide a "snapshot" of infections in a LTCF but are less timely and less accurate than concurrently collected incidence data.

SURVEILLANCE ELEMENTS—THE HOW

Definitions

Written and approved definitions of infections need to be established in the facility for surveillance to have a solid basis.[3] McGeer's definitions of infection for surveillance in long-term care facilities provide descriptions of infections by body site adapted to the LTCF.[4] These definitions, published in 1991, are reproduced in this chapter's appendix. It should be remembered that definitions are only guidelines to help meet the needs of each facility.

Although definitions of infections for acute care hospitals have been available for many years,[5] no standard definitions of infections specific to the LTCF have been universally agreed upon, and even McGeer's definitions have not yet been validated in the field. Traditional hospital definitions depend on laboratory and radiologic data that are often unavailable in the LTCF. Thus they lack sensitivity when applied there. However, clinically based definitions lack sensitivity in this setting, due to the atypical symptoms in the elderly, lack of symptoms in demented patients, infrequent documentation of symptoms in the medical record, and other factors.[6]

The use of specific criteria for nosocomial infections provides uniformity in determining nosocomial origins and prevents biased individual decisions. The definitions of infection also assist the ICP in deciding if an infection is present and whether it is nosocomial or community-acquired, and in differentiating infection from colonization (see Chapter 1). Once criteria have been established they should be used consistently because changes in definitions will hinder comparison studies (e.g., last month's rates to this month's rates).

Procedure

How surveillance is accomplished in a facility will vary. It is essential that a brief written procedure be developed so that if emergencies arise surveillance can continue on a consistent basis. This procedure should list exactly how the surveillance is done.

Example

1. Review sources for possible infections
   - Medication book
   - Treatment book
   - Shift reports
   - Laboratory and x-ray reports
   - Charge personnel (question them for further information)
   - Caregivers (question them for further information)
   - Resident examination
2. Complete forms (possible infections and those that meet criteria)
3. Collect and analyze data weekly/monthly
4. Report results
5. Decide what situations/problems require action

Collection of Data

No single method for data collection has been found to identify all infections or risks in a hospital or LTCF, so a combination of methods is recommended. Committment and participation by the nursing staff are essential for comprehensive and efficient data retrieval. A staff nurse familiar with the residents can help identify the designated risks, symptoms, and treatments for infection. This important use of staff nurses may eliminate some chart and medication/treatment book review by the ICP, although "walking rounds" with visits to nursing stations is an extremely important part of surveillance.

In a LTCF, actual review of all the charts and medication/treatment books in search of new orders and infectious conditions may be too time-consuming even in a small facility. An alternative method of surveying is usually employed; for example, a resident review can be done daily by a charge nurse on each nursing unit. This method will provide a current, timely, and cost-efficient system of collecting data. Alternatively, the ICP may find clues to infection from the nursing staff and may selectively review charts. Clues that suggest an infection include fever, purulent drainage, abnormal x-rays, antibiotic administration, isolation, and the obtaining of cultures.

Forms

A data collection form may be used by the ICP to help find clues to infection in residents. An *infection information form* may be completed by the charge nurse and given to the ICP at designated intervals—e.g., daily or weekly (Fig. 10.1). The ICP then reviews these forms from all nursing areas.

Symptoms of infection are identified on the infection information form (see Fig. 10.1, column 2). Cloudy urine, fever, drainage from a wound, cough, nausea, vomiting, or diarrhea could be clues to the development of an infection or an outbreak within the facility. Other potential sources of information are progress notes, laboratory information, and radiology reports. Identifiable risks of infection in geriatric populations (Fig. 10.1, column 3) include the presence of a bladder catheter, intravenous administration, feeding tubes, and pressure sores.

If a culture is ordered, the physician obviously suspects infection; any resident who has had a culture done will need to be assessed for transmission of the suspected infection (see Fig. 10.1, column 4). Isolation precautions may be necessary while the culture is incubating (see Chapter 19). The mode of transmission of the suspected infection must be determined and the appropriate isolation or precaution immediately instituted. Any resident who receives an antibiotic should be evaluated for evidence of infection, particularly of nosocomial origin.

When the ICP suspects an infection in a LTCF resident (e.g., from reviewing forms completed by the nursing staff or from clues noted on walking rounds), data collection is initiated. An *infection worksheet,* seen in Fig. 10.2, is to be initiated by the ICP for any resident suspected of having a new infection. Some practitioners prefer 8 1/2 x 11 paper for a three-ring looseleaf notebook; others choose a 5 x 8 card to be placed in a card file. In small-scale programs, the looseleaf forms are more easily stored and filed. The sheets can be duplicated with a conventional copy machine in quantities as needed without the use of professional services for preprinting cards. The 5 x 8 cards, on the other hand, are easier to handle and somewhat more durable.

The worksheet form should be initiated by the ICP from the infection information. An infection worksheet such as the one seen in Fig. 10.2 can be designed to provide data specific to each resident's suspected nosocomial and community acquired infections. The form should be

Figure 10.1 *Infection Information Form*   *Week of* _____

Resident Name and Room #	Symptoms/Indications of Infection	Predisposing Factors	Cultures, X-Rays, Treatment Initiated	Comments/Nurse Initials

FLOOR_____

Figure 10.2   *Infection Worksheet*

Date _____

Resident _____

ID # _____

Room _____

Age _____ Sex M_____ F_____

Date of Admission _____

Nosocomial Infection _____

Community–Aquired Infection _____

Date of Onset _____

M.D. Diagnosis Yes _____ No _____

Procedure Related YES _____ NO _____

Prodedure _____

INFECTION SITE

SIGNS & SYMPTOMS

UTI (Urinary Tract) _____

_____

SST (Skin/Soft Tissue) _____

_____

LRT (Lower Resp Tract)_____

_____

GI (Gastrointestinal)_____

_____

EENT (Ear, Eye, Nose, Throat)_____

_____

Other _____

_____

Culture Yes _____ No _____

Culture Date _____

Specimen _____

Culture Results _____

Isolation/Prec._____

Date In _____ Date Out _____

Treatment _____

Expired Yes _____ No _____

Comments _____

_____

Update Info._____

_____

_____

designed to collect only the data that will be useful in determining nosocomial infections and causes.

Most of the information and assessments needed to complete the worksheet will be available from the resident's chart. It is very important for the ICP to review all microbiology and radiology reports. Data collected on community-acquired infections will be useful in tracking secondary infection cases needing isolation and in identifying potential epidemics.

The form itself is not a part of the resident's medical record; rather, it is a worksheet to help the ICP collect and analyze data. The form is used for any resident who has an infection, any resident confined to isolation precautions, any resident with a communicable or reportable disease, and any resident who has a culture ordered. Each resident's nosocomial infection becomes a statistic for the monthly infection report.

Nosocomial Determination

When an infection is found, the ICP must decide whether or not that infection is nosocomial. Nosocomial determinations can be made once all the data related to the resident's infection are gathered. However, in complicated cases the ICP may request assistance from the medical director or another physician. Such assistance will often involve differentiating between infection and colonization or determining a feasible incubation period for the resident's infection. The ICP must keep in mind that a nosocomial infection is one that was not present or incubating at the time of admission to the LTCF. It is critical that the date of onset of the resident's signs and symptoms be specifically identified. This date (and sometimes hour) must be considered along with the known incubation period of the infection. If the incubation period is unknown and the infection developed more than 48 hours after admission, it is called *nosocomial*. Any infection with obvious signs and symptoms noted upon admission is easily classified as *community-acquired*.

Analysis of infection initially involves determining if the resident is truly infected or merely colonized. Information necessary for this decision is based on the signs and symptoms; for example, residents who are merely colonized rarely have fever or wound drainage. Culture results are beneficial in identifying true infections. Most LTCFs use a commercial laboratory outside the institution. Specimens must be transported outside the building where inocula-

tion of culture media is done. Obtaining accurate results from the culture depends upon correct technique in culturing the body site and appropriate transportation of the specimen to the laboratory. Culture techniques are reviewed in Chapter 1.

The ICP should be able to recognize possible superinfection in the resident already infected. A resident compromised by infection is vulnerable to invasion by other microorganisms in that same or another body site. Similarly, a resident may have more than one infection at the same time. Therefore, each infection should be recorded and counted as a separate nosocomial infection.

The worksheet should be kept in the ICP's notebook until all information is obtained and the determination is made. This worksheet should be used until the resident's infection resolves, the resident transfers, or death occurs.

DATA ANALYSIS

Record Keeping

A continuous record of all infections present within the institution must be kept. The information recorded on the infection worksheet is then transferred to a line-listing. In order to meet the individual needs of the ICP, a *line-listing form* can be developed (Fig. 10.3).

This form is kept for quick reference and to provide an overview of the infections present within the LTCF for a given month. Sometimes in an outbreak or cluster of infections the index case (first case of an outbreak) may be community-acquired. However, the other cases caused by this infection will be nosocomial. For this reason, all infections occurring within the facility, both nosocomial and community-acquired, should be line-listed.

The form can be hand-printed and lined. It can be duplicated by a conventional copying machine using 8 1/2 x 14–inch paper in order to provide adequate space for data.

Computing Nosocomial Infection Rates

In Chapter 1, it was pointed out that numbers of infections are not as useful for analysis as infection *rates*. The infection rate takes into account fluctuation in resident base (denominator). Infection rates are used within an institution to provide a common basis for evaluating surveillance data. In acute care hospitals in the United States, about 5% to 10% of all patients develop nosocomial infections. Thus,

Figure 10.3 *Line Listing Form*

Month _____ Year _____

ROOM	NAME	AGE	SEX	SITE	PROCEDURE RELATED	SIGNS/ SYMPTOMS	M.D. DIAGNOSIS	DATE OF ONSET	CULTURE DATE	CULTURE RESULTS	TREAT- MENT	COM- MENTS	COMMUNITY ACQUIRED	EXPIRED

the incidence rate for nosocomial infections is 5% to 10%. Similar rates have been found in LTCF populations (see Chapter 4). During the first 12 months of a surveillance program, infection rates can be determined in order to develop a data base for future comparison. Comparison to the facility's own prior rates is the most valid standard for evaluating change.

Most acute care hospitals calculate rates based on infections per 100 discharges or infections per 1,000 patient days.[6] Because the number of resident discharges from a LTCF is usually low, the average census per month or the number of resident-days is a more significant figure. These figures can be obtained from the administration of the facility.

To begin the task of computing a nosocomial infection rate, the ICP must accumulate infection worksheets and count the new nosocomial infections. The total becomes the numerator for the computation. This number is placed over the denominator (e.g., resident-days/month).

For example, assume a facility has an average daily census of 140 for July (31 days in July). The ICP finds 14 new nosocomial infections during this month. The nosocomial infection rate is

$$\frac{14}{(140 \times 31)} \times 1,000 = 3.2 \text{ (infections per 1,000 resident - days)}$$

or

$$\frac{14}{140} \times 100 = 10 \text{ infections / 100 residents / month}$$

The same method of calculation is used to compute monthly infection rates per nursing unit or area.

Examples

Oak Hall: Four nosocomial infections for July; census = 46. The nosocomial infection rate is

$$\frac{4}{46 \times 31} \times 1,000 = 2.8 \text{ infections / 1,000 resident days}$$

Walnut Hall: Seven nosocomial infections for July; census = 47. The nosocomial infection rate is

$$\frac{7}{47} \times 100 = 14.9 \text{ infections / 100 residents / month}$$

Incidence rates, as exemplified above, reflect the number of new infections occurring in the LTCF. A *prevalence* rate may also be used; this is the percentage of persons in a population who have a nosocomial infection at any given time. For example, if a one-day study reveals 7 residents with active nosocomial infections and the facility has 140 residents, then the nosocomial infection prevalence rate is

$$\frac{7}{140} \times 100 = 5\%$$

The prevalence rate identifies the number of infections at a particular point in time. Such a rate is usually determined with data accumulated over a single 24-hour period. All available charts of residents within the facility are systematically reviewed, and any resident with an infection is identified and documented. The criteria for infection (infection definitions) used in surveillance can be used in prevalence studies also (see the appendix). Prevalence infection rates may have value for a LTCF infection control program. Prevalence rates may be done at regular intervals in order to test the validity of monthly incidence rates; they may also help to establish priorities for infection control efforts. Prevalence studies will obviously require more surveillance time and personnel, and should be carefully undertaken and planned.

Whatever rate is used in the analysis of infection data, several points should be kept in mind. First, rates should be consistent (i.e., use the same collection methods and denominator data) so that comparisons are valid. Second, nosocomial infection rates should be used by the ICP to look for deviations from normal that may suggest an outbreak or to solve infection control problems.[7]

Analysis of Nosocomial Infection Rates

As surveillance data are accumulated and organized, the ICP should be continually searching for clusters of infections either at the same body site or with the same microorganism (see Chapter 11). Clusters of residents with similar symptoms should also be noted. Surveillance data should be evaluated at the end of each week and at the end of the month, when infection rates and statistics are made available. The weekly review will be a brief assessment of developing trends.

Seasonal trends should also be noted. These are annual variations in occurrence of particular diseases that increase when circumstances facilitate transmission. An example of a seasonal trend is an increase in respiratory infections occurring during the cold winter months.

Caution should be used when comparing statistics such

as monthly nosocomial infection rates with other LTCFs or acute care hospitals. Each facility has its own acuity level and individualized method of calculating statistics, so to compare rates outside an institution is dangerous and may lead to erroneous conclusions. For this reason, infection rates are usually confidential information for the facility. An exception to this rule might be a situation where a group of LTCFs is managed collectively; comparison among the individual facilities may be requested by administration. This comparison is valid only if all facilities use the same method of calculating infection rates and serve comparable resident populations.

Comparison is one of the major reasons for surveillance, however. The most beneficial and significant comparison is the comparison of the infection rate for one month with that of the same month last year. This analysis deemphasizes seasonal trends. A similar evaluation is the comparison of the rate for one month with that of the previous month. Another potential comparison is the comparison of one nursing unit with another unit, although this is significant only if the units have comparable resident populations and nursing staffing. A desired outcome of surveillance is to generate comparison in order to change the behavior of persons or change environmental factors, with the ultimate goal to minimize the infection rate.

Reporting of Results

A report summarizing the nosocomial infection rates should be prepared, reported, and discussed with administration, the medical director, department heads, and nursing staff each month. The ultimate goal of surveillance is to improve resident care; infection rates therefore become a progress report for staff and others concerned with the quality of care. An example of an *infection control monthly report form* is seen in Figure 10.4.

Infection data may be presented in a more visually appealing form with the use of visual aids such as graphs or charts. Simple, concise graphs will outline trends that can be visualized and understood by most employees, even those unfamiliar with surveillance methods and computation of statistics. Examples of graphs are shown in Figure 14.1.

Reporting nosocomial infection rates to the staff can provide positive as well as negative feedback. Infection statistics and reports should not merely be filed, because behavior does not change without knowledge of the need for change. In-service education topics may be derived from the reports to influence resident care practices (see Chapter 14). Employee input into possible factors for increases or decreases in specific infection rates is a valuable resource and will facilitate learning. The LTCF ICP has a great deal of opportunity to influence resident care techniques that impact on infection control.[8]

The availability and use of computer infection control software programs have enabled the ICP to enter and retrieve data more efficiently. Computer-generated charts and graphs may provide the ICP with additional visual aids but are not necessary for a workable surveillance program.

Use of Surveillance Data in Infection Control

The goal of surveillance is to use infection control data to prevent infections. Data can be used to identify problems and develop and monitor control efforts (as in any quality improvement program). Surveillance data are also useful for detecting epidemics, directing educational programs, and identifying individual resident infection problems that may need treatment.

SUMMARY

A surveillance program must be individually developed for each LTCF. It should be simple and basic at first. After acceptance has been established within the institution, the program can be extended. Data collection should be done continually. Weekly, monthly, quarterly, and annual evaluations of data to detect trends provide the most benefit for the time spent in data collection. Ongoing, prospective surveillance is more beneficial than retrospective methods (e.g., chart reviews) because it permits earlier detection of infection control problems such as epidemics.

Surveillance can be organized efficiently through the use of forms. After information is collected it must be analyzed. The relationship among admission date, onset of symptoms of infection, and any predisposing factor is critical for the determination of nosocomial origin.

LTCF surveillance efforts should include (1) documentation of baseline levels, (2) detection of infectious disease outbreaks, (3) identification of residents who require follow-up, and (4) utilization of data regarding actual conditions to further education of staff members.[9]

Figure 10.4 *Infection Control Monthly Report - _____*

(Month)

DATE: _____, _____

    Month   Year

Total Number New Nosocomial Infections: _____

Resident Days per Month: _____

Infection Rate: _____ (Infections/1,000 Resident-Days)

Incidence Rate Formula:

$$\frac{\text{\# New Infections / Month}}{\text{Resident - Days/ Month}} \times 1,000 = \text{Infections /1,000 Resident - Days}$$

SITE	*NOSOCOMIAL INFECTIONS*	*COMMUNITY-AQUIRED INFECTIONS*
UTI (Urinary Tract)	_____	_____
SST (Skin Soft Tissue)	_____	_____
LRT (Lower Respiratory)	_____	_____
GI (Gastrointestinal)	_____	_____
EENT (Eye, Ear, Nose, Throat)	_____	_____
Other	_____	_____
Total	_____	_____

Infection Rate/Resident Care Area

	INFECTIONS	*RESIDENT-DAYS*	*INFECTIONS/1,000 RESIDENT DAYS*
Area 1	_____	_____	_____
Area 2	_____	_____	_____
Area 3	_____	_____	_____

Quality Improvement Conclusions/Actions:_____

_____

_____

_____

_____

_____

APPENDIX

DEFINITIONS OF INFECTION FOR SURVEILLANCE IN LONG-TERM CARE FACILITIES*

Principles

The definitions presented here are not all-inclusive. They focus on infections for which surveillance is expected to be useful (i.e., infections that are common and can be acquired in and detected by the facility). Three important conditions apply to all the definitions:

1. All symptoms must be new or acutely worse. Many residents have chronic symptoms, such as cough or urinary urgency, that are not associated with infection. However, a change in the resident's status is an important indication that an infection may be developing.
2. Noninfectious causes of signs and symptoms should always be considered before a diagnosis of infection is made.
3. Identification of infection should not be based on a single piece of evidence. Microbiologic and radiologic findings should be used only to confirm clinical evidence of infection. Similarly, physician diagnosis should be accompanied by compatible signs and symptoms of infection.

Respiratory Tract Infection

Common Cold Syndromes/Pharyngitis

The resident must have at least two of the following signs or symptoms: (a) runny nose or sneezing, (b) stuffy

nose (i.e., congestion), (c) sore throat or hoarseness or difficulty in swallowing, (d) dry cough, (e) swollen or tender glands in the neck (cervical lymphadenopathy).

Comment. Fever may or may not be present. Symptoms must be new, and care must be taken to ensure that they are not caused by allergies.

Influenza-Like Illness

Both of the following criteria must be met:

1. Fever (≥38°C)—a single temperature of ≥38°C. taken at any site.
2. The resident must have at least three of the following signs or symptoms: (a) chills, (b) new headache or eye pain, (c) myalgias, (d) malaise or loss of appetite, (e) sore throat, (f) new or increased dry cough.

Comment. This diagnosis can be made only during influenza season. If criteria for influenza-like illness and another upper or lower respiratory tract infection are met at the same time, only the diagnosis of influenza-like illness should be recorded.

* Adapted from: McGeer A, et al: Definitions of infection for surveillance in long-term care facilities. Am J Infect Control 1991;1:1–7 (with permission).

Pneumonia

Both of the following criteria must be met:

1. Interpretation of a chest radiograph as demonstrating pneumonia, probable pneumonia, or the presence of an infiltrate. If a previous radiograph exists for comparison, the infiltrate should be new.
2. The resident must have at least two of the signs and symptoms described under "other lower respiratory tract infections."

Comment. Noninfectious causes of symptoms must be ruled out. In particular, congestive heart failure may produce symptoms and signs similar to those of respiratory infections.

Other Lower Respiratory Tract Infections (Bronchitis, Tracheobronchitis).

The resident must have at three of the following signs or symptoms: (a) new or increased cough, (b) new or increased sputum production, (c) fever ($\geq 38°C$), (d) pleuritic chest pain, (e) new or increased physical findings on chest examination (rales, rhonchi, wheezes, bronchial breathing), (f) one of the following indications of change in status or breathing difficulty: new/increased shortness of breath or respiratory rate >25 per minute or worsening mental or functional status. The latter is defined as significant deterioration in the resident's ability to carry out the activities of daily living or in the resident's cognitive status, respectively.

Comment. This diagnosis can be made only if no chest film was obtained or if a radiograph failed to confirm the presence of pneumonia.

Urinary Tract Infection

Urinary tract infection includes only symptomatic urinary tract infections. Surveillance for asymptomatic bacteriuria (defined as the presence of a positive urine culture in the absence of new signs and symptoms of urinary tract infection) is not recommended, as this represents baseline status for many residents.

Symptomatic Urinary Tract Infection

One of the following criteria must be met:

1. The resident does not have an indwelling urinary catheter and has at least three of the following signs and symptoms: (a) fever ($\geq 38°C$) or chills, (b) new or increased burning pain on urination, frequency or urgency, (c) new flank or suprapubic pain or tenderness, (d) change in character of urine, (e) worsening of mental or functional status (may be new or increased incontinence). Change in character of urine may be clinical (e.g., new bloody urine, foul smell, or amount of sediment) or as reported by the laboratory (new pyuria or microscopic hematuria). For laboratory changes, this means that a previous urinalysis must have been negative.
2. The resident has an indwelling catheter and has at least two of the following signs or symptoms: (a) fever ($\geq 38°C$) or chills, (b) new flank or suprapubic pain or tenderness, (c) change in character of urine, (d) worsening of mental or functional status.

Comment. It should be noted that urine culture results are not included in the criteria. However, if an appropriately collected and processed urine specimen was sent and if the resident was not taking antibiotics at the time, then the culture must be reported as either positive or contaminated.

Because the most common occult infectious source of fever in catheterized residents is the urinary tract, the combination of fever and worsening mental or functional status in such residents meets the criteria for a urinary tract infection. However, particular care should be taken to rule out other causes of these symptoms. If a catheterized resident with only fever and worsening mental or functional status meets the criteria for infection at a site other than the urinary tract, only the diagnosis of infection at this other site should be made.

Eye, Ear, Nose, and Mouth Infection

Conjunctivitis

One of the following criteria must be met:

1. Pus appearing from one or both eyes, present at least 24 hours.

2. New or increased conjunctival redness, with or without itching or pain, present for at least 24 hours (also known as "pink eye").

Comment. Symptoms must not be due to allergy or trauma to the conjunctiva.

Ear Infection

One of the following criteria must be met:

1. Diagnosis by a physician of any ear infection. This requires a written note or a verbal report from a physician specifying the diagnosis. Usually implies direct assessment of the resident by a physician. An antibiotic order alone does not fulfil this criterion. In some facilities, it may be appropriate also to accept a diagnosis made by other qualified clinicians (e.g., nurse practitioner, physician associate).
2. New drainage from one or both ears. (Nonpurulent drainage must be accompanied by additional symptoms, such as ear pain or redness).

Mouth and Perioral Infection

Oral and perioral infections, including oral candidiasis, must be diagnosed by a physician or a dentist.

Sinusitis

The diagnosis of sinusitis must be made by a physician.

Skin Infection

Cellulitis/Soft Tissue/Wound Infection.

One of the following criteria must be met:

1. Pus present at a wound, skin, or soft tissue site.
2. The resident must have four or more of the following signs or symptoms: (a) fever ($\geq 38°C$) or worsening mental/functional status; *and/or*, at the affected site, the presence of new or increasing (b) heat, (c) redness (d) swelling, (e) tenderness or pain, (f) serous drainage.

Fungal Skin Infection

The resident must have both (a) a maculopapular rash and (b) either physician diagnosis or laboratory confirma-

tion. For *Candida* or other yeast, laboratory confirmation includes positive smear for yeast or culture for *Candida species.*

Herpes Simplex and Herpes Zoster Infection

For a diagnosis of cold sores or shingles, the resident must have both (a) a vesicular rash and (b) either physician diagnosis or laboratory confirmation (positive electron microscopy or culture of scraping or swab).

Scabies

The resident must have both (a) a maculopapular and/or itching rash and (b) either physician diagnosis or laboratory confirmation (positive microscopic examination of scrapings).

Comment. Care must be taken to ensure that a rash is not allergic or secondary to skin irritation.

Gastrointestinal tract infection

Gastroenteritis

One of the following criteria must be met:

1. Two or more loose or watery stools above *what is normal* for the resident within a 24-hour period.
2. Two or more episodes of vomiting in a 24-hour period.
3. Both of the following: (a) a stool culture positive for a pathogen (*Salmonella, Shigella, E. coli* 0157:H7, *Campylobacter*) or a toxin assay positive for *C. difficile* toxin and (b) at least one symptom or sign compatible with gastrointestinal tract infection (nausea, vomiting, abdominal pain or tenderness, diarrhea).

Comment. Care must be taken to rule out noninfectious causes of symptoms. For instance, new medications may cause both diarrhea and vomiting; vomiting may be associated with gallbladder disease.

Systemic Infection

Primary bloodstream infection

One of the following criteria must be met:

1. Two or more blood cultures positive for the same organism.

2. A single blood culture documented with an organism thought not to be a contaminant and at least one of the following: (a) fever (≥38°C), (b) new hypothermia (<34.5°C, or does not register on the thermometer being used), (c) a drop in systolic blood pressure of >30 mm Hg from baseline, or (d) worsening mental or functional status.

Comment. Bloodstream infections related to infection at another site are reported as secondary bloodstream infections and are not included as separate infections.

Unexplained Febrile Episode

The resident must have documentation in the medical record of fever (≥38°C) on two or more occasions at least 12 hours apart in any 3-day period, with no known infectious or noninfectious cause.

REFERENCES

1. Thacker SB, Keewhan C, Brachman PS: The surveillance of infectious diseases. *JAMA* 1983;249:1181–1185.
2. Smith PW, Rusnak PG: APIC guideline for infection prevention and control in the long-term care facility. *Am J Infect Control* 1991;19:196–215.
3. Smith PW: Infections in long-term care facilities (editorial). *Am J Infect Control* 1985;6:435.
4. McGeer A, et al: Definitions of infection for surveillance in long-term care facilities. *Am J Infect Control* 1991;1:1–7.
5. Garner JS, Jarvis WR, Emori TG, et al: CDC definitions for nosocomial infections, 1988. *Am J Infect Control* 1988;16:128–140.
6. Smith PW: Infection surveillance in long-term care facilities. *Infect Control Hosp Epidemiol* 1991;12:55–58.
7. Latham EK, Standfast SJ, Baltch AL, et al: The prevalence survey as an infection surveillance method in an acute and long-term care institution. *Am J Infect Control* 1981;9:76–81.
8. Satterfield N: Infection control in long-term care facilities: The hospital-based practitioner's role. *Infect Control Hosp Epidemiol* 1993;14:40–47.
9. Vlahov D, Tenney T, Cervino K, et al: Routine surveillance for infection in nursing homes: Experience at two facilities. *Am J Infect Control* 1987;15:47–53.

CHAPTER

11

EPIDEMIC INVESTIGATION

Philip W. Smith

This chapter is devoted specifically to outbreaks that have been reported in nursing homes and a discussion of the general approach to a nursing home epidemic. Epidemics may be classified broadly into *common-vehicle* outbreaks and outbreaks spread by *cross-contamination*. The latter refers to outbreaks propagated by person-to-person spread, whereas common-vehicle outbreaks occur when a number of individuals are exposed to the same epidemic source.

Many common vehicles have been responsible for transmission of infections, including food, water, medications, and even air. The infection may disseminate by contact (with an object such as a bronchoscope transmitting the infection), by airborne spread (e.g., suspension of particles by coughing), or by a vector (e.g., spread of encephalitis by mosquitoes). Some epidemics have features of both types of outbreaks. Salmonellosis, for example, may initially involve persons from a foodborne common source and spread secondarily to others by cross-contamination (fecal-oral route).

EPIDEMICS IN NURSING HOMES

Most nosocomial infections in the nursing home are endemic, but an important percentage occur in epidemics. These are theoretically more preventable than endemic nosocomial infections. LTCF epidemics are significant because of (a) the threat of morbidity and mortality to residents and employees, (b) the cost of investigation and treatment of cases, and (c) the potential adverse publicity for the nursing home.

Garibaldi[1] noted clustering of cases of upper respiratory tract infections, diarrhea, conjunctivitis, and urinary tract infections, suggesting that outbreaks of these infections occur frequently in the nursing home. In a survey of Nebraska nursing homes, 60% reported the occurrence of at least one infectious disease epidemic, most commonly respiratory tract infections, during the preceding year. An average of 30 residents and 13 staff were estimated to be involved in each epidemic.[2] Subsequent surveys have documented the great variety of epidemics in this setting. Personnel need to consider their potential role in the evolution of epidemics and constantly consider the decreased resistance of the institutionalized elderly resident to infectious diseases.

Respiratory Disease Outbreaks

Most respiratory disease outbreaks in nursing homes are spread by cross-infection involving airborne particle spread (see Table 11.1).

Reported Outbreaks

Influenza spreads rapidly among susceptible persons and causes mortality predominantly among the elderly and the chronically ill. Many severe outbreaks of influenza A in the nursing home have been reported.[3–9] In one, 25% of the 120 residents in a nursing home developed an influenza-like illness, nine of the residents died (a case fatality ratio of 30%), and the median duration of illness was nine days.[5] Of the 13 residents hospitalized during the outbreak, 12

Table 11.1.   *Causes of Respiratory Tract Outbreaks in Nursing Homes*

Tuberculosis

Influenza A

Influenza B

Parainfluenza

Respiratory syncytial virus (RSV)

Streptococcus, group A

Hemophilus influenzae

Pertussis

Psittacosis

---

had clinical pneumonia on physical examination or chest x-ray. An influenza A virus was isolated from eight residents, most of whom had a fourfold rise in complement fixation antibody titer.

In the influenza B outbreak described by Hall, the attack rate was 36%, the mean duration of illness was 4.5 days, and temperatures as high as 40.9°C were noted.[4] Five residents were hospitalized for treatment of pneumonia, and one resident expired. In searching for epidemiologic clues to their outbreak, it was found that residents requiring only self-care nursing experienced higher attack rates, which may reflect the increased contact among ambulatory residents resulting in a greater opportunity for spread of the influenza virus. Also noted was an increased attack rate with increasing age, an increased attack rate associated with residents on a closed (locked) intermediate care ward, and a temporal association with residents who ate the majority of their meals in a common dining room.

Reported outbreaks demonstrate that influenza is a very contagious disease, with attack rates averaging 30% to 60% of unvaccinated residents. Complications are also significant, with an average 10% mortality rate noted in nursing home outbreaks, and residents frequently requiring hospitalization.

An outbreak at a skilled nursing facility in New York demonstrated the potential for *respiratory syncytial virus* (RSV) to cause illness in the institutionalized elderly as well as the potential for concurrent epidemics with more than one respiratory virus.[3] Residents usually recover in three to seven days without major complications.[10]

Another virus, *parainfluenza*, has been shown to cause respiratory illness among the elderly in extended care facilities.[11] Both residents and employees were involved in the outbreaks. Rhinoviruses, coronaviruses, and adenoviruses may also cause respiratory tract infections in nursing homes.[12]

Although *bacterial pneumonia* in the elderly is common, outbreaks in residential homes are quite unusual. Two cases of *Streptococcus pyogenes* pneumonia, a rare infection, were encountered in a nursing home and felt to be transmitted by respiratory spread in one case and foodborne spread in another case.[13] In both instances, the infections were suspected to have spread from personnel to residents. One of the residents expired. Outbreaks of *Hemophilus influenzae* respiratory tract disease in the elderly have occurred,[14,15] as have outbreaks of *pertussis*.[16] These pathogens reflect the declining immunity of the elderly nursing home resident. Even *psittacosis* can cause long-term care facility epidemics, traced to birds in a pet therapy program.[17]

Tuberculosis (TB) is a mycobacterial disease of low to moderate contagiousness that is the classic example of airborne spread of disease. This disease is more common among the elderly than among any other segment of the population. Stead reported a prevalence of positive TB skin tests of 12% when he tested entering residents in a nursing home in Arkansas.[18]

Although TB is not highly contagious, a case of contagious pulmonary disease may be clinically silent and spread to many residents before being diagnosed. Nursing home outbreaks are traced to a single, usually ambulatory resident who spreads infection to a significant number of residents and staff before being detected. Serious outbreaks of tuberculosis in nursing homes have been reported with some frequency,[18–24] involving both residents and staff. In one typical epidemic, 49 (30%) of 161 tuberculin-negative residents became infected after exposure to an infectious resident, as did 21 (15%) of 138 employees.[19] Progressive primary tuberculosis developed in eight infected residents, one of whom died.

Control Measures

A number of general control measures for terminating or preventing outbreaks of respiratory infections in nursing homes are suggested from the experience of nursing home respiratory epidemics described earlier:

1. Maintaining good health among employees is essential. In outbreaks in nursing homes as well as in hospitals, staff-to-resident transmission of infection has been involved. One needs to keep in mind that a staff member with mild or subclinical infection (e.g., an asymptomatic influenza case) may be the source of severe or even fatal disease in the relatively debilitated and immunocompromised elderly population. Hence, one needs to maintain an effective employee health program with tuberculosis screening and annual influenza vaccination. The nursing home should educate employees about the hazard of infection transmission to residents and encourage them to report potentially infectious diseases to an employee health nurse and maintain good personal hygiene. Employee health programs are discussed in greater detail in Chapter 16.

2. Simply alerting the staff or the nursing home to the presence of an outbreak and emphasizing standard infection control practices may terminate an outbreak. The staff should be reminded to wash hands before and after contact with every resident, especially during an outbreak.

3. During influenza outbreaks, some have recommended[5,8,25] barring the admission of residents from the community with a diagnosis of influenza, restricting high-risk residents' visitors during community outbreaks, and cohorting residents with influenza (separating residents with influenza from those who are not infected). Residents should receive the influenza vaccine annually (see Chapter 17). In some situations,

antiviral prophylaxis with amantadine may be appropriate during an institutional epidemic,[26,27] although amantadine resistance can occur.[9]

4. For outbreaks of influenza or other viral respiratory illnesses, it may be wise to undertake measures that will decrease contact between residents, such as discontinuing social activities, restricting acutely ill residents to one area, serving meals in residents' rooms instead of in a common dining room, and restricting resident-to-resident visitation.

5. When there is an outbreak of tuberculosis in a nursing home one needs to undertake a rapid and diligent search for an index case or source among residents and personnel. Available recommendations[21–24] also suggest screening residents and staff for TB with the appropriate skin test, respiratory isolation of pulmonary TB cases, and chemotherapy of infected residents (see Chapter 5).

Outbreaks of Gastrointestinal Disease

Epidemic gastrointestinal infections may be classified by the type of reservoir. The reservoir for *Shigella*, amoebae, typhoid fever, *Staphylococcus aureus*, *Giardia*, toxin-producing *Escherichia coli*, hepatitis A, hepatitis B, *Clostridium difficile* and viral gastroenteritis is people. Spread is generally from person to person, and when a foodborne outbreak occurs, it can usually be traced to an infected food handler. The source for *Clostridium perfringens*, *Bacillus cereus*, *Clostridium botulinum*, and non-typhoid *Salmonella* is food items, such as poultry, meat, or custard products.

Reported GI Epidemics

The most important gastrointestinal infections in nursing homes are listed in Table 11.2. The leading causes of person-to-person epidemic GI illnesses are viral gastroenteritis agents, whereas most foodborne outbreaks in nursing homes are caused by Salmonella species, Staphylococcus aureus, and Clostridium perfringens.[28]

Viral gastroenteritis is usually relatively mild clinically. The leading causes are Norwalk virus[29] and rotavirus.[30,31] In a study by the Centers for Disease Control and Prevention (CDC), 11 outbreaks of gastroenteritis due to Norwalk virus were described that resulted in two deaths in nursing home residents.[29] In the outbreak reported by Marrie, 19 of

Table 11.2   *Causes of Gastroenteritis Outbreaks in the Nursing Home*

Viral gastroenteritis
Salmonellosis
Shigellosis
Staphylococcus aureus
Giardiasis
Clostridium perfringens
Clostridium difficile colitis
Amebiasis
E. coli 0157:H7

34 geriatric residents and 4 of 23 staff assigned to the ward developed gastroenteritis, suggesting staff involvement in transmission of the disease.[31] Other viruses have also been reported.[32-34] The attack rate among both residents and staff is high in viral gastroenteritis outbreaks, not a surprising observation in view of the high frequency of fecal incontinence in nursing homes.

The *hepatitis A* (infectious hepatitis) virus is excreted in stool, and the risk of spread is significantly increased in the incontinent resident, although many residents have had hepatitis A and thus are immune. Institutional hepatitis A can occur in large epidemics, especially in mental institutions. *Hepatitis B* is rarely seen in nursing homes. A minor epidemic of hepatitis B at a home for the aged was described in which 6 of 59 residents at a nursing home developed hepatitis B, and the source was felt to be bath brushes that resulted in cross-contamination. One resident died in that outbreak, and the hepatitis virus was demonstrated in a decubitus ulcer.[35]

Shigellosis is an uncommon cause of person-to-person outbreaks in nursing homes, but shigellosis is clinically much more severe than viral gastroenteritis.

Two parasitic diseases have the potential to cause outbreaks of gastrointestinal illness in nursing homes. Outbreaks of *amebiasis* occur in institutions,[36] where person-to-person spread is usually involved. *Giardia lamblia* is a parasite that causes a milder disease than amebiasis. *Giardiasis* has occurred in mental institutions, and in one outbreak there was evidence for both foodborne and secondary person-to-person spread.[37]

Recently a number of outbreaks of *Clostridium difficile* diarrhea have been described in nursing homes.[38-40] The diarrhea is facilitated by antibiotic use (see Chapter 12), with spread of the organism by person-to-person means. High carriage rates and environmental contamination are often seen, and the outbreaks may be difficult to control.[38]

Reported Epidemics: Foodborne Gastroenteritis

Food poisoning, foodborne gastroenteritis occurring in nursing home epidemics, is most often due to nontyphoid *Salmonella, C. perfringens*, or *Staphylococcus aureus*.[28] Nursing home residents in this study accounted for 2.4% of the foodborne illness in the United States during those years but nearly 20% of the deaths.

Perhaps the most important type of infectious gastroenteritis occurring in the nursing home setting is *salmonellosis*.

Between 1963 and 1972, 112 of 395 outbreaks in the United States occurred in institutions.[41] Salmonellosis in this study was unusually severe in institutionalized persons, as evidenced by an overall case fatality ratio of 8.7% in nursing homes. A total of 48 deaths occurred in the 25 nursing home outbreaks over this period, and the mean number of residents ill with each outbreak was 22.

Outbreaks of nursing home–associated salmonellosis have been reported with some frequency. In one outbreak a total of 38 residents, 5 staff members, and 2 domiciliary contacts of one of the residents were found to be infected.[42] Residents may excrete *Salmonella* in their stool for weeks to months, increasing the chance for secondary person-to-person spread and prolongation of an epidemic. Most cases in the nursing home setting are traced to common vehicles such as poultry, poultry products, ungraded eggs, and milk products.

Most epidemics of food poisoning in the geriatric setting caused by *Clostridium perfringens* were related to preheated meat and poultry dishes that had been cooked one day and inadequately cooled or stored before serving on the following day. Such foods as stews, pies, rolled and minced meats, and chicken dishes are involved in the outbreaks. Nursing home outbreaks account for about 3% of all reported epidemics.[43] *Staphylococcus aureus* enterotoxin results in nausea and vomiting one to six hours after ingestion; baked goods, custard products, and prepared salads are most often implicated. *Bacillus cereus, Aeromonas, E. coli* 0157:H7, and *Campylobacter jejuni* cause occasional foodborne outbreaks in nursing homes.[28,44-46]

Control Measures

The outbreaks just described suggest a number of control measures for prevention and control of gastrointestinal outbreaks in nursing homes:

1. Promptly evaluate clusters of residents with diarrhea (see Chapter 8).
2. Bacterial isolates from stool should be saved by the nursing home or by the reference microbiology lab in the event that future studies of epidemiologic import are required. Leftover foods should be saved for culture.
3. It may be appropriate to suspect a human carrier, either a resident or staff member, in an outbreak of viral gastroenteritis, shigellosis, hepatitis A, *S. aureus*, amebiasis, or typhoid fever. Carriers may be asymptomatic.
4. During outbreaks of hepatitis A, salmonellosis, shigel-

losis, giardiasis, *Clostridium difficile* colitis, or viral gastroenteritis, enteric precautions may be appropriate for infected residents (see Chapter 19). Handwashing needs to be emphasized.

5. Ill residents should be treated appropriately. Antibiotics have no place in the treatment of viral gastroenteritis and are rarely helpful in the treatment of *Salmonella* infections, but they should be seriously considered for residents with amebiasis, giardiasis, shigellosis, *Salmonella typhi* infection or *Clostridium difficile* diarrhea.

6. Elective admission of residents to a nursing home during an epidemic should be deferred. In addition, all new residents should be questioned with regard to recent diarrhea, and when such a history is positive, stool cultures should be obtained.

7. In a foodborne outbreak, knowledge of the agent involved in the outbreak of gastroenteritis may give a clue as to the type of food to be investigated, such as looking for contaminated custard products in an outbreak of *Staphylococcus aureus* food poisoning or for eggs and poultry products in an outbreak of salmonellosis.

8. Proper food-handling and preparation practices should be specifically outlined and followed (see Chapter 18).

Diseases Spread by Contact

Bacterial Diseases

The reservoir of *gram-negative bacteria* is either residents (e.g., infected bladder or wound) or the environment (e.g., whirlpool tub). Examples of gram-negative bacteria of importance in the nursing home are *E. coli, Klebsiella, Proteus* and *Pseudomonas* (see Table 1.2). Gram-negative bacteria are the leading cause of nosocomial urinary tract infections in the nursing home and frequently are involved in infections of decubitus ulcers.

The reservoir of *gram-positive bacteria*, on the other hand, is generally people, either those infected with the bacteria or those carrying the organism without apparent harm (colonization). *Staphylococcus aureus* is a cause of skin infections such as cellulitis and abscesses as well as deep infections of decubitus ulcers and wounds. Staphylococci may be spread by the hands by personnel or by individuals who have staphylococcal skin infections. Asymptomatic persons may be nasal carriers of S. aureus and may spread the organism. Residents with staphylococcal skin infection frequently require isolation to prevent spread of this organism to others.

The group A beta-hemolytic *streptococcus* is a virulent gram-positive bacteria that causes serious skin infections. Like *S. aureus*, the reservoir for this organism is persons who are infected or who are carriers of the bacteria.

Cross-infection with any of these bacteria may occur in the nursing home. Both *S. aureus* and various gram-negative bacilli may cause infections of decubitus ulcers, gastrostomy tube sites, the urinary tract, or vascular access sites. Clusters of group A streptococcal infections in the nursing home have been well described and cause pneumonia, cutaneous infections, or toxic-shock-like syndrome.[13,47–49] Spread is from resident to resident or from a staff person. Control measures for residents with bacterial infections involve primarily good handwashing by personnel and physical separation of residents with infected lesions.

Resistant Bacteria

Outbreaks of infections caused by unusually resistant bacteria have occurred in nursing home facilities. There are reports of spread of multiply antibiotic-resistant gram-negative bacilli, particularly in residents with urinary tract infections who have indwelling bladder catheters.[50,51] Antibiotic usage contributes to selection of resistant bacteria.[51]

The greatest problem in nursing homes is *methicillin-resistant Staphylococcus aureus (MRSA)* infection.[52–57] The spread of resistant bacteria appears to occur primarily by the hands of personnel. MRSA results in clinical infections similar to sensitive *S. aureus*, but can be treated only with parenteral vancomycin, a toxic and expensive drug. The organism is extremely difficult to eradicate from infected or colonized individuals, and nursing homes with an established MRSA problem have great difficulty with control of spread. A number of measures have been used to terminate outbreaks in hospitals and nursing homes (see Chapter 12).

Other Problems

Conjunctivitis due to bacteria or viruses may be quite contagious. Secretion precautions are appropriate (see Chapter 19). *Scabies* has occurred in nursing home outbreaks.[58,59] Topical treatment is available (see Chapter 4). A thorough cleaning of the environment is also indicated and should include drapes, floors, walls, and bedding. The

---

Table 11.3   *Steps in Epidemic Investigation*

1. Verification of the epidemic
2. Proper communication
3. Case analysis
4. Formation of a tentative hypothesis
5. Institution of control measures
6. Completing the investigation

---

standard laundering and drying cycle should be adequate to kill mites in clothing and bedding.

STEPS IN INVESTIGATING AN EPIDEMIC

Epidemics in nursing homes affect residents and staff alike. An effective infection surveillance program as described in Chapter 10 permits early detection and control of epidemics. An orderly sequence of steps should be followed when evaluating a possible outbreak (see Table 11.3).

Verification of the Epidemic

Before spending time investigating an epidemic, one needs to confirm whether or not there indeed is an epidemic. An *epidemic* is defined as the excessive prevalence of an infectious disease in a community. In this case, the community is the nursing home population. It is frequently not easy to determine (a) if an infectious disease is present, (b) the incidence or prevalence rate of the disease, and (c) whether the rate exceeds the baseline rate. Pseudoepidemics due to misdiagnoses or erroneous analysis of data can occur in the nursing home and are often costly.[60]

Confirming the Diagnosis

In some instances, as in an outbreak of staphylococcal wound infections or *Shigella* gastroenteritis, one may readily confirm the diagnosis by a positive culture. The diagnosis of influenza and viral gastroenteritis, however, is primarily clinical, and many different etiologies pre-sent with an identical clinical picture. Hence, in order to carry out an objective investigation, one needs a case definition.

Case Definition

A good case definition will assist in the evaluation of an epidemic. Case definitions may be assigned with differing degrees of stringency, with differing results. For instance, let us assume that there is an outbreak of *Salmonella* gastroenteritis on a nursing home ward. If one defines a case as "a nursing home resident who developed fever and diarrhea on ward A of a nursing home in October," then one has a definition that is specific geographically and temporally, but based on a clinical diagnosis of gastroenteritis. Included in this definition will be the vast majority of the cases of *Salmonella* gastroenteritis that occurred during the epidemic, but other cases, such as residents with viral gastroenteritis or diarrhea related to medication, may be included coincidentally. The epidemic may thus be overestimated.

On the other hand, a very specific definition such as "a nursing home resident on ward A with a positive stool culture for *Salmonella* during October" may be used. In this case, however, one may be excluding from the investigation a number of cases of salmonellosis that were not cultured or were improperly cultured and thus did not fit the microbiologic definition of the disease. The epidemic may thus be underestimated.

One may stratify definitions into definite, probable, and possible cases or classify them according to whether or not they are outbreak-related. It is acceptable to refine a case definition as the investigation goes along. As an example, the initial case definition may encompass "nursing home residents with fever, cough, and a pulmonary infiltrate," but when the involved residents are found to have a positive tuberculosis (PPD) skin test, the case definition may be refined to include only "residents with fever, pulmonary infiltrate, and a positive PPD skin test."

Case Finding

Early in the course of the investigation of a potential epidemic, one needs to search for inapparent cases. A number of resources may be used, including the nursing home nurses, physicians who care for the residents, the reference microbiology laboratory (particularly when a specific organism has been identified), and local or state public health officials, who may be aware of outbreaks in other institutions.

The ability to characterize an outbreak depends on complete case finding. An epidemic may be larger than it first appears. A broad search may find cases earlier in time, in other areas of the nursing home, or even in other facilities.

Comparison to Normal Frequency

Knowledge of the baseline frequency of occurrence of an infectious problem is necessary in order to determine whether or not an epidemic exists. The decision as to whether an epidemic is occurring depends on the disease in question and the context. For instance, 20 urinary tract infections in a large nursing home may be a relatively normal occurrence, whereas a single new case of tuberculosis represents a worrisome finding. The presence of MRSA might be expected in a large hospital intensive care unit but would be quite significant in most nursing homes.

Two additional points need to be made here. First, the comparison to normal frequency is much easier if one deals with *rates* rather than raw numbers. Incidence and prevalence rates (see Chapter 1) facilitate objective decisions.

Example 1:

An observer feels that there are more urinary tract infections (UTIs) at nursing home A than usual. A prevalence survey revealed 15 UTIs compared to 9 during a prevalence survey three months ago. However, the nursing home census was 140 then and is 223 now. The prevalence rates are 15/223 = 6.7% and 9/140 = 6.4%, not significantly different.

It is hazardous to compare rates *between* institutions. A higher UTI rate, for example, may reflect the fact that a nursing home has a more accurate data collection system, performs more urine cultures, or has more residents with indwelling urinary catheters, rather than reflecting any deficiency in infection control practices.

As we have seen, the normal incidence and prevalence of disease varies tremendously depending on the disease itself and the setting. As a rough rule, if the incidence or prevalence of a given infectious disease has *doubled* from

the baseline incidence or prevalence, one should suspect an epidemic. A second point to be emphasized is that an epidemic may not become apparent until a more detailed analysis of the data is completed.

Example 2:

Further analysis of the UTIs in Example 1 is done by examining the bacteria causing the infections. Nine of the 15 current UTIs are found by urine culture to be caused by multiply antibiotic-resistant *Pseudomonas aeruginosa*, which was not seen in any urine samples in the previous survey. This definitely suggests an outbreak.

The microbiology laboratory can be of great assistance in analysis of organisms to prove whether bacterial isolates in an outbreak are identical or unrelated. Examples of such tests that can be done include antibiotic-sensitivity patterns, phage typing (*S. aureus*), pyocin typing (*Pseudomonas*), serotyping (streptococci), plasmid analysis (resistant bacteria), and restriction enzyme analysis (viruses). These tests are generally available only at reference laboratories.[61]

Proper Communication

Once it has been decided that there is an epidemic, it is important to communicate to the appropriate individuals early in the course of the investigation. There are several reasons for this. First of all, communication to appropriate physicians, nursing personnel, and nursing home administrators is courteous and avoids misunderstanding and confusion. Misinformation about an epidemic may cause panic. Second, this communication may lead to discovery of additional cases that can be included in the epidemic investigation. Finally, communication with public health officials is important because it may lead to recognition of an epidemic that extends beyond the boundaries of the individual nursing home and thereby has public health impact.

Case Analysis

Line Listing of Cases

An appropriate first step during an epidemic is to perform a line listing of cases that involves listing all cases involved in the epidemic in a column with a few key

Table 11.4   *Sample Line Listing: Outbreak of Diarrhea in a Nursing Home*

CASE NO.	PATIENT	AGE	DATE OF ONSET	ROOM
1	JS	84	6/2	A-16
2	RB	71	6/2	A-16
3	GS	59	6/2	A-19
4	AY	92	6/4	A-24
5	LL	68	6/10	B-3
6	TR	69	6/11	B-5

information bits on each case (see Table 11.4). Examples of baseline information include resident name, room number, age, date of onset of symptoms, and culture results. The line listing permits very rapid assessment of the extent and general nature of the outbreak. Line listings can be expanded to include other relevant data that may have bearing on the cause of the outbreak. For instance, in a respiratory disease outbreak, one may want to list information on chest x-rays or TB skin tests. In an outbreak of gastroenteritis, one may wish to list whether the resident eats in the room or in the common dining area and whether the resident is incontinent. In an outbreak of urinary tract infection, one needs to know whether residents have indwelling bladder catheters or are sharing rooms with residents who have indwelling bladder catheters.

Making an Epidemic Curve

Often it is easier to characterize an epidemic when results are in graphic form. The epidemic curve should be plotted with the number of cases on the vertical axis and time on the horizontal axis (see Fig. 11.1). The shape of the curve may facilitate classification of the epidemic in terms of exposure and method of spread. A *person-to-person* epidemic, for instance, is suggested by bimodal curves with a larger first peak and a smaller secondary wave of disease due to spread from the group of residents who were primarily infected to other susceptibles. This may be seen in influenza outbreaks. Another type of outbreak is a *common-source* outbreak, which may be further divided into single- or continuous-exposure epidemics. A sharply rising and falling

EPIDEMIC CURVES

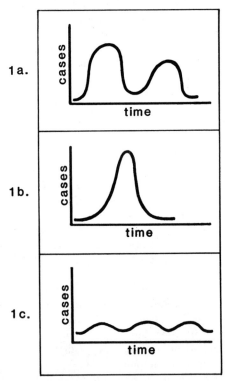

Figure 11.1   *Epidemic curves for typical person-to-person (1a), point exposure-common source (1b), and continuous exposure-common source (1c) outbreaks.*

Table 11.5 *Sample Frequency Listing: Outbreak of Respiratory Disease in a Nursing Home*

WARD LOCATION	NO. OF RESPIRATORY DISEASE CASES	NO. OF INFLUENZA CASES
1E	4	0
1W	8	1
2E	10	2
2W	12	9
3E	7	0
3W	10	2

curve suggests a *single-point exposure*, as in a staphylococcal food poisoning outbreak. A flat or undulating curve suggests *continuous exposure*, such as an outbreak of Legionnaires' disease related to a contaminated cooling tower.

Demographic Analysis

A demographic analysis involves the continued search for clues to the underlying cause. After the initial line listing and epidemic curve have been done, demographic analysis may be as simple as a more complex line listing looking for other common factors. A resident's medical history, geographic location in the nursing home, or contact with other residents or staff may provide information that gives a clue to the outbreak. Detailed food histories are necessary when investigating a foodborne outbreak.

Another aspect of demographic analysis is preparation of frequency distributions and graphs by time, place, and person. Listing or plotting locations of cases geographically may be useful when person-to-person spread is suspected (see Table 11.5). Such a case map may detect a focal outbreak.

Statistical Analysis

A refinement of the data collection process is the calculation of statistical rates. Outbreaks can usually be solved without complex statistics, but some statistical analysis may help the investigation. Basic statistics such as incidence rate, prevalence rate, and attack rate are useful tools (see Chapter 1).

Formation of a Tentative Hypothesis

At this point, one hopes to have characterized the outbreak thoroughly with regard to time, place, person, and possible mode of spread. It may be possible to estimate the incubation period by measuring the time from a common-source exposure to the mean date of onset of cases or by measuring the distance between primary and secondary epidemic curves in a person-to-person epidemic.

In order to form a hypothesis, reference sources must be consulted. Background information is gathered from studying the literature or consulting with others who have experience with the problem. Texts are available that describe diseases in terms of contagiousness, mode of spread, incubation period, period of communicability, symptoms, diagnosis, and control measures.[62,63] The literature may also reveal clues to the etiology by describing associations of organisms with certain vehicles, such as *Salmonella* and egg products.

Example 3:

In a published outbreak of *Acinetobacter* infections,[64] the epidemic curve displayed peaks in winter months. The institution was located in a cold climate, which led the authors to suspect and investigate room humidifiers as a source of airborne spread (see Fig. 11.2).

Example 4:

The data in Table 11.5 suggest an influenza cluster on ward 2W, probably originating from an infected

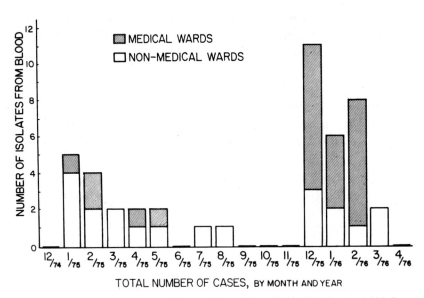

Figure 11.2   *Epidemic curve—Acinetobacter infections (From Smith PW, Massanari RM: Room humidifiers as the source of Acinetobacter infections. JAMA 1977; 237: 795-797. Copyright 1977, American Medical Association)*

resident, staff member, or visitor. A general list of respiratory diseases did not provide as much information as a specific listing of influenza cases.

Institution of Control Measures

Testing the Hypothesis

The hypothesis should be tested either by intervening with appropriate control measures to see if the epidemic disappears or by instituting further steps in data collection and analysis. In Example 3, the contaminated room humidifiers were removed and the epidemic ceased. More data were gathered by doing laboratory tests on bacterial colonization of room humidifiers as well as the potential of humidifiers to disperse airborne bacteria. It was found that humidifiers in infected patients' rooms were colonized with *Acinetobacter calcoaceticus* and that the contaminated humidifiers could spray the organism up to 10 meters.[64]

Other examples of data collection include culturing equipment or personnel, typing of organisms, and sending out questionnaires to gather more information. As a general rule, cultures of personnel and environment

should not be performed hastily or early in the investigation but selectively, after a hypothesis for possible spread of the epidemic organism has been developed. Indiscriminate culturing is expensive and may cause panic on the part of personnel or residents. However, collection and saving of specimens for future study is wise.

Implementing Control Measures

The goal of an epidemic investigation is, of course, to control or terminate the epidemic. In addition, the best test of the hypothesis frequently is to intervene (e.g., to remove humidifiers, to eliminate the suspected food, to treat the staphylococcal carrier) and then to see if the epidemic stops. Sometimes epidemics are terminated even if a precise cause is not pinpointed. This may be because the investigation itself reminds personnel of correct procedures (e.g., handwashing or cleaning instruments) about which they may have become lax. A reminder is often enough to improve performance and terminate the epidemic. Alternatively, ancillary control measures (such as isolation for tuberculosis cases) may stop an outbreak. These common sense measures to protect residents and personnel should be instituted early in the investigation and not await final results.

Causality

Because of the occasional random disappearance of epidemics during investigation, one must be cautious about ascribing credit to any particular individual control measure. In addition, it must be remembered that statistical association does not prove causality. For example, a nurse who is a staphylococcal nasal carrier may not be responsible for an outbreak of staphylococcal infection among residents. The nurse may have a different strain of *S. aureus* than the one that caused the epidemic. Alternatively, even if the nurse has the epidemic strain, she may have acquired it from a resident with an infected decubitus ulcer rather than the reverse (staff-to-resident transmission). Statistical or microbiological association should not necessarily imply guilt or causality.

Testing Effectiveness of Control Measures

Control measures, even if they seem logical, may not stop an epidemic. The search for new cases must go on. Failure of control measures requires reconsideration of the hypothesis.

Completing the Investigation

When recommendations to implement certain control measures are made, they should be made specifically and in writing. One may recommend modification of the environment, personnel changes, procedural or policy changes, or implementation of an educational program. Sometimes it is necessary to make interim recommendations until the exact cause of an outbreak has been defined.

During the investigation, one needs to save as much information as possible. All bacterial isolates collected during the investigation should be saved in the event that serotyping, phage typing, or antibiotic sensitivity testing is required. These tests may help to determine whether strains of bacteria cultured during an epidemic investigation are identical to the epidemic strain. All records, questionnaires, interviews, and line listings should be filed for further reference.

During the course of an investigation, appropriate persons should be informed of developments; this includes nursing home administrators, physicians, and public health officials.

Good records should be kept during the entire epidemic. At that conclusion of an epidemic, a complete and thorough report should be made and sent to all appropriate individuals. This report should include when and how the investigation was initiated, persons involved in the investigation, persons notified during the investigation, all data collected, the control measures implemented, and the effectiveness of these control measures.

ILLUSTRATIVE EXAMPLE: SALMONELLOSIS IN A NURSING HOME

The following relates the events during an actual epidemic of salmonellosis in a Nebraska nursing home that demonstrates appropriate investigation techniques.[*]

Background

The nursing home involved is a 72-bed community facility that employs about 60 employees. A single kitchen prepares food for all residents, and all but the bed feeders consume meals in a central dining room. The home has three wings that share one nursing station adjacent to the lounges and the dining room. The investigation was carried out by the state epidemiologist, Nebraska State Health Department. He was contacted initially by a physician from the nursing home area when it was noted that during a five-day period, 16 residents and 2 staff members of the nursing home became ill with diarrhea, fever, and vomiting.

Verification of the Outbreak

The records of all suspected cases were reviewed in order to confirm the presence of diarrhea. A case definition was developed. By this time, a number of residents had *Salmonella enteritidis* isolated from their stools. Hence, a case was

[*] The author wishes to thank Paul A. Stoesz, M.D., former Director, Disease Control Division, Nebraska State Health Department, for providing him with this case study.

Table 11.6   *Characteristics of Cases of Salmonellosis: Illustrative Example*

Case No.	Age	Sex	Onset of Illness	Diarrhea	Fever	Vomiting
1	83	F	9/11	+	+	–
2	71	F	9/12	+	+	–
3	90	F	9/12	+	+	–
4	–	F	9/12	+	+	–
5	74	F	9/11	+	+	–
6	88	F	9/11	+	+	–
7	96	F	9/11	+	+	+
8	91	F	9/11	+	+	–
9	80	F	9/11	+	+	–
10	94	F	9/11	+	+	–
11	66	F	9/11	+	+	–
12	89	F	9/12	+	+	–
13	83	F	9/11	+	+	–
14	82	F	9/10	+	+	–
15	101	F	9/11	+	+	–
16	97	F	9/13	+	+	–
17*	–	F	9/14	+	+	–
18*	–	F	9/14	+	+	+

*Staff members

defined as "a resident having a positive stool culture for *Salmonella* and any two of the following symptoms: abdominal pain, diarrhea, and fever."

Cases were collected by interviews with appropriate nursing home staff, including administrative staff, nurses, and physicians. The records of all suspected cases were reviewed to determine if each met the formulated case definition. It was determined that during a 5-day period, 16 residents and 2 staff members of the nursing home had become ill with diarrhea, and 12 of the 16 cases were found to be stool culture–positive for *Salmonella enteritidis*. Two of the 12 infected residents expired.

No precise baseline statistics had been kept at the nursing home during the previous years. However, all were in agreement that the number of cases of diarrhea in general and *Salmonella* in particular were greatly increased over normal.

Communication

The investigating team communicated with state public health officials and with all appropriate administrative and medical interests at the nursing home and in the local community.

Analysis of the Cases

A line listing of cases was completed (see Table 11.6). The nurses' notes were reviewed to determine the level of nursing care each resident required, type of diet, and other information. An epidemic curve was drawn (see Fig. 11.3). The shape of the curve suggested a common-vehicle outbreak with a single-point source exposure.

An investigation of the food service area was conducted to evaluate the role of sanitation. Food service personnel

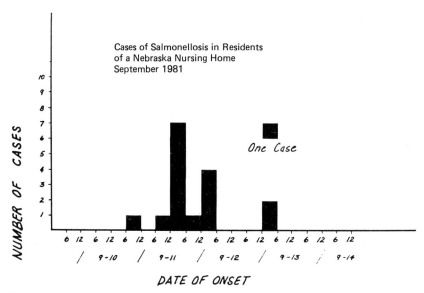

Figure 11.3   *Epidemic curve—Salmonella cases in a nursing home*

were interviewed in order to determine the sources of food served and the techniques of handling, storing, preparing, and serving food to the residents. The menus listing the food served at each meal for 72 hours prior to the first case were also reviewed. Food service personnel were questioned about their own prior gastrointestinal illness history.

At this point, selective stool cultures were performed on all residents suspected of being involved in the epidemic and all food service employees. Some of the food service equipment and several food samples were also cultured. All isolates of *Salmonella* obtained during this outbreak were sent to the Bureau of Laboratories at the Centers for Disease Control for serotyping.

Early in the investigation it was noted that a total of 18 residents were on pureed food and that 15 of the 16 cases fell in this group. Furthermore, none of those who were well had eaten the pureed diet. A review of menus for the 72 hours prior to the first case revealed four foods that were frequently associated with the transmission of *Salmonella*. When each of these foods was served in the pureed state, it was not served to the other residents. All of the food ingredients were from commercial sources, and three were leftovers from previous meals. The suspected foods were pureed in a blender just prior to serv-

ing. Roast beef and chicken were contained in the suspected foods. Only one food was available for culturing and was negative for *Salmonella*.

Investigation of the methods used to clean and sanitize food service equipment revealed no written protocol for kitchen workers to follow. There was a lack of supervision in the kitchen at all times, lack of monitoring of internal temperatures of foods during cooking and reheating, and lack of knowledge of the proper temperatures. No food service personnel had a history of gastrointestinal illness. All submitted stool cultures, and all were negative for *Salmonella*. Stool cultures on the 12 cases that were positive for *Salmonella enteritidis* were all confirmed as being serotype montevideo.

Formation of a Tentative Hypothesis

Several facts were evident at this point:

1. There was an outbreak of febrile diarrheal illness due to a certain *Salmonella* strain.
2. *Salmonella* outbreaks are usually foodborne, and deficiencies in food handling and preparation practices were noted.
3. The epidemic curve suggested a single-exposure, common-vehicle outbreak.

4. The only mode of transmission shared by all cases was food, suggesting a foodborne outbreak.

5. The food histories among the residents who had acquired salmonellosis suggested that the food was contaminated during the puree process.

6. It is known that the incubation period of *Salmonella* is 6 to 72 hours. The median onset of illness was 3:00 P.M. September 11. Hence the range of possible infected meals was 3:00 P.M. on September 8 through 9:00 A.M. on September 11.

Control Measures

It was impossible to test the impact of control measures on the epidemic curve because the point-source exposure period had passed without the occurrence of additional cases. The hypothesis was tested statistically when investigation revealed that 15 of 16 cases had eaten a pureed diet 72 hours prior to the onset of illness compared to none ill who had not eaten the pureed diet. This is highly statistically significant. An effort was made to confirm the theory microbiologically by culturing the blender, but this had been cleaned in the interim, and cultures were negative.

Interim control measures were immediately recommended by the Health Department at the initiation of the investigation. These included cohorting of staff members who treat residents, moving all infected cases into one wing of the nursing home, and recommending that no double rooms be shared by well and ill residents. It was decided that there would be no interchange of staff with resident contact from one wing to another, that no new residents would be allowed into the nursing home until the epidemic was resolved, and that all cases would be placed in enteric precautions. These control measures prevented secondary person-to-person propagation of the epidemic.

Completing the Investigation

A detailed final report was made that included a number of suggested control measures designed to prevent recurrence of the outbreak:

1. Food should be obtained from sources that comply with all laws relating to food inspection and labeling.

2. In food service areas, all food should be protected against contamination during storage, preparation, and serving. Potentially hazardous food requiring cooking should be cooked to heat all parts of the food to a temperature of at least 140°F. However, poultry, poultry stuffings, stuffed meats, and stuffings containing meat should be cooked to heat all parts of the food to at least 165°F, and pork or any food containing pork should be cooked to heat all parts of the food to at least 150°F.

3. A metal stem-type thermometer should be used in order to assure the attainment and maintenance of proper internal cooking, holding, or refrigeration temperatures of all potentially hazardous foods.

4. Potentially hazardous foods requiring refrigeration after preparation should be rapidly cooled to an internal temperature of 45°F or below. Potentially hazardous foods of large volume or prepared in large quantities should be rapidly cooled, utilizing such methods as shallow pans, agitation, quick chilling, or water circulation external to the food container so that the cooling period does not exceed four hours.

5. Food service equipment and utensils should be washed, rinsed, and sanitized after each use in order to prevent cross-contamination in the kitchen and to prevent the accumulation of food residue that may decompose or support the development of bacterial pathogens or toxins.

6. Food contact surfaces of equipment and utensils should be easily cleanable, smooth, and free of breaks and open seams that make such a surface impossible to clean and sanitize.

7. All operations of the food service should be supervised at all times. The supervisor should instruct the staff in their responsibilities through in-service training. In order to prevent contamination of food and food contact surfaces, employees must comply with strict standards of cleanliness and personal hygiene. This would include handwashing, clean clothing, and hair restraints.

8. The development of an infection control committee should be initiated considering the population of the nursing home. The committee could perform surveillance of infections in the facility to assist early epidemic control.

Control measures addressed washing, rinsing, and sanitizing of the kitchen equipment as well as proper food handling, holding, reheating, and serving. Cultures of all food service workers were negative. In view of this and the known epidemiology of *Salmonella* infections, it was suspected that the source was not a food service worker, but rather contaminated poultry, eggs, or meat that had been brought into the kitchen and, through inadequate cooking and reheating, led to infection of those who ate the food. The final report and recommendations were written clearly and specifically, as is ideal.

REFERENCES

1. Garibaldi RA, Brodine S, Matsumiya S: Infections among patients in nursing homes: Policies, prevalence and problems. *N Engl J Med* 1981;305:731–735.
2. Chaulk P: Infection control practices in Nebraska nursing homes. Presented at Consensus Conference on Nosocomial Infections in Long-Term Care Facilities. Omaha, NB, May 19–20, 1986.
3. Mathur U, Bentley DW, Hall CB: Concurrent respiratory syncytial virus and influenza A infections in the institutionalized elderly and chronically ill. *Ann Intern Med* 1980;93(Part 1):49–52.
4. Hall WN, Goodman RA, Noble GR, et al: An outbreak of influenza B in an elderly population. *J Infect Dis* 1981;144:297–302.
5. Goodman RA, Orenstein WA, Munro TF, et al: Impact of influenza A in a nursing home. *JAMA* 1982;247:1451–1453.
6. Centers for Disease Control. Control of influenza outbreaks in nursing homes: Amantadine as an adjunct to vaccine—Washington, 1989–1990. *MMWR* 1991;40:841–844.
7. Centers for Disease Control. Outbreak of influenza in a nursing home: New York, December 1991–January 1992. *MMWR* 1991;41:129–131.
8. Gravenstein S, Miller BA, Drinka P: Prevention and control of influenza outbreaks in long-term care facilities. *Infect Control Hosp Epidemiol* 1992;13:49–54.
9. Degelau J, Somami SK, Cooper SL, et al: Amantadine-resistant influenza A in a nursing facility. *Arch Intern Med* 1992;52:390–392.
10. Garvie DG, Gray J: Outbreak of respiratory syncytial virus infection in the elderly. *Br Med J* 1980;281:1253–1254.
11. Centers for Disease Control: Parainfluenza outbreaks in extended-care facilities: United States. *MMWR* 1978;27:475–476.
12. Falsey AR: Noninfluenza respiratory virus infection in long-term care facilities. *Infect Control Hosp Epidemiol* 1991;12:602–608.
13. Barnham M, Kerby J: *Streptococcus pyogenes* pneumonia in residential homes: Probable spread of infection from the staff. *J Hosp Infect* 1981;2:255–257.
14. Patterson JE, Madden GM, Krisiunas EP, et al: A nosocomial outbreak of ampicillin-resistant *Haemophilus influenzae* type B in a geriatric unit. J Infect Dis 1988;157:1002–100

15. Smith PF, Stricof RL, Shayegani M, et al: Cluster of *Haemophilus influenzae* type B infections in adults. JAMA 1988;260:1446–1449.
16. Addiss DG, Davis JP, Meade BD, et al: A pertussis outbreak in a Wisconsin nursing home. *J Infect Dis* 1991;164:704–710.
17. Robson D, Frederick H, Speerman G, et al: Avian psittacosis outbreak in a geriatric wing of a tertiary care hospital (abstract). Presented at Association for Practitioners in Infection Control 16th Annual Conference, Reno, NV, 1989.
18. Stead WW, Lofgren JP, Warren E, et al: Tuberculosis as an epidemic and nosocomial infection among the elderly in nursing homes. *N Engl J Med* 1985;312:1483–1487.
19. Stead WW: Tuberculosis among elderly persons: An outbreak in a nursing home. *Ann Intern Med* 1981;94:606–610.
20. Narain JP, Lofgren JP, Warren E, et al: Epidemic tuberculosis in a nursing home: a retrospective cohort study. *J Am Geriat Soc* 1985;33:258–263.
21. Bentley DW: Tuberculosis in long-term care facilities. *Infect Control Hosp Epidemiol* 1990;11:42–46.
22. Price LE, Rutala WA: Tuberculosis screening in the long-term care setting. *Infect Control* 1987;8:353–356.
23. Centers for Disease Control. Prevention and control of tuberculosis in facilities providing long-term care to the elderly: Recommendations of the Advisory Committee for Elimination of Tuberculosis. *MMWR* 1990;39:7–20.
24. Stern JK, Smith PW: Tuberculosis in the long-term care facility. *Geriatr Focus Infect Dis* 1991;1:6–10.
25. Arden NH, Kendal AP, Patriarca PA: *Managing an Influenza Vaccination Program in the Nursing Home.* U.S. Department of Health and Human Services, Centers for Disease Control, 1987.
26. Arden NH, Patriarca PA, Fasano MB, et al: The roles of vaccination and amantadine prophylaxis in controlling an outbreak of influenza A (H3N2) in a nursing home. *Arch Intern Med* 1988;148;865–868.
27. Patriarca PA, Arden NH, Koplan JP, et al: Prevention and control of type A influenza infection in nursing homes—benefits and costs of four approaches using vaccinations and amantadine. *Ann Intern Med* 1987;107:732–740.
28. Levine WC, Smart JF, Archer DL, et al: Foodborne disease outbreaks in nursing homes, 1975–1987. *JAMA* 1991;266:2105–2109.

29. Kaplan JE, Gary GW, Baron RC, et al: Epidemiology of Norwalk gastroenteritis and the role of Norwalk virus in outbreaks of acute nonbacterial gastroenteritis. *Ann Intern Med* 1982;96(Part 1):756–761.

30. Cubbit WD, Holzel H: An outbreak of rotavirus infection in a long-stay ward of geriatric hospital. *J Clin Path* 1980;33:306–308.

31. Marrie TJ, Lee SHS, Faulkner RS, et al: Rotavirus infection in a geriatric population. *Arch Intern Med* 1982;142:313–316.

32. Gelbert GA, Waterman SH, Ewert D, et al: An outbreak of acute gastroenteritis caused by a small round structured virus in a geriatric convalescent facility. *Infect Control Hosp Epidemiol* 1990;11:459–464.

33. Reid JA, Breckon D, Hunter PR: Infection of staff during an outbreak of viral gastroenteritis in an elderly persons' home. *J Hosp Infect* 1990;16:81–85.

34. Gordon SM, Oshiro LS, Jarvis WR, et al: Foodborne snow mountain agent gastroenteritis with secondary person-to-person spread in a retirement community. *Am J Epidemiol* 1990;131:702–710.

35. Braconier JH, Nordenfelt E: Serum hepatitis at home for the aged. *Scand J Infect Dis* 1972;4:79–82.

36. Krogstad DJ, Spencer HC Jr, Healy GR, et al: Amebiasis: Epidemiologic studies in the United States, 1971–1974. *Ann Intern Med* 1978;88:89–97.

37. White KE, Hedberg CW, Edmonson LM, et al: An outbreak of giardiasis in a nursing home with evidence for multiple modes of transmission. *J Infect Dis* 1989;160:298–304.

38. Bentley DW: *Clostridium difficile*-associated disease in long-term care facilities. *Infect Control Hosp Epidemiol* 1990;11:432–438.

39. Thomas DR, Bennett RG, Laughon BE, et al: Postantibiotic colonization with *Clostridium difficile* in nursing home patients. *J Am Geriatr Soc* 1990;38:415–420.

40. Brooks SE, Veal RO, Kramer M, et al: Reduction in the incidence of *Clostridium difficile*-associated diarrhea in an acute care hospital and a skilled nursing facility following replacement of electronic thermometers with single-use disposables. *Infect Control Hosp Epidemiol* 1992;13:98–103.

41. Baine WB, Gangarosa EJ, Bennett JV, et al: Institutional salmonellosis. *J Infect Dis* 1973;128:357–360.

42. Anand CM, Finlayson MC, Garson JZ, et al: An institutional outbreak of salmonellosis due to lactose-fermenting *Salmonella* newport. *Am J Clin Pathol* 1980;74:657–660.

43. Shandera WX, Tacket CO, Blake PA: Food poisoning due to *Clostridium perfringens* in the United States. *J Infect Dis* 1983;147:167–170.

44. DeBuono BA, Brondum J, Kramer JM, et al: Plasmid, serotypic and enterotoxin analysis of *Bacillus cereus* in an outbreak setting. *J Clin Microbiol* 1988;26:1571–1574.

45. Bloom HG, Bottone EJ: Aeromonas hydrophila diarrhea in a long-term care setting. *J Am Geriatr Soc* 1990;38:804–806.

46. Ryan CA, Tauxe RV, Hosek GW, et al: *Escherichia coli* 0157:H7 diarrhea in a nursing home: Clinical, epidemiological and pathological findings. *J Infect Dis* 1986;154:631–638.

47. Auerbach SB, Schwartz B, Williams D, et al: Outbreak of invasive group A streptococcal infections in a nursing home—lessons on prevention and control. *Arch Intern Med* 1992;152:1017–1022.

48. Harkness GA, Bentley DW, Mottley M, et al: *Streptococcus pyogenes* outbreak in a long-term care facility. *Am J Infect Control* 1992;20:142–148.

49. Schwartz G, Ussery XT: Group A Streptococcal outbreaks in nursing homes. *Infect Control Hosp Epidemiol* 1992;13:742–747.

50. Shlaes DM, Lehman MH, Currie-McCumber CA, et al: Prevalence of colonization with antibiotic resistant gram-negative bacilli in a nursing home care unit: the importance of cross-colonization as documented by plasmid analysis. *Infect Control* 1986;7:538–545.

51. Rice LB, Willey SH, Papanicolaou GA, et al: Outbreak of ceftazidime resistance caused by extended-spectrum β-lactamases at a Massachusetts chronic-care facility. *Antimicrobial Agents Chemother* 1990;34:2193–2199.

52. Hsu CCS, Macaluso CP, Special L, et al: High rate of methicillin-resistance of *Staphylococcus aureus* isolated from hospitalized nursing home patients. *Arch Intern Med* 1988;140:569–570.

53. Thomas JC, Bridge J, Waterman S, et al: Transmission and control of methicillin-resistant *Staphylococcus aureus* in a skilled nursing facility. *Infect Control* 1989;10:106–110.

54. Kauffman CA, Bradley SF, Terpenning MS: Methicillin-resistant *Staphylococcus aureus* in long-term care facilities. Infect Control Hosp Epidemiol 1990;11:600–603.

55. Hsu CCS: Serial survey of methicillin-resistant *Staphylococcus aureus* nasal carriage among residents in a nursing home. *Infect Control Hosp Epidemiol* 1991;12:416–421.

56. Muder RR, Brennen C, Wagener MM, et al: Methicillin-resistant staphylococcal colonization and infection in a long-term care facility. *Ann Intern Med* 1991;114:107–112.

57. Strausbaugh LJ, Jacobson C, Sewell DL, et al: Methicillin-resistant *Staphylococcus aureus* in extended care facilities: experience in a Veterans' Affairs nursing home and a review of the literature. *Infect Control Hosp Epidemiol* 1991;12:36–45.

58. Scabies in institutions. *J Iowa Med Soc* 1981;71:78–79.

59. Degelau J: Scabies in long-term care facilities. *Infect Control Hosp Epidemiol* 1992;13:421–425.

60. Poulin C, Schlech WF: A pseudo-outbreak in a nursing home. *Infect Control Hosp Epidemiol* 1991;12:521–522.

61. McGowan JE: New laboratory techniques for hospital infection control. *Am J Med* 1991;91(suppl):245–251.

62. Benenson AS (ed): *Control of Communicable Diseases in Man*, 15th ed. Washington DC, American Public Health Association, 1990.

63. Wehrle PF, Top FH Sr: *Communicable and Infectious Diseases*, 9th ed. St. Louis, Mosby, 1981.

64. Smith PW, Massanari RM: Room humidifiers as the source of *Acinetobacter* infections. *JAMA* 1977;237:795–797.

CHAPTER

ANTIBIOTICS

Jane S. Roccaforte and Philip W. Smith

OVERVIEW OF ANTIBIOTICS

Mechanisms of Action

The term *antibiotic* includes agents active against microorganisms ranging from viruses to parasites. The most commonly used agents are antibacterial drugs.

Antibacterial drugs generally act by one of five mechanisms: interference with cell wall synthesis, damaging the bacterial cell membrane, inhibition of DNA synthesis, inhibition of protein synthesis, or interference with bacterial metabolism.

Penicillins, cephalosporins, and vancomycin are drugs that act by interfering with bacterial cell wall synthesis. Penicillin itself is an extremely useful drug against streptococci, *Streptococcus pneumoniae, Neisseria meningitidis,* syphilis, and anaerobic infections. Because most strains of *Staphylococcus aureus* have become resistant to penicillin, members of the family of drugs that includes oxacillin, nafcillin, and dicloxacillin have become the drugs of choice for treatment of *S. aureus* infections. Ampicillin and amoxicillin are penicillin derivatives that are very useful against enterococci, *Hemophilus influenzae, Salmonella, Shigella, Escherichia coli,* and *Proteus mirabilis* infections. There are several broad-spectrum penicillins used parenterally against *Pseudomonas aeruginosa.* Included in this group are ticarcillin, mezlocillin, and piperacillin.

Clavulanate and sulbactam are beta-lactamase inhibitors that expand the spectrum of beta-lactam antibiotics when used in combination with them. Examples include amoxicillin/clavulanate, ticarcillin/clavulanate, and ampicillin/sulbactam.

The family of antibiotics known as cephalosporins is of great importance in treating staphylococcal and other infections in patients who are allergic to penicillins. Broad-spectrum cephalosporins, available in injectable and oral forms, are active against many of the gram-negative bacteria found in hospitals and long-term care facilities, but are expensive. Certain cephalosporins such as ceftazidime and cefoperazone are particularly useful against *Pseudomonas aeruginosa.*

Other beta-lactam antibiotics are available for clinical use. Imipenem is a very broad-spectrum agent active against gram-positive, gram-negative, and anaerobic organisms. In contrast, aztreonam, a monobactam, has a narrower focus and is quite useful in the treatment of infections due to aerobic gram-negative bacilli (see Table 1.2).

Bacterial protein metabolism is affected by a number of agents, including the aminoglycosides, clindamycin, chloramphenicol, and the macrolides. Aminoglycosides are effective against the great variety of gram-negative bacteria found in the hospital and long-term care facility environments. They can be given only parenterally; the most widely used aminoglycosides are gentamicin, tobramycin, and amikacin. Clindamycin is an appropriate drug for treating anaerobic infections, and erythromycin may be used for *Mycoplasma* pneumonia, for Legionnaires' disease, and as an alternative to penicillin for streptococcal infections. Newer macrolides such as azithromycin and clarithromycin expand the coverage that erythromycin provides to include organisms such as *H. influenzae* and *M. catarrhalis,* bacteria of importance in respiratory tract infections.

Sulfonamides are examples of antibiotics that act by interfering with bacterial metabolism. Sulfonamides, pyrimethamine, and trimethoprim interfere with folate metabolism in microorganisms. Sulfonamides and trimethoprim are used orally alone or in combination primarily for the treatment of urinary tract infections.

Quinolones are bactericidal drugs that act by inhibiting the function of DNA in bacterial cells. This class of antimicrobial agents shows greatest activity against gram-negative organisms. Examples include norfloxacin, ciprofloxacin, ofloxacin, and lomefloxacin. These agents are of interest in the LTCF because of long half-lives and the fact that all can be given orally. They are the only oral compounds active against *Pseudomonas.*

The development of effective antiviral agents has been limited by the difficulty in killing the virus without damaging the human cell in which it lives. As a result, a limited number of antiviral agents are available. Acyclovir can be used intravenously, orally, or topically for herpes simplex infections and severe herpes zoster/varicella infections such as shingles. Amantadine and rimantadine are available for prophylaxis and treatment of influenza A infections. These drugs interfere with the penetration of viruses into human cells or with viral nucleic acid replication. A number of agents, such as zidovudine, have activity against HIV.

Antifungal agents generally alter the fungal cell membrane. Amphotericin B can be administered only intravenously in the therapy of fungal infections. Three oral drugs of assistance in the treatment of fungal infections are ketoconazole, fluconazole, and itraconazole. They are indicated for moderate to severe fungal infections such as mucocutaneous candidiasis, cryptococcosis, and histoplasmosis.

Pharmacokinetics

Patients not requiring hospitalization are usually treated with oral antibiotics. Food, antacids, and malabsorptive disorders often interfere with drug absorption. Intramuscular administration should be avoided in the presence of shock and bleeding disorders. Intravenous administration assures reliable blood levels but requires the presence of an intravenous cannula.

Antibiotics may also be classified by their route of elimination (see Table 12.1). Drugs excreted by the kidney should be used with extreme caution in the presence of renal disease. Drug elimination is measured by the half-life ($t_{1/2}$), the time it takes a normal person to lower the level of antibiotic in blood by 50%. The longer the $t_{1/2}$, the fewer daily doses of antibiotic needed for adequate therapy.

Side Effects

Toxicity

Toxicity is defined as a dose-related or expected side effect of a drug. This will inevitably occur if a drug is used long enough and at a high enough dosage. Examples of antibiotic toxicity include renal failure and deafness (aminoglycosides), vertigo (streptomycin), hepatitis (ketoconazole), and seizures (imipenem/cilastatin). Antibiotic toxic effects may or may not be reversible. Aminoglycoside nephrotoxicity is generally reversible when the drug is discontinued, whereas aminoglycoside ototoxicity is often irreversible. Toxicity can be minimized by a knowledge of drug side effects (see Table 12.1) as well as an awareness of appropriate length of therapy. Adverse reactions to antimicrobial agents have been shown to occur in about 5% of all antibiotic courses and are often severe.[1] The elderly appear to be at greater risk of adverse drug reactions.[2]

Allergy

Allergic or hypersensitivity reactions are generally less common, unexpected side effects of antibiotics that do not occur in all persons. Examples of hypersensitivity reactions include rash, serum sickness, anaphylaxis, asthma, and allergic vasculitis. These are most commonly seen with penicillins, cephalosporins, and sulfonamides, but may be seen with almost any antibiotic. Immediate hypersensitivity, which occurs shortly after administration of an antibiotic, can be life-threatening. Urticaria, anaphylaxis, and shock comprise the syndrome. A hypersensitivity reaction to any antibiotic requires discontinuation of the offending drug and avoidance of all related drugs in the future. The medical record should clearly document the presence and nature of a drug allergy; a labeled medical bracelet may be appropriate.

Superinfection

Antibiotics are never completely specific for the intended pathogenic organism but have varying degrees of effect on normal bacterial flora. If the normal flora of the body is disturbed by antibiotic therapy, the host becomes more susceptible to other pathogens. Broad-spectrum antibiotics, such as the broad-spectrum penicillins, third-generation

Table 12.1 *Antibiotics*

Drug	Half-Life	Primary Route of Elimination	Major Side Effects
Penicillins	30–60 min	Renal	Hypersensitivity
Cephalosporins	1–8 h	Renal	Hypersensitivity
Imipenem	1 h	Renal	GI intolerance, rash
Aztreonam	2 h	Renal	GI intolerance, rash
Aminoglycosides	2–3 h	Renal	Nephrotoxicity, citotoxicity
Tetracyclines	6–20 h	Renal, hepatic	Dental staining, rash, GI intolerance
Macrolides	1.4–40 h	Hepatic	Cholestatic hepatitis, GI intolerance
Clindamycin	4 h	Hepatic	Diarrhea, colitis
Sulfonamides	6–18 h	Renal, hepatic	Hypersensitivity, crystalluria
Trimethoprim	11 h	Renal	Anemia, rash
Vancomycin	6 h	Renal	Nephrotoxicity, phlebitis
Metronidazole	7 h	Renal	GI intolerance
Quinolones	3–11 h	Renal	GI intolerance, neurologic

Adapted from Smith PW: Infectious Diseases, in Kochar MS, Kutty K (eds): *Concise Textbook of Medicine,* 2nd ed. Norwalk, CT, Appelton & Lange, 1990. Used with permission.

cephalosporins, and carbapenams, exert a profound influence on normal bacterial flora of the host and are associated with a higher incidence of superinfection. Organisms commonly responsible for superinfections include resistant gram-negative bacteria, yeasts (especially *Candida albicans*), and *Clostridium difficile*, the organism responsible for antibiotic-associated colitis (see Chapter 8).

Cost

In an era of increasing cost awareness, a potential undesirable consequence of antibiotic use is expense. The cost of new antibiotics, in particular, is great. For instance, a 10-day course of therapy with a third-generation cephalosporin at maximal dosage would cost thousands of dollars. In view of the marginal therapeutic benefits of many of the new antibiotics, a physician must consider cost when making an antibiotic selection.

Resistance Development

Widespread use of antibiotics has resulted in the emergence and selection of many antibiotic-resistant strains of microorganisms (see below).

ANTIBIOTIC RESISTANCE

The Extent of the Problem

Antibiotic resistance is a worldwide problem of great public health import.[3] The most serious problem is bacterial resistance, especially hospital strains of gram-negative bacilli resistant to multiple antibiotics and methicillin-resistant *Staphylococcus aureus* (MRSA). Other examples of important bacterial resistance include penicillin-resistant gonorrhea, ampicillin-resistant *Hemophilus influenzae*, cephalosporin-resistant gram-negative bacilli, and quinolone-resistant *Pseudomonas aeruginosa.*

Resistance problems are not confined to common bacteria, however, as demonstrated by dapsone-resistant leprosy, multidrug-resistant tuberculosis, chloroquine-resistant malaria, and herpes simplex strains resistant to acyclovir.

Nosocomial antibiotic resistance problems are no longer seen only in hospitals. Reported problems in long-term care facilities have included antibiotic-resistant gram-negative bacilli, particularly associated with urinary tract infections, and MRSA. These bacteria have caused major outbreaks in the LTCF.

Gram-negative bacilli such as *E. coli, Proteus mirabilis, Klebsiella pneumoniae,* and *Pseudomonas aeruginosa* are leading causes of urinary tract infections (UTIs) in the long-term care facility resident, especially the catheterized resident. These bacteria are frequently resistant to multiple antibiotics. Gram-negative bacteria causing UTIs in the nursing home are generally more resistant than those found in the community[4,5] and may occur in clusters suggesting epidemic spread.[6] MRSA is discussed later.

LTCF infections and colonization with antibiotic-resistant gram-negative bacteria are relatively common and may spread by cross-infection to cause an outbreak.[7-9] Risk factors for these infections include use of urinary catheters, inappropriate antibiotics, incontinence, and large LTCFs. Resistant enterococci have also been seen in the LTCF setting.[10]

Measuring Antibiotic Sensitivity/Resistance

Antibiotic sensitivity testing for bacteria is commonly performed by the Bauer-Kirby method. This involves measuring the zone of inhibition of bacterial growth around an antibiotic-impregnated disk. The size of the zone indicates sensitivity or resistance (see Fig. 12.1), the larger zones correlating with greater antibiotic sensitivity.

Broth or agar dilution methods enable the laboratory to quantitatively determine the minimum concentration of an antibiotic that is inhibitory (minimum inhibitory concentration, MIC) or bactericidal (minimum bactericidal concentration, MBC) for an organism. Automated MIC measurements are used instead of the disk sensitivity method by many laboratories. Comparison to achievable antibiotic levels enables the laboratory to provide a convenient "sensitive" or "resistant" interpretation.

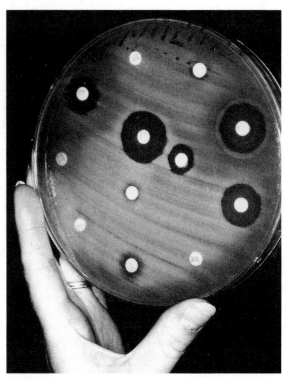

Figure 12.1 *Antibiotic disk sensitivity testing (From Smith PW: Infectious diseases. In: Kochar MS, Kutty K: Concise Textbook of Medicine, 2nd Edition, Appleton & Lange, Norwalk, CT. Used with permission).*

Mechanisms of Resistance

Some degree of resistance has eventually been seen with virtually every antibiotic developed. Organisms have devised a number of ways to circumvent antibiotics. The most common biochemical mechanism is production of an enzyme that inactivates the antibiotic. An example of this is the penicillinase produced by *Staphylococcus aureus, Neisseria gonorrhoeae,* and *Hemophilus influenzae,* which cleaves the penicillin molecule. Aminoglycosides also are enzymatically inactivated. Other mechanisms of resistance include evolution of a target site that is less susceptible to antibiotic action (erythromycin) and decreased uptake or transport of an antibiotic (tetracycline).

Bacteria have several genetic mechanisms for spreading drug resistance. Resistance that is coded for in the bacterial chromosome is passed on to daughter cells, but bacteria have evolved a much more rapid system for transferring drug resistance. A *plasmid* is an extrachromosomal piece of DNA that codes for a number of genetic traits, including drug resistance. Multiple copies of a plasmid may be present per cell, and plasmids may be spread between bacteria of the same or different species. Plasmids greatly increase the genetic adaptability of bacteria and enable resistance to be spread from bacterium to bacterium very rapidly.

Another point to be kept in mind is that antibiotic resistance that develops to a given antibiotic is often "linked" to antibiotic resistance to other drugs. Administration of a particular antibiotic often encourages development of resistance not just to that antibiotic, but to many other antibiotics as well.

Causes of Resistance

Numerous studies have demonstrated that the extent of resistance can be correlated directly with the extent of antibiotic use. Antibiotic resistance can appear rapidly; in fact, resistance may appear after a single exposure to an antibiotic. Under the selective pressure of antibiotic administration, resistant bacteria become prominent when antibiotic-sensitive bacteria are eliminated.

Once resistance develops, spread occurs. This is particularly true in the hospital and LTCF environment, where one encounters a population of persons with multiple medical illnesses in close proximity, many of whom are receiving antibiotics. The final common pathway for spread is usually the hands of personnel. Person-to-person spread of antibiotic-resistant bacteria on the hands of personnel has been implicated in several outbreaks.[11]

Solutions

Solutions to the problem of antibiotic resistance can be aimed either at preventing development of antibiotic-resistant bacteria or at blocking their spread.

Because antibiotic use correlates directly with the extent of antibiotic resistance, one potential solution is to decrease the amount of antibiotics used. Studies have consistently demonstrated a great deal of inappropriate antibiotic use (see below). Errors in administration of antibiotics include inadequate documentation of indications for antibiotic administration, errors in antibiotic dosing, administration of an antibiotic despite documented resistance on sensitivity testing, and even

administration of antibiotics when no indication exists, such as in the patient with a viral upper respiratory tract infection.

Education

It is clear that more accurate and conservative administration of antibiotics would result in better medical care, less antibiotic resistance, and considerable cost savings. One proposed solution is increased education of physicians. Although this is a very logical first step, results have been somewhat mixed.[12] Some have advocated using the pharmacist to present an objective review of antibiotics to the practitioner.

Antibiotic Control

When education fails, more drastic measures may be required. Deletion of certain drugs from the formulary is one way to decrease abuse of the substances. Some hospitals require that physicians justify in writing in the hospital record the indication for antibiotic administration, or require use of an antibiotic order form before an antibiotic can be administered.[13] Even these simple restraints may substantially decrease the use of antibiotics. Automatic stop orders on antibiotics have been used. Hospitals and LTCFs may also restrict the use of an antibiotic or require infectious disease consultation prior to use of certain widely abused or toxic antibiotics.[14]

Isolation

Other measures may be employed in the LTCF setting to interrupt the spread of antibiotic-resistant bacteria from resident to resident or from environment to resident. Isolation methods have been found to be effective in terminating a number of epidemics. In one outbreak, patients who were infected with multiply resistant *Pseudomonas aeruginosa* were admitted to a single room and placed in isolation for resistant bacteria.[15] Others have found that similar measures have effectively terminated outbreaks.[11,16]

METHICILLIN-RESISTANT *STAPHYLOCOCCUS AUREUS* (MRSA)

Overview

The majority of *S. aureus* isolates in the United States, particularly those acquired in health care facilities, are resistant to penicillin. Therefore, the development and release of methicillin in the early 1960s was welcome; it and related compounds such as oxacillin and nafcillin have become the drugs of choice for treatment of *S. aureus* infections. Unfortunately, MRSA was described very soon after the release of methicillin. It first appeared about 1960, then gradually increased, so that by the mid-1960s 20% to 40% of *S. aureus* isolates in some facilities in Europe were MRSA.[17] The first outbreak in the United States was in 1968, but this country was largely spared until the late 1970s.[18]

The determinant of MRSA resistance is located on the chromosome. This is in contrast to the mechanism of resistance for penicillin among *S. aureus* isolates (see above). In methicillin resistance, an enzyme is not involved. Rather, resistance involves alteration of the target sites for the antibiotic.

Risk Factors

The prevalence of MRSA is highest in tertiary care hospitals that are associated with medical schools. Patients in these places are more likely to have invasive procedures, placement of several intravenous lines and broad-spectrum antibiotics, and to be immunosuppressed. There is no question that smaller hospitals and LTCFs have MRSA, too. The most important mechanism by which MRSA is introduced is by transfer of a patient who is either colonized or infected with MRSA. This "spillover effect" accounts for a significant percentage of MRSA seen in centers other than tertiary care hospitals.

Residents, medical personnel, and the environment are known reservoirs for MRSA. Both infection and colonization are important. Sites that are commonly colonized with MRSA in the LTCF resident include nares, tracheostomy, gastrostomy-tube site, rectum, and the surface of pressure sores. MRSA is not more virulent than methicillin-sensitive *S. aureus*, but it can cause serious infections such as cellulitis, infected pressure sores, pneumonia, and bacteremia. Spread in the facility seems to be mainly by hands.

Studies of MRSA in the LTCF

Several articles describing the occurrence of MRSA infection and colonization in LTCFs have been published.[19-30] MRSA can be spread from the hospital to the LTCF and vice versa by means of an infected or colonized patient.[19]

Colonization with MRSA occurs in 9% to 34% of residents of LTCFs; higher rates are seen in facilities associated with Veterans' Affairs Hospitals in some studies.[20,22,24,25,27] The carriage rate in personnel in two studies was 7%.[20,24]

Risk factors associated with MRSA colonization of LTCF residents include nasogastric intubation, prior antibiotic therapy, recent hospitalization, presence of pressure sores, poor functional status, and the bedridden state.[19,22,27,28]

In one survey of 75 LTCFs in western New York, 81% had housed at least one MRSA colonized or infected resident.[29] Facility bed size was a predictor of the number of residents with MRSA. Interestingly, only 21% of facilities surveyed felt that an infection control problem existed in their facility.

Infection Control Issues

85% of facilities that have had a significant cluster of MRSA infections will be unable to get rid of the organism. Eradication is unusual, but some measure of control is possible (see Table 12.2). Central to all programs is the isolation of infected or colonized residents from noncarriers. This can consist of strict isolation or contact isolation, or the isolation technique can be tailored to the body site where MRSA is found (see Chapter 19).

Although hospitals generally select strict or contact isolation, LTCF resources may make strict isolation impractical. Several state guidelines for approaching MRSA have been developed, but not all are in agreement. It is advisable to

---

Table 12.2   *MRSA Control Techniques in the LTCF*

Isolation of infected and colonized residents

In-service education

Antibiotic treatment of infected residents

Surveillance cultures

Antibiotic restriction

Cohorting of colonized and infected residents

Antibiotic eradication regimens for colonized
   residents and personnel

have MRSA infected or colonized residents in a single room, or rooming with another MRSA resident, and to emphasize handwashing and wearing gloves for contact with body secretions. Because of the difficulty in eradicating this organism, MRSA isolation is continued indefinitely.

Surveillance cultures of residents and staff are not routinely necessary, but they may be performed if a nosocomial MRSA case is found and the source is sought. Cohorting, or confining MRSA cases to one area of the LTCF, is recommended to limit spread. Finally, continuous education is an important part of MRSA control, both to reinforce handwashing and to control staff fears about the hazards of MRSA.

Treatment

Treatment choices for MRSA infection are limited. MRSA is resistant to all penicillins and all cephalosporins. Also, it is usually resistant to a variety of other antibiotics, none of which can be used for MRSA infections. Most MRSA isolates are sensitive to rifampin, and all strains so far reported are sensitive to vancomycin. Vancomycin is the drug of choice in treating MRSA infections.[31] It has been as successful in treating severe MRSA infection as it is in treating methicillin-sensitive *S. aureus* infection. Unfortunately, vancomycin must be administered intravenously, and it has been associated with side effects such as ototoxicity and nephrotoxicity. Also, although vancomycin cures the infection, it does not eradicate the carrier state.

Treatment of staff members who are colonized is controversial, as is their removal from resident care. Fortunately, most studies have shown that it is uncommon for LTCF personnel to acquire MRSA in the course of caring for infected or colonized residents.[20,24] The real concern is staff members picking up MRSA on their hands and then transferring the organism directly to nearby residents.

Systemic and local antibiotics have been used to try to eradicate the carrier state.[32–36] Rifampin is a major element of this treatment. Advantages include exquisite sensitivity of the MRSA to the drug, low toxicity with short-term use, and good penetration into nasopharyngeal secretions. However, when rifampin is used alone, rapid emergence of resistance is a problem. Therefore, trimethoprim/sulfamethoxazole (TMP/SMZ) is added to eradication regimens. One approach to eradication is to give rifampin 300 mg by mouth twice daily and TMP/SMZ one double-strength

tablet by mouth twice daily for 5 to 10 days, although success rates for eradicating MRSA from nursing home and hospital patients are low. The use of mupirocin, a topical antistaphylococcal agent, may also be tried in eradicating the MRSA carrier state.

ANTIBIOTICS: ASPECTS OF IMPORTANCE IN THE ELDERLY

Drug Use in the Elderly

Because of age-related diseases, the elderly use more drugs in general and more antibiotics in particular than younger persons. The population over the age of 65 years comprises about 11% of the total population of the United States, yet they spend approximately 21% of the total national budget for drugs.[37] Residents in long-term care facilities are frequently recipients of multiple drugs; in one survey, 73% of nursing home residents received at least three prescription medications daily. Two nursing home surveys found that 7% to 10% of residents were receiving antibiotics, and almost half were receiving sedatives or tranquilizers.[6,38,39]

Pharmacology

The pharmacokinetics and metabolism of drugs are different in the elderly.[2,40,41] Perhaps the most important change is the decrease in renal function with age, which results in altered elimination of drugs excreted by the kidney. Glomerular filtration rate declines with age, with a mean 35% reduction in the elderly compared with the young. Most commonly used antimicrobial agents are excreted by the kidney; hence, one may expect higher levels and delayed excretion in the elderly.

In the elderly, in general, lean body mass declines and adipose tissue mass increases relative to total body weight, resulting in an altered distribution of drugs. There may be a decrease in serum level of proteins that bind drugs, resulting in a greater level of free antibiotic in the serum. The elderly may also have decreased drug absorption from the intestine or altered hepatic metabolism of drugs.

A number of practical points for antibiotic usage based on an altered metabolism of drugs in the elderly have been proposed, including using smaller doses for the elderly and simplifying the drug regimen.[37,42] Potentially toxic drugs need to be monitored especially closely. For example, gentamicin pharmacokinetics are quite variable in the elderly, which makes frequent measurement of gentamicin levels prudent. Also, amantadine is administered once daily to the elderly, instead of the usual twice daily dosing.

Adverse Drug Reactions

Adverse drug reactions appear to occur more frequently in the elderly. Several studies have found an adverse reaction rate of 10% to 20% in patients over the age of 60, a figure that is considerably higher than the corresponding rate for patients between the ages of 40 and 50.[2,43]

One reason for the increase in adverse reactions among the elderly may be the altered excretion or metabolism of drugs in this population group. This is felt to explain the increased nephrotoxicity of aminoglycoside antibiotics in the elderly patient.[44] Altered hepatic metabolism with age may explain the observation that isoniazid hepatotoxicity increases steadily with age.[37,45]

Other factors contributing to the problem of increased adverse drug reactions in LTCFs include medication errors and inappropriate therapy (see below). Thus, the elderly appear to be more susceptible to adverse drug reactions intrinsically and have an increased risk of such adverse occurrences by virtue of requiring multiple medications.

Drug Interactions

In view of the great number of drugs used by the elderly patient, the risk of adverse interactions among the drugs is significant.[46] The risk of adverse interaction increases exponentially with increasing numbers of drugs. The interactions between antibiotics and other drugs have been categorized:[46,47]

1. One type of interaction is the displacement of a drug from a protein binding site by an antibiotic that is also protein-bound. An example of this is the displacement of tolbutamide or warfarin from a serum carrier site by sulfonamides, resulting in hypoglycemia or bleeding, respectively, due to increased levels of free (i.e., active) drug.
2. A second type of mechanism is competition for renal tubular secretion. In this instance, probenecid competes with antibiotics such as penicillins and cephalosporins for renal elimination, resulting in elevated antibiotic levels. This is used to advantage by physicians when higher serum drug levels are desirable.
3. Antibiotics may affect hepatic enzymes that control elimination of other drugs. As an example, isoniazid inhibits the hepatic enzymes responsible for diphenylhydantoin (dilantin) elimination, resulting in dilantin toxicity. Similarly, some of the quinolone antibiotics can interfere with theophylline metabolism, increasing its serum concentration. Reduction of the dose of theophylline compounds and/or monitoring the serum concentration is in order.[48,49]
4. Drugs may interact at tissue sites to potentiate toxicity, as exemplified by the increased nephrotoxicity associated with the use of aminoglycosides with furosemide.
5. Miscellaneous types of interactions that are possible include the effect of one drug on another by alterations of urinary acidity, decreased absorption (e.g., of oral tetracycline or ciprofloxacin by oral antacids and iron), and reactions similar to that with disulfiram (Antabuse) when alcohol is ingested with metronidazole.
6. Finally, a special category of potential adverse interactions among antibiotics occurs when multiple antibiotics are used together. Antagonism may result, especially when bactericidal and bacteristatic antibiotics are used in combination.

RATIONAL APPROACH TO ANTIBIOTIC USE

Antibiotic Use in the LTCF

Prerequisites of good antibiotic utilization include a knowledge of the underlying infectious disease, an appropriate indication for antibiotic administration, knowledge of the antibiotic properties (mechanisms, pharmacokinetics, side effects, and cost), selection of the least toxic antibiotic, knowledge of patient allergies, use of narrow-spectrum antibiotics, and periodic reassessment of antibiotic efficacy and side effects during treatment. Health care personnel should be aware of marketed antibiotic products that are ineffective and to be avoided.[50] Finally, the unique aspects of drug pharmacology and toxicity in the elderly must be kept in mind.

Articles describing the appropriate (and inappropriate) use of antibiotics in LTCFs have been published, as have explicit criteria which may be used in future studies.[51-56] Using an overview panel of infectious diseases specialists and a pharmacist, less than half of the antibiotic courses for presumed infections in residents at two LTCFs were deemed appropriate.[52] In a New York study, the majority of antibiotic prescriptions (54%) were made by telephone order.[53]

Vestal has suggested some basic principles for prescribing to geriatric patients,[37] some of which are particularly relevant to prescription of antibiotics for the LTCF resident: (a) use smaller doses for the elderly; (b) simplify the therapeutic regimen; (c) explain the treatment plan to both the resident and a friend or relative and give concise, written directions; (d) choose a dosage form that is appropriate to the resident; (e) suggest the use of a diary or calendar to record daily drug administration; (f) label the drug container clearly; (g) encourage the return and destruction of old or unused medications; (h) regularly review drugs in the treatment plan and discontinue those not needed; and (i) keep in mind potential adverse effects and interactions of the antibiotics.

Another option to improve antibiotic utilization and effectiveness in the LTCF setting is involvement of LTCF consultant pharmacists. Consultant pharmacists have been queried most often about antibiotic side effects, generic equivalence, contraindications, and drug interactions.[57] In

Table 12.3 *Sample Criteria: Monitor of UTI Therapy in the LTCF*

Methods: The LTCF infection control practitioner will review infection control records for the last three months, analyzing all nosocomial urinary tract infections (UTIs). All residents in the LTCF during those three months will be included. This monitor is a follow-up monitor; a similar monitor six months ago revealed an increase in *Pseudomonas* UTIs.

ELEMENTS	STANDARD	EXCEPTIONS	INSTRUCTIONS FOR DATA RETRIEVAL
1. Diagnosis of UTI: 100,000 bacteria/ml urine on culture or	100%	—	Review lab sheets (cultures)
Fever *and* dysuria or pyuria	—	—	Review clinical notes, lab sheets (urinalysis)
2. Foley catheter present?	Information only	—	Review nurses' notes
3. Antibiotic therapy:			
a. Organism sensitive	100%	Culture negative	Review lab sheets (cultures)
b. No less toxic or expensive drug available	100%	Resident allergic to preferred drug	Review lab sheets (antibiotic sensitivities), history
c. Length of therapy			Review medication orders

Table 12.4   *Sample Results: Monitor of UTI Therapy in the LTCF*

	STANDARD	RESULTS

1. 200 Residents:
    18 met criteria for
    UTI (9%)
   a. Urine culture done
   b. Culture positive, sensitivity done
	100%
	 —
		18/18 = 100%
		 16/18 = 89%

2. Bladder catheter present	—	15/18 = 83%

3. Antibiotic therapy:
   a. Organism sensitive
   b. No less toxic or
     expensive drug
     available
   c. Length of therapy
	100%
	 100%
	
	 —
		16/16 = 100%
		 13/16 = 81%
		
		 mean = 9 days

Conclusions: Both the incidence of UTIs (9%) and the percent of infected residents with indwelling bladder catheters (83%) are within the expected range for a large LTCF for this period of time. Appropriate urine cultures were obtained prior to therapy frequently (100%) and were almost always positive. The organisms cultured were:

Proteus mirabilis: 6
Escherichia coli: 5
Pseudomonas aeruginosa: 2
Enterococci: 2
Klebsiella species: 1

The increase in *Pseudomonas* isolates noted in the facility six months ago has subsided.

   All physicians selected drugs for therapy that were appropriate to sensitivities of the organism, although in three instances (19%) a less toxic or less expensive drug could have been used. In two cases this involved use of an expensive cephalosporin rarely indicated for UTIs. A number of antibiotic courses were for greater than 10 days, which is not routinely necessary.
Plan: Distribute results of survey to all facility physicians and LTCF personnel. Continue to monitor results from urine cultures and consider a future study of length of antibiotic therapy for UTI.

some instances, the use of consultant pharmacists may decrease the average number of drugs used per LTCF resident.[58]

Antibiotic Monitoring

   One of the duties of the infection control practitioner or infection control program is the monitoring of antibiotic utilization and resistance in the LTCF. The latter can be done without much difficulty by inspecting the results of all cultures obtained on residents at the facility. A cluster of isolates of the same bacterium (with identical antibiotic sensitivity pattern) suggests an outbreak (see Chapter 11). An increase in antibiotic resistance, particularly MRSA or aminoglycoside-resistant gram-negative bacilli, poses a real hazard to residents and may be an indication for isolation.

   A survey of antibiotic utilization may provide useful information for the infection control team about antibiotic use and potential overuse in a LTCF. An area for investigation is generally selected on the basis of high antibiotic cost (such as the new cephalosporins), extensive antibiotic use, or well-known potential misuse (such as quinolones). Examples of potential surveys include antibiotic therapy of urinary tract infections in residents with urinary catheters, documentation of infection in medical records, monitoring antibiotic toxicity during therapy, and obtaining proper cultures prior to therapy. Topics of local interest should be selected.

The next step is determination of criteria. Criteria should be objective and nonthreatening. Standard criteria have been suggested.59 Although the referenced criteria were developed primarily for hospital antibiotic surveys, they are relevant to LTCFs as well. The LTCF should develop its own criteria (see Table 12.3).

Data are then collected[60] and performance at the LTCF is compared to an ideal standard (see Table 12.4). Deficiencies are identified, and corrective action is taken, usually in the form of an educational program, newsletter, or further monitoring of antibiotic use. The most valid comparison of performance is internal, such as comparison of results before and after an educational program.

Antibiotic utilization studies are commonly performed in the LTCF[61] and may have significant benefit in terms of improving quality of care, decreasing the risk of selecting resistant bacteria, and controlling costs.

REFERENCES

1. Caldwell JR, Cluff LE: Adverse reactions to antimicrobial agents. *JAMA* 1974;230:77–80.
2. Montamat SC, Cusack BJ, Vestal RE: Management of drug therapy in the elderly. *N Engl J Med* 1989;321:303–308.
3. Levy SB: Microbial resistance to antibiotics: An evolving and persistent problem. *Lancet* 1982;ii:83–88.
4. Gleckman R, Blagg N, Hibert D, et al: Catheter-related urosepsis in the elderly: A prospective study of community-derived infections. *J Am Geriatr Soc* 1982;30:255–257.
5. Sherman FT, Tucci V, Libow LS, et al: Nosocomial urinary tract infections in a skilled nursing facility. *J Am Geriatr Soc* 1980;28:456–461.
6. Garibaldi RA, Brodine S, Matsumiya S: Infections among patients in nursing homes: Policies, prevalence, and problems. *N Engl J Med* 1981;305:731–735.
7. Bjork DT, Pelletier LL, Tight RR: Urinary tract infections with antibiotic resistant organisms in catheterized nursing home patients. *Infect Control* 1984;5:173–176.
8. Gaynes RP, Weinstein RA, Chamberlin W, et al: Antibiotic-resistant flora in nursing home patients admitted to the hospital. *Arch Intern Med* 1985;145:1804–1807.
9. Shlaes DM, Lehman MH, Currie-McCumber CA, et al: Prevalence of colonization with antibiotic resistant gram-negative bacilli in a nursing home care unit: The importance of cross-colonization as documented by plasmid analysis. *Infect Control* 1986;7:538–545.
10. Zervos MJ, Terpenning MS, Schaberg DR, et al: High-level aminoglycoside-resistant enterococci: Colonization of nursing home and acute care hospital patients. *Arch Intern Med* 1987;147:1591–1594.
11. Weinstein RA: Resistant bacteria and infection control in the nursing home and hospital. *Bull N Y Acad Med* 1987;63:337–344.
12. Schroeder SA, Myers LP, McPhee SJ, et al: The failure of physician education as a cost controlled trial at a university hospital. *JAMA* 1984;252:225–230.
13. Echols RM, Kowalsky SF: The use of an antibiotic order form for antibiotic utilization review: Influence on physicians' prescribing patterns. *J Infect Dis* 1984;150:803–807.
14. Seligman SJ: Reduction in antibiotic cost by restricting use of an oral cephalosporin. *Am J Med* 1981;71:941–944.
15. Smith PW, Rusnak PG: Aminoglycoside-resistant *Pseudomonas aeruginosa* urinary tract infections: Study of an outbreak. *J Hosp Infect* 1981;2:71–75.
16. Gardener P, Bennett JV, Burke JP, et al: Nosocomial management of resistant gram-negative bacilli. *J Infect Dis* 1980;141:415–417.
17. Jessen O, Rosendal K, Bulow P, et al: Changing staphylococci and staphylococci infections: A ten-year study of bacteria and causes of bacteremia. *N Engl J Med* 1969;281:627–635.
18. Barrett FF, McGehee RF, Finland M: Methicillin-resistant *Staphylococcus aureus* at Boston City Hospital. *N Engl J Med* 1968;279:441–448.
19. O'Toole RD, Drew WL, Dahlgren BJ, et al: An outbreak of methicillin-resistant *Staphylococcus aureus* infection. *JAMA* 1970;213:257–263.
20. Storch GA, Radliff JL, Meyer PL, et al: Methicillin-resistant *Staphylococcus aureus* in a nursing home. *Infect Control* 1987;8:24–29.
21. Hsu CC, Macaluso CP, Special L, et al: High rate of methicillin-resistance of *Staphylococcus aureus* isolated from hospitalized nursing home patients. *Arch Intern Med* 1988;148:569–570.
22. Thomas JC, Bridge J, Waterman S, et al: Transmission and control of methicillin-resistant *Staphylococcus aureus* in a skilled nursing facility. *Infect Control Hosp Epidemiol* 1989;10:106–110.
23. Kauffman CA, Bradley SF, Terpenning MS: Methicillin-

resistant *Staphylococcus aureus* in long-term care facilities. *Infect Control Hosp Epidemiol* 1990;11:600–603.

24. Strausbaugh LJ, Jacobson C, Sewell DL, et al: Methicillin-resistant *Staphylococcus aureus* in extended care facilities: Experiences in a Veteran's Affairs nursing home and a review of the literature. *Infect Control Hosp Epidemiol* 1991;12:36–45.

25. Muder RR, Brennan C, Wagener MM, et al: Methicillin-resistant staphylococcal colonization and infection in a long-term care facility. *Ann Intern Med* 1991;114:107–112.

26. Boyce JM: Methicillin-resistant *Staphylococcus aureus* in nursing homes: Putting the problem in perspective. *Infect Control Hosp Epidemiol* 1991;12:413–415.

27. Hsu CC: Serial survey of methicillin-resistant *Staphylococcus aureus* nasal carriage among residents in a nursing home. *Infect Control Hosp Epidemiol* 1991;12:416–421.

28. Bradley SF, Terpenning MS, Ramsey MA, et al: Methicillin-resistant *Staphylococcus aureus*: Colonization and infection in a long-term care facility. *Ann Intern Med* 1991;115:417–422.

29. Mylotte JM, Karuza J, Bentley DW: Methicillin-resistant *Staphylococcus aureus*: Questionnaire survey of 75 long-term care facilities in western New York. *Infect Control Hosp Epidemiol* 1992;13:711–718.

30. Boyce JM: Methicillin-resistant *Staphylococcus aureus* in hospitals and long-term care facilities: Microbiology, epidemiology and preventive measures. *Infect Control Hosp Epidemiol* 1992;13:725–737.

31. Brumfitt W, Hamilton-Miller J: Methicillin-resistant *Staphylococcus aureus*. *N Engl J Med* 1989;320:1188–1195.

32. McAnally TP, Lewis MR, Brown DR: Effect of rifampin and bacitracin on nasal carriers of *Staphylococcus aureus*. *Antimicrob Agents Chemother* 1984;25:442.

33. Ellison RT, Judson FN, Peterson LC, et al: Oral rifampin and trimethoprim/sulfamethoxazole therapy in asymptomatic carriers of methicillin-resistant *Staphylococcus aureus* infections. *West J Med* 1984;140:735–740.

34. Casewell MW, Hill RLR: Elimination of nasal carriage of Staphylococcus aureus with mupirocin (pseudomonic acid)—a controlled trial. *J Antimicrob Chemother* 1986;17:365–372.

35. Cederna JE, Terpenning MS, Ensberg M, et al: *Staphylococcus aureus* nasal colonization in a nursing home: Eradication with mupirocin. *Infect Control Hosp Epidemiol* 1990;11:13–16.

36. Strausbaugh LJ, Jacobson C, Sewell DL, et al: Antimicrobial therapy for methicillin-resistant *Staphylococcus aureus* colonization in residents and staff of a Veteran's Affairs nursing home care unit. *Infect Control Hosp Epidemiol* 1992;13:151–159.

37. Vestal RF: Pharmacology and aging. *J Am Geriatr Soc* 1982;30:191–200.

38. Cohen ED, Hierholzer WJ Jr, Schilling CR, et al: Nosocomial infections in skilled nursing facilities: A preliminary survey. *Publ Health Rep* 1979;94:162–165.

39. Zimmer JG, Bentley DW, Valenti WM, et al: Systemic antibiotic use in nursing homes. *J Am Geriatric Soc*

1986;34:703–710.

40. Koch-Weser J: Drug distribution in old age. *N Engl J Med* 1982;306:1081–1087.

41. Lamy PP: Comparative pharmacokinetic changes and drug therapy in an older population. *J Am Geriatr Soc* 1982;30:S11–S19.

42. Ljungberg B, Nilsson-Ehle I: Pharmacokinetics of antimicrobial agents in the elderly. *Rev Infect Dis* 1987;9:250–262.

43. Seidl LG, Thornton GF, Smith JW, et al: Studies on epidemiology of adverse drug reactions: Reactions in patients on a general medical service. *Bull Johns Hopkins Hosp* 1966;119:299–315.

44. Ristuccia AM, Cunha BA: The aminoglycosides. *Med Clin North Am* 1982;66:303–312.

45. Mitchell JR: Isoniazid liver injury: Clinical spectrum, pathology, and probable pathogenesis. *Ann Intern Med* 1976;84:181–192.

46. Lamy PP. The elderly and drug interactions. *J Am Geriatr Soc* 1986;34:586–592.

47. Adverse interactions of drugs. *Med Lett* 1981;5:17–28.

48. Wijnands WJA, Vree TB, van Herwaarden CLA: The influence of quinolone derivatives on theophylline clearance. *Br J Clin Pharmacol* 1986;22:677–683.

49. Gregoire SL, Grasela TH Jr, Freer JP, et al: Inhibition of theophylline effects. *Antimicrob Agents Chemother* 1987;31:375–378.

50. *Prescription Drug Products Currently Classified by the Food and Drug Administration as Lacking Adequate Evidence of Effectiveness.* Rockfield, MD, U.S. Department of Health and Human Services, Food and Drug Administration, 1980.

51. Bergman HD: Prescription of drugs in a nursing home. *Drug Intell Clin Pharm* 1975;9:365–368.

52. Jones SR, Parker DF, Liebow ES, et al: Appropriateness of antibiotic therapy in long-term care facilities. *Am J Med* 1987;83:499–502.

53. Katz PR, Beam TR, Brand F, et al: Antibiotic use in the nursing home. *Arch Intern Med* 1990;150:1465–1468.

54. Beers MH, Ouslander JG, Rollinger I, et al: Explicit criteria for determining inappropriate medication use in nursing home residents. *Arch Intern Med* 1991;151:1825–1831.

55. Warren JW, Palumbo FB, Fitterman L, et al: Incidence and characteristics of antibiotic use in aged nursing home patients. *J Am Geriatr Soc* 1991;39(10):963–972.

56. Beers MH, Ouslander JG, Fingold SF, et al: Inappropriate medication prescribing in skilled-nursing facilities. *Ann Intern Med* 1992;117:684–689.

57. Evens RP, Guernsey BG, Hightower WL: Nursing home consultant pharmacists: Drug information services, opinions, and activity study. *Hosp Formulary* 1982;17:408–420.

58. Cooper JW Jr, Bagwell CG: Contribution of the consultant pharmacist to rational drug usage in the long-term care facility. *J Am Geriatr Soc* 1978;26:513–520.

59. Marr JJ, Moffet HL, Kunin CM: Guidelines for improving the use of antimicrobial agents in hospitals: A statement by the Infectious Diseases Society of America. *J Infect Dis*

1988;157:869–876.

60. Latorraca R, Bartons R: Surveillance of antibiotic use in a community hospital. JAMA 1979;242:2585–2587.

61. Crossley KB, Irvine P, Kaszar DJ, et al: Infection control practices in Minnesota nursing homes. *JAMA* 1985;254:2918–2921.

CHAPTER

REGULATIONS, POLICIES, AND PROCEDURES

Patricia G. Rusnak and Mary C. Boehle

REGULATIONS

Infection prevention and control have always been important components of health care. Physicians, nurses, sanitarians, and other health professionals have established professional standards regarding infection prevention and control as part of their daily practice.

A number of agencies, private and governmental, have established guidelines over the years for the control and prevention of infections in health care institutions. The Joint Commission for Health Care Organizations (JCAHO)[1] along with the Centers for Disease Control and Prevention (CDC),[2] the Association for Practitioners in Infection Control (APIC),[3] and the Occupational Safety and Health Administration (OSHA)[4] are just a few.

Regulations may have varying purposes. For example, the OSHA regulations are designed primarily to protect the employee, whereas other federal regulations (see below) are designed primarily to protect the LTCF resident.

State and Local Standards

Depending on its location, state and local standards governing an individual facility will vary. One survey found that state regulations regarding infection control issues in the LTCF were variable and often inconsistent with current scientific knowledge.[5] It is necessary to secure copies of state regulations and standards from the appropriate state agency, most commonly the state department of health.

Local standards for sanitation and infection control can be obtained from the local health department. These agencies are generally excellent resources, not only for written materials but also for consultation with the long-term care facility (LTCF) regarding individual questions pertaining to regulations and standards.

Federal Regulations

In 1987, Congress passed the Omnibus Budget Reconciliation Act (OBRA), which was a result of a Supreme Court decision mandating the Health Care Finance Administration (HCFA) to develop a survey process that would ensure that the residents of LTCFs receive the highest quality of care possible and that these residents maintain their highest practicable level of functioning. In order to execute this mandate, all the rules and regulations governing these facilities were rewritten.[6] The regulatory emphasis was placed on the outcome of any given situation rather than on the process or structural components.

Several structural changes occurred as a result of these regulations. The differentiation between skilled nursing facilities and intermediate care facilities was discarded. The care given to residents of either type of facility was to be the same, and the staff providing the care was to be adequately trained and qualified.

The requirement for an infection control committee was dropped and replaced by the new requirement for a quality assurance committee, which is to function on a broader scale. The committee is to identify problems in all areas of the facility, address ways to correct them, and develop a mechanism for follow-up or evaluation. With the implementation of OBRA, all facilities are also required to employ a medical director who is responsible for the implementation of resident care policies and who must monitor the quality of care rendered to residents in the facility.

Survey Process

The new survey process requires the surveyors to select a percentage of residents from four main categories: (a) residents who are interviewable and require minimal care, (b) residents who are interviewable but require considerable care and assistance from the nursing staff, (c) light care, noninterviewable residents, and (d) heavy care, noninterviewable residents. One of the factors weighing heavily in the decision-making process is to select residents from these categories who are at risk for infections of any kind.

After residents are selected from each of the categories, the surveyors briefly review the resident record, medications, and care plan. The majority of the survey time should be spent observing all aspects of the resident's care. This includes toileting, perineal care, bathing, treatments, meals, physical therapy, restorative therapy, and administration of medications as well as the social aspects of the resident's daily life.

The surveyors pay particular attention to the infection control techniques the staff utilize in the provision of all the aforementioned categories of care to residents. Through direct observation and interviews with the staff, families, and the residents, the surveyors make a determination of whether quality care has been rendered to the residents.

The federal regulations for infection control,[6] cited under the regulatory number 483.65, cover such areas as basic infection control program design, isolation, dietary services, urinary catheters, pressure sores, and environmental cleanliness.

HCFA Regulations

Infection Control

The facility must establish and maintain an infection control program designed to provide a safe, sanitary, and comfortable environment and to help prevent the development and transmission of disease and infection.

a) Infection control program (see Chapter 9).

The facility must establish an infection control program under which it:

- Investigates, controls, and prevents infections in the facility;
- Decides what procedures, such as isolation should be applied to an individual resident; and
- Maintains a record of incidents and corrective actions related to infections.

In conjunction with the regulations themselves, the surveyors are provided with additional guidance referred to as the "interpretive guidelines." These assist the surveyors by providing information regarding the intent of the regulations, areas of specific concern, and probes to use in further investigating each requirement. Although the interpretive guidelines are not regulatory, they reflect minimum standards of care.

Interpretive Guidelines: 483.65-a

The facility's infection control program must have a system to monitor and investigate causes of infection (nosocomial and those present on admission) and manner of spread (see Chapter 10). A facility should, for example, maintain a separate record on infections that identifies each resident with an infection and describes what cautionary measures were taken to prevent the spread of the infection within the facility. The system should enable the facility to analyze clusters or significant increases in the rate of infection (see Chapter 11).

Surveillance data should be routinely reviewed and recommendations made for the prevention and control of additional cases.

The infection control program may include such observable practices as:

- The direct care staff routinely washing their hands according to facility policy
- The consistent use of aseptic techniques, when appropriate
- An active training program that ensures that individuals receive adequate information to prevent the acquisition and spread of infections (see Chapter 14)
- Routine monitoring of staff infection control practices.

The facility should also address prevention of infections common to nursing home residents (e.g., vaccination for influenza and pneumococcal pneumonia as appropriate). Resident health programs are discussed in Chapter 17.

The infection control program should be able to identify new infections quickly, paying particular attention to residents at high risk of infection (e.g., residents who are immobilized, have invasive devices or procedures, have pressure sores, have been recently discharged from a hospital, are mentally retarded or mentally ill, have decreased mental status, are nutritionally compromised, or have altered immune systems).

For nonsporadic, facility-wide infections that are difficult to control, the infection control program should have procedures to inform and involve a local or state epidemiologist.

During the survey, surveyors will observe staff providing care to residents identified at high risk of infection and may interview staff to determine what has been done to prevent or reduce these residents' risk of infection.

The surveyors may also wish to evaluate how the facility disposes of its infectious waste (see Chapter 19) and determine if the staff are following the facility policies and procedures.

b) Preventing Spread of Infection

- When the infection control program determines that a resident needs isolation to prevent the spread of infection, the facility must isolate the resident (see Chapter 19).
- The facility must prohibit employees with a communicable disease or infected skin lesions from direct contact with residents or their food, if direct contact will transmit the disease (see Chapter 16).
- The facility must require staff to wash their hands after each direct resident contact for which handwashing is indicated by accepted professional practice.

Interpretive Guidelines: 483.65-b

Procedures must be followed to prevent cross-contamination, including handwashing or changing gloves after providing personal care or when performing tasks that provide the opportunity for cross-contamination among individuals. Facilities for handwashing must

exist and be available to staff. Handwashing is discussed in Chapters 18 and 19.

The facility should isolate infected residents only to the degree needed to isolate the infecting organism. The method used should be the least restrictive possible that maintains the integrity of the process. Universal precautions for prevention of transmission of bloodborne pathogens is discussed in Chapter 15. The resident in the communicable stages of an infection should also be isolated. Skin lesions should be considered to be infected if they have purulent drainage or are red and hot without purulent drainage. State law defines communicable diseases for the purposes of defining facility policies.

The surveyors will observe staff to assure that proper handwashing and preventative procedures are consistently followed by all personnel. If a resident is isolated, the surveyor will examine the appropriateness of the isolation and observe how the staff control the spread of infection.

The surveyors will also note if staff providing care to residents have communicable diseases or infected skin lesions.

If residents have developed communicable diseases as defined by state law while in the facility, the surveyors will note whether appropriate barriers or isolation precautions have been followed.

c) Linens

Personnel must handle, store, process, and transport linens so as to prevent the spread of infection.

Interpretive Guidelines: 483.65-c

Soiled linens should be handled to contain and minimize exposure to any waste products. Soiled linen storage areas should be well ventilated and maintained under a relative negative air pressure. The laundry should be designed to eliminate crossing of soiled and clean linen (see Chapter 18).

d) Urinary Catheters and Pressure Sores

The regulations regarding urinary catheters and the treatment of pressure sores are in the Quality of Care section under 483.25-c-2.

A resident having pressure sores should receive necessary treatment and services to promote healing, prevent infection, and prevent new sores from developing (see Chapter 7).

The surveyors will include residents with pressures sores in the selected survey sample. This includes residents who developed these sores in the hospital.

The surveyors will observe staff techniques during treatments to determine that they observe proper handwashing and clean or sterile technique as appropriate. Clean technique is adequate for noninfected wounds.

483.25-d-2

A resident who is incontinent of bladder should receive appropriate treatment and services to prevent urinary tract infections and to restore as much normal bladder function as possible (see Chapter 6).

Interpretive Guidelines

For purposes of this regulation, "urinary tract infection (UTI)" is defined as colonization (growth of bacteria) of the urinary tract with signs and symptoms of UTI. Asymptomatic colonization is not a UTI.

If the resident has an indwelling catheter, the staff will be monitored to determine if they are following the facility's protocol and/or written procedures for catheterization. Personnel will also be monitored to be sure that they wash their hands before and after caring for the catheter/tubing/collection bag.

e) Dietary Services

Dietary departments represent another area of potential infections (see Chapter 18). During the course of the standard survey, the surveyors will observe all aspects of food storage, handling, preparation, and distribution.

483.35

The facility must:

- Procure food from sources approved or considered satisfactory by Federal, state, or local authorities. The surveyors will observe the milk and milk products, frozen and fresh fish and shellfish, fresh and pasteurized eggs, canned foods, fresh produce, meat, and poultry to determine that they are from approved sources. (Examples of food items not from approved sources would be farm fresh eggs from a distributor who does not possess a current license, or home canned food items.)

- Store, prepare, distribute, and serve food under sanitary conditions.

Interpretive Guidelines

"Sanitary conditions" means storing, preparing, distributing, and serving food properly to prevent foodborne illness. Prevention of foodborne illness focuses on potentially hazardous food (foods subject to continuous time and temperature controls in order to prevent the rapid and progressive growth of infectious or toxigenic microorganisms). Potentially hazardous food includes animal products such as milk, eggs, poultry, fish, meat, and synthetic food ingredients. Some fruits and vegetables (e.g., cantaloupe and baked potatoes) as well as specialty foods (e.g., garlic in oil) are also potentially hazardous foods.

Hot foods should leave the kitchen (or steam table) above 140°F and cold foods below 45°F Refrigerator temperatures should be maintained at 45°F or below.

During the survey of the dietary services the surveyors will observe the storage of food items in the store room and kitchen to assure that food items are stored off the floor and on clean surfaces in a manner to protect them from contamination.

Refrigerators and freezers will be checked to determine that they are maintaining safe storage temperatures.

The surveyors will observe food preparation and will pay particular attention to the treatment of leftovers and handling of foods to assure that safe temperatures are maintained during preparation.

During the distribution of food, all items should be covered during transportation.

The dietary areas of the facility will be observed for evidence of rodent or insect infestation.

The surveyors will also observe how dishes are sanitized and that adequate precautions are taken to assure that the water is hot enough (according to manufacturers' specifications) or that there is sufficient sanitizing solution in the water.

Handwashing facilities should be conveniently located and properly equipped for dietary staff to use. Staff should use good hygienic practices, and staff with communicable diseases or infected skin lesions should not have contact with food if that contact will transmit the disease.

The facility should be equipped with a portable water supply and a sewage system constructed and operated in accordance with state or local laws.

Toxic items (such as insecticides, detergents, and polishes) should be properly stored, labeled, and used.

- Dispose of garbage and refuse properly.

Interpretive Guidelines

Observe garbage and refuse container construction, and outside storage receptacles. They should be in good condition (no leaks), with waste properly contained in dumpsters or compactors with lids or otherwise covered.

f) Physical Environment

Physical environment regulations are located at 483.70. The facility must be designed, constructed, equipped, and maintained to protect the health and safety of residents, personnel, and the public.

During the survey, the surveyors will observe the physical environment to determine if the facility is clean.

The facility must maintain an effective pest control program so that the facility is free of pests and rodents.

Interpretive Guidelines

An "effective pest control program" means measures to eradicate and contain common household pests (e.g., roaches, ants, mosquitoes, flies, mice, and rats).

As a part of the overall review of the facility, the surveyors will look for signs of vermin. Evidence of pest infestation in particular is only a potential indicator of non-compliance. The surveyors will consider the scope of the pest problem (i.e., facility-wide, isolated to one area, isolated to a single resident's room) and the facility's efforts to control the problem before citing a deficiency.

Summary: Regulations

Regulations for infection control in LTCFs have increased as the problem of infections in that setting has been increasingly recognized. Because regulations change, infection control programs need to be aware of new and current regulations.

The federal regulations set minimum standards of care for long term care facilities. This in no way precludes a facility from exceeding those minimum guidelines. A well-informed, well-educated, and well-trained staff is the long-term care resident's best defense against infection. The surveyors are in the facility for a relatively short time. Staff performance should be the same regardless of whether or not a survey is in progress. To be truly effective, the facility staff must provide quality care in a consistent manner for all residents at all times.

POLICIES AND PROCEDURES

One of the most important aspects of the infection control program is the developing, implementing, and updating of infection control policies and procedures. Several surveys of LTCFs have found that although the majority of nursing homes have written policies and procedures, these policies (e.g., isolation policies, urinary catheter care policies) are often incomplete or at variance with current recommendations.[7,8]

Areas of Application

There are many policies and procedures related to an infection control program that a facility must establish. These policies and procedures should be based on standards (i.e., federal, state, and local) regarding infection control. Policies and procedures are the means to implement the standards. A *policy* reflects standards and the principles upon which decisions governing the operation of the facility are based; a *procedure*, also reflecting standards, is the method by which that policy is carried out. Infection control policies and procedures direct the facility as to how they will help minimize the transmission and spread of pathogenic microorganisms within the facility, and control them if an outbreak should occur.

The administrator of each facility must decide, as part of its infection control program, whether to have a separate infection control policy and procedure manual or whether all infection control policies and procedures will be integrated into the facility's overall general policy and procedure operations manual. For example, a very small LTCF may decide not to have a separate manual, whereas a larger facility may have one. Whichever format option is chosen, the policies and procedures should be based on the same principles of infection prevention and control.

Whether or not a separate manual or an integrated manual is incorporated, many areas should be considered

Table 13.1   *Sample List of Long-Term Care Facility Policies and Procedures for Infection Control*

1. Role of administration in infection control
2. Admission to the LTCF
3. Transfer to an acute care facility
4. Disease reporting to the health department
5. Surveillance and data collection
6. Housekeeping (e.g., cleaning schedules)
7. Isolation/precautions
8. Food service (e.g., food preparation and storage)
9. Laundry (e.g., collection of dirty linen)
10. In-service training/staff development
11. Visitors
12. Employee health (e.g., TB screening)
13. Disinfectants/antiseptics
14. Handwashing
15. Bloodborne pathogen plan (universal precautions)
16. Resident care practices (e.g., urinary catheter insertion)

when establishing infection prevention and control policies and procedures. These areas might include, but are not limited to those listed in Table 13.1. Resources are available to assist in the development of policies and procedures in general,[9] the overall infection control program,[3,10] and specific areas of interest, such as laundry,[11] physical therapy,[12] and handwashing.[13,14]

Writing Policies

In writing policies, begin by looking at the standards that need to be conveyed. Use previous wording as a guideline, and make any necessary changes that address the individual facility's situation. Always keep in mind that a policy reflects standards and is the principle upon which decisions governing the operation of the facility are based.

Another way to explain the definition of a policy is to think of a policy as defining *who, what, when,* and *where.* Usually a policy is written to correct a single repetitive problem, to clarify the limitations on future actions, and to define specific results desired.

The example in Figure 13.1 shows the *who, what, when,* and *where* that needs to be reflected in a policy, using the housekeeping department as an example.

Another example, a handwashing policy, is shown in Chapter 19.

Writing Procedures

After policies are developed, it is usually necessary to develop *how* and *why* the policy will be carried out—in other words, procedures. Procedures should be specific, clearly stated, current, and accessible to the people for who they are intended. It is difficult for procedures to be carried out unless the responsible individuals know how to effect them and the proper equipment and supplies are available as stated in the procedure. Procedures reflect standards, just as policies do. In general terms, a *procedure* is a standardized method of performing specified work, usually a single task. Several examples of infection control procedures are given here. Figure 13.2 depicts the *how* and *why* needed in writing a procedure. A separate column may be added to explain the *why,* if needed; such a column could be titled "Rationale." As additional examples, a handwashing procedure is shown in Table 19.1 and a surveillance procedure is shown in Chapter 10.

Forms

The format used for policies and procedures is an institutional decision. Usually a very simple format is chosen because of easier use and understandability. It is important to remember that policies and procedures need to be reviewed constantly, usually on an annual basis, and revised accordingly.

Review Date and Signature

The review date should be on each policy and procedure as a reminder when last reviewed (see Figures 13.1 and 13.2). Revising on an annual basis will eliminate extensive work, shorten the amount of time needed for review, and assure timely policies and procedures.

References

If policies and procedures are questioned or challenged as to accuracy or completeness, it will save considerable time and frustration if references are included. In addition, references provide sources where more detailed explanations may be found.

Distribution

Policy and procedure manuals need to be distributed to the appropriate areas and persons. A short, written explana-

---

SunnyVale Villa

Policy: *Housekeeping Department Supervisor Responsibilities*

Responsible Person: Housekeeping Department Supervisor

It is the policy of this facility that the Housekeeping Department will be headed by a full-time employee who will be responsible for all housekeeping services as well as the supervision, training, and evaluation of all personnel in the department. The housekeeping supervisor will review handwashing and safety practices with all staff annually, with assistance from the infection control practitioner as needed.

Reference: *Housekeeping Supervisor USA,* Volume 3, page 411

Review Date:_____ **Signature**_____

Figure 13.1 *Housekeeping Policy*

SunnyVale Villa

Procedure: *Annual Review of Infection Control Manual*

Responsible Person: Infection Control Practitioner (ICP)

Jan–Mar: Review manual, updating policies and procedures to be in compliance with current standards and regulations.
Apr–May: Rewrite those policies and procedures needing changes.
June: Present changes to administrator and department head, requesting approval.
July: Present revised manual to administrator and department head.

Reference: *The ICP Today,* Volume 19, page 6

Review Date:_____ **Signature**_____

Figure 13.2 *Infection Control Manual Review Procedure*

tion or list of revised policies and procedures should be given to each department head. The placement of manuals is vital for the employee. Manuals should be available twenty-four hours a day for anyone to review, not locked in an office.

Monitoring Compliance/Continuous Quality Improvement

The effectiveness of infection control policies and procedures is evidenced by the quality of care given to the resi-

dent or employee. Monitoring the compliance with policies and procedures is part of the responsibility of the ICP as well as that of the quality improvement committee.

Summary: Policies and Procedures

Infection control policies and procedures are necessary for quality care in LTCF. Each one should be easily understood, available at all times, and in compliance with current standards and regulations. Compliance with policies and procedures needs to be measured.

REFERENCES

1. Joint Commission on Accreditation of Healthcare Organizations. *Long-Term Care Standards Manual.* Chicago, Joint Commission on Accreditation of Healthcare Organization, 1990.
2. Centers for Disease Control and Prevention. Guideline for isolation precautions in hospitals. *Infect Control* 1983;4:245–325.
3. Smith PW, Rusnak PG. APIC guideline for infection prevention and control in the long-term care facility. *Am J Infect Control* 1991;19:198–215.
4. Occupational Safety and Health Administration. Occupational exposure to bloodborne pathogens, final rule. *Federal Register* 1991;56:64004–64182.
5. Crossley K, Nelson L, Irvine P. State regulations governing infection control issues in long-term care. *J Am Geriatr Soc* 1992;40:251–254.
6. Health Care Financing Administration: CFR Part 431. Medicare and Medicaid: Requirements for long term care facilities, final rules. *Federal Register* 1991;56:48826–48880.
7. Crossley KB, Irvine P, Kaszar DJ, Loewenson RB. Infection control practices in Minnesota nursing homes. *JAMA* 1985;254:2918–2921.

8. Khabbaz RF, Tenney JH. Infection control in Maryland nursing homes. *Infect Control Hosp Epidemiol* 1988;9:159–162.
9. Soule BM, Berg R. *The APIC Curriculum for Infection Control Practice*, Vol. I, II and III. Dubuque, IA: Kendall Hunt, 1983, 1988.
10. Health Care Financing Administration: *Long Term Care Survey Process Training Manual.* National Technical Information Service, 1986. Springfield, VA, U.S. Department of Commerce, 1986.
11. Joint Committee on Healthcare Laundry Guidelines: *1993 Guidelines for Healthcare Linen Services*. Richmond, KY: National Association of Institutional Laundry Management, 1993.
12. Centers for Disease Control: Disinfection of Hydrotherapy Pools and Tanks, in Training Bulletin, Microbiological Control Section, Bacterial Diseases Branch, Centers for Disease Control, Public Health Service, Atlanta, GA. 1972.
13. Larson E. Guideline for use of topical antimicrobial agents. *Am J Infect Control* 1988;16:253–266.
14. Rutala WA, APIC guideline for selection and use of disinfectants. *Am J Infect Control* 1990; 18:99–117.

CHAPTER

INFECTION CONTROL STAFF TRAINING AND MANAGEMENT

Pamela B. Daly

Educating personnel has long been recognized as an important component of hospital infection control (IC) programs and is an important facet of long-term care facility (LTCF) IC efforts as well. Both federal regulations[1] and other infection control guidelines[2] require regular in-service education of LTCF staff. Traditional IC education, however, has suffered from lack of measurement of results and a perception of lack of efficacy, leading to a greater focus on other behavior management tactics.[3] For the infection control practitioner (ICP) who is concerned that staff learn and use IC practices, a program that includes both educational and behavioral management procedures is required. This chapter outlines a program based on this principle and designed specifically for the LTCF ICP.

The particular configuration of the procedures proposed here should be viewed as guidelines to be modified and adapted according to the IC needs of the particular LTCF. It is based on considerations of the limited time and resources most multirole ICPs in LTCFs have to devote to such an undertaking and the need for "how-to" steps and procedures that can be incorporated into day-to-day activities. Many of the procedures are derived from research findings from the fields of applied behavior analysis, organizational behavior management, and total quality management.[4–7]

APPROACH TO STAFF TRAINING AND MANAGEMENT

The ICP can rarely devote the time necessary to carry out all aspects of an effective staff training and management program. A self-managed or self-directed team approach offers advantages in both time invested over the long term and effectiveness. Under the leadership of the ICP, team members can become more knowledgeable and skilled in IC issues and can multiply the impact of the ICP in promoting correct use of IC practices throughout the facility. Members could serve as "IC liaisons" to their various units and departments in addition to helping to develop and conduct training, evaluation, and feedback activities. A self-managed team composed of members who are expected to use the various IC practices as part of their daily work is more likely to know what the obstacles to proper use of these practices are and to produce more innovative and acceptable solutions than one person working alone. Although a thorough treatment of work teams is beyond the scope of this chapter, a number of resources are available that provide practical guidance in how to build and use work teams.[8–10] In the remainder of the chapter the term *IC team* should be substituted for *ICP* for those who elect to use the team approach.

Program Components

Though often labeled the ICP's "educational role," training activities are only one of three components necessary for increasing personnel use of IC practices. These are:

- Clearly specifying the expected IC practices of each job category so their occurrence can be easily observed
- Instructing staff in the practices they are expected to employ
- Managing ongoing staff performance

Table 14.1   *IC Practices Sample Training and Management Plan*

STAFF	IC PRACTICE	TRAINING METHOD	FREQ/ (LAST DATE)	LEARNING EVALUATION	ON-THE-JOB EVALUATION	FEEDBACK METHOD
RN LPN CSM Aides	Handwashing	Learning station	9/yr (Oct)	Demo	Self-record	Grp—Graph
	Universal precautions	In-service	3/yr (Jan)	Demo	Direct observation	Ind—Graph
	Perineal care	Videotape	AA*	Demo	Direct observation	Ind—Verbal
	Feeding residents	During rounds	6/yr (Aug)	Demo	Survey Q.	Grp—Graph
	Recognizing infection signs and symptoms	In-service case studies	2/yr (Apr)	Pre-post vignettes	Charting & surveillance	Grp—Graph
	Routine skin care	Learning station	4/yr (Feb)	Demo	Product use	Grp—Graph
	Specimen collection	Program learning	AA	Demo	Lab feedback	Peer—Verbal
	Soiled laundry care	Learning station	2/yr (Sept)	Quiz	Survey Q.	Grp—Graph
RN, LPN CSM	Pressure sore care	Program learning videotape during rounds	AA	Multiple choice test	Direct observation	Individual Verbal
RN LPN	Tracheostomy care/ suctioning	Videotape Return demo Team learning	1/yr (July)	Demo Oral quiz	Survey Q. with reliability check	Group Graph
	Foley catheter insertion					
	Tube feeding					
RN	IV starting/ care	In-service	1/yr (Aug)	Demo	Direct observation	Ind—Verbal
Housekeeping	Facility cleaning practices	Posted instructions	AA	Oral quiz	Work sample	Checklist summary
	Handwashing	During rounds	1/mo (Apr)	Demo	Self-record	Grp—Graph
Dietary Service	Food prepara- tion practices	Program learning	AA	Multiple choice test	Survey Q	GroupGraph

Table 14.1   *(continued)*

STAFF	IC PRACTICE	TRAINING METHOD	FREQ/ (LAST DATE)	LEARNING EVALUATION	ON-THE-JOB EVALUATION	FEEDBACK METHOD
	Handwashing	During rounds	6/yr (Mar)	Demo	Self-record	
	Cleaning practices	Manual	AA	Quiz	Product use	
Activities Staff	Handwashing	During rounds	2/yr (Jan)	Demo	Self-record	Ind—Graph
	Equipment cleaning	Manual	AA	Quiz	Product use	Ind—Verbal
All Staff	Basic personal hygiene and health practices	Learning station	3/yr (Jan)	Pre post quiz	Survey Q.	Group graph

** AA - Always Available

Whether or not the ICP creates a formal self-managed team, the success of this model of management will depend on explicitly involving all levels of staff in the activities of each component. The collaboration and support of administrators and managers is critical if the goal is truly to affect staff behavior, as opposed to just meeting regulatory requirements. The ICP should attempt to continuously increase their involvement in all facets of the IC program.

The chart in Table 14.1 is a sample planning chart that outlines the major program elements addressed in this chapter. When completed by the ICP or team for a particular facility, it will not only organize the training and management tasks but will also provide documentation of IC staff activities in the facility for licensing surveyors, the IC committee, and administrators. In the sections that follow, the reader will be referred to the particular columns of this chart that relate to the program component being discussed.

COMPONENT 1: SPECIFYING THE EXPECTED BEHAVIORS

Columns of the planning chart in Table 14.1 relevant to this section are "Staff" and "IC Practice."

Determining what IC practices each staff role is expected to perform is the place to begin in constructing a behav-

ioral change program. This provides a more focused foundation for future efforts at instruction and performance assessment than beginning with general IC topics that may not target a LTCF's actual employee activities. Defining IC behaviors is an ongoing process that is affected by many factors including changing federal and state regulations, scientific discoveries, the particular resident population, and the judgment of the ICP and the IC committee. The skills required of staff will vary according to the facility's size, type (skilled vs. intermediate care), resident activity, and nursing intensity. Devising such a list is not always easy (an excellent task for the self-managed team), but it will serve to guide and streamline the other training and management tasks.

Areas of focus for training should be timely and relevant: Staff suggestions will be useful in defining topics. General suggested IC areas include handwashing, resident assessment, transmission of infections, basic hygiene, and employee health.[11] Within each relevant topic area, one should look for behaviors that could be modified and that would be likely to impact infection rates. A systematic review of the facility's policies and procedures will often reveal the majority of IC practices that should be implemented. Another good reference for specific staff practices is the *APIC Guideline for Infection Prevention and Control in the Long-Term Care Facility*.[2]

Table 14.2 *Sample Training Curriculum Card for Aides*

INFECTION CONTROL TRAINING CURRICULUM CARD FOR AIDES

IC PRACTICE	LEARNING RESOURCE	RESOURCE SCHEDULE	LEARNING EVALUATION			MANAGER ENDORSED
			METHOD	DATE COMPLETED	SCORE	
Handwashing	Learning station	First Thurs-Sun, each month except Dec, May, Aug	Demonstration			
Universal precautions	In-service	Last Friday, Jan,May, Sept	Demonstration			
Perineal care	Videotape	Always Available - ICP or IC liaison	Demonstration			
Feeding residents	Feeding residents	Schedule anytime with ICP or IC liaison	Demonstration			
Recognizing inf. signs	In-service case studies	Offered April, November	Pre-post test			
Routine skin care	Learning station	Fourth week, Jan,Apr, Jul, Oct,	Demonstration			
Specimen collection	Programmed learning manual	Always Available—ICP	Demonstration			
Soiled laundry care	Learning station	Second week, Feb, Sept	Quiz			

Once a list of all staff IC practices is developed, they can be grouped according to use by the different job titles. The criterion for grouping is similarity of conditions under which the practice is expected to be performed. For example, there are a number of practices that should be performed under similar conditions for all staff who provide direct nursing care. These practices would then be grouped with those staff—typically, aides, certified staff members (CSMs), LPNs, and RNs. The first two columns of Table 14.1 illustrate a potential grouping scheme. Note that handwashing is listed separately for direct care givers, housekeeping staff, and dietary staff because the conditions for handwashing vary for each job category.

COMPONENT 2: TEACHING

Columns of the planning chart in Table 14.1 relevant to this section are "Training Method," "Freq/(Last Date)" and "Learning Evaluation."

After creating a list of specific staff IC practices, the ICP needs to ensure that all staff receive instructions on the practices they are expected to perform, when and how to perform them, and why they are important. Limited time, shift schedules, staff turnover, and poor in-service attendance are often cited as obstacles for the ICP in carrying out "teaching responsibilities." A large part of the problem, however, lies in the underlying premise that it is the ICP's responsibility to get staff to learn. Such an assumption, often conditioned by our educational histories, leads staff to adopt the passive, uninvolved role of information receivers, waiting for the teacher to come to them rather than seeking out the teacher. The ICP's responsibility could be better defined as providing the resources for staff to teach themselves. Responsibility for using those resources to learn needed job skills should be given to staff and established by managers as a clear job expectation. A way to operationalize this expectancy is to provide each employee with a personal "training curriculum card" that lists expected IC skills along with a description and schedule of the available instructional resources. An example of such a card, using the aide's position, is shown in Table 14.2. In the column labeled "Learning Evaluation," the trainer can indicate how well the employee learned a skill, and in the last column, the manager's endorsement ensures that the employee receives credit for educational objectives that have been met.

Methods of Instruction

Instruction methods range from simply telling staff what to do, either verbally or in writing, to more formal in-service programs.

Written Instructions

Memos, posting of responsibilities, scheduling staff assignments, setting goals, and specifying policies are examples of relatively simple instructions that often can be used to communicate the *what*, *when*, and *how* of an IC practice. Uncomplicated practices such as handwashing and many cleaning practices can be taught with these simpler means. This low-cost method for teaching skills is usually underused, possibly because there is little confidence in its effectiveness. As with any instructional method, however, its effectiveness depends on how it is used. Posting handwashing instructions over sinks, for example, will by itself produce little change. Attracting staff attention to written or posted instructions requires the support of direct supervisors, who must underscore their importance, ensure that

they are understood, and prompt and monitor staff compliance. Using a system such as the training curriculum card (Table 14.2), which includes a skill demonstration sign-off, will also enable the ICP to determine the effectiveness of the instructional method.

Teaching on the Job

Occasions for informal instruction occur whenever the ICP interacts with other staff. Answering direct questions, modeling proper IC technique while others are observing, and prompting by giving brief instructions while a behavior is ongoing are ways in which the ICP and managers can teach on a daily basis in the learner's work environment. This type of on the job instruction can be more effective than classroom instruction: Interest in learning a skill that can be applied to solve an immediate work problem is usually high, and the learner is more apt to remember a skill taught within the context of the familiar cues of the work environment. Surveillance rounds provide excellent opportunities for teaching IC practices. The key to capitalizing on their teaching potential is to *consciously look for teaching opportunities*.

To maximize the effectiveness of these interactions, the ICP needs to remember to maintain a teaching role, not the "doer" role. For example, if a nurse needs help cleaning a pressure sore, the ICP should resist the tendency to do it alone, and instead should verbally guide the nurse, prompting only when needed. On those occasions that call for the actual intervention of the ICP, teaching demonstration techniques should be used. An efficient, silent performance may be lost on the onlooking staff. The ICP should make sure staff can see the movements, clearly explain each step, and have the staff return the demonstration whenever possible.

Self-Instruction

Learning stations, videotapes, and programmed instruction manuals are all teaching methods that can be developed for flexible access and self-paced learning. Such modules can often be obtained from pharmaceutical or medical supply companies, from professional associations, or through contacts at other facilities. Learning stations are particularly useful ways of teaching a wide array of skills. These can be constructed on a nursing cart in a format similar to a conference poster presentation. The cart can then

---

Table 14.3   *Sample In-service Preparation Form*

IN-SERVICE PLANNING OUTLINE

Topic: _____
Objectives: _____
_____
_____
_____

Trainees: _____
Location: _____
Date, Time: _____

Presentation Components	Teaching Method/Aids
	(Lecture, videotape, slides, overheads, flipcharts, discussion, case study, etc.)
Why is it important? (Value of skill to residents and employees)	
Description of major steps/points	
Demonstration or example case	
Skill practice or other exercise	
Evaluation methods	

be moved from place to place as needed, and topics can be easily changed or updated.

For optimal effectiveness, self-instruction methods should include:

- A logical sequence of information beginning with clear communication of learning objectives
- Step-by-step pictorial illustration of the skill with brief written explanations
- A method for testing learning such as a skill demonstration session or paper and pencil test.

The evaluation component is especially needed to provide both learning review and motivational functions. Managers should collect tests or observe skill demonstrations before giving credit for completing a learning objective. This provides one more way of placing accountability for learning at the individual employee and department level.

In-service Presentations

A number of related skills or some of the more complex skills such as starting IVs or catheterization may be taught more efficiently in the in-service training format. Designing a formal presentation is an opportunity to exercise creative energies and expand one's boundaries. Many ICPs are intimidated by this teaching method, perhaps because of the unfortunately widespread belief that a background in educational theory or experience is necessary to successfully conduct more formal instructional programs. For some, the anxiety of speaking in front of a group is incapacitating. Both of these fears can often be overcome with repeated in-service teaching efforts and advanced preparation. An outline format, such as the one presented in Table 14.3, helps to structure the preparation process. A description of each of its major areas follows.

a. What new behaviors *should participants be able to do after the presentation?*

The first step is to list the learning objectives, which clearly define the observable behaviors that participants should be able to perform after the training session. These should be limited to three or four per major topic area and should be used to evaluate the learning outcome. Well-conceived objectives work like a homing device for both teacher and learner, providing a clear signal to guide the teaching and learning process along the most direct route. They are especially helpful in affording learners a means of classifying and incorpo-

rating the material to be learned into their present knowledge base. Jackson and Lynch[12] provide a detailed treatment of educational objectives including how to construct objectives and distinguish between cognitive (e.g., analysis of a problem) and psychomotor (e.g., starting an IV) skills.

b. Who should the participants be and how many should be trained at once?

The mix of staff positions should be limited to those who will use the information or skills under the same conditions. The more heterogeneous the participant mix, the more general the presentation must be in order to keep the material relevant to each staff role. "General topic" presentations tend to be boring and rarely result in information staff find useful.[13] The number of participants should ideally be no more than 12 in order to promote active participation. Whenever possible, small group exercises (skill practice, problem solving, etc.) should be planned with five or six participants each. The larger the size of the total group, the more facilitators will be needed for these break-out groups.

c. Where should I conduct the training, and how can I optimize the learning setting?

The environment can have a powerful influence on the learning experience. Consider room size, lighting, temperature, noise interference, and space for group activities. Avoid row seating, which fosters the passive learner role. A horseshoe-shaped seating arrangement permits more immediate contact among all participants and the presenter. Practice "stations" set up around a room allow groups to practice different skills simultaneously but should be far enough apart to minimize noise and movement interference. Attention should also be given to such details as how to darken a room and the location of outlets so that audio-visual aids can be used effectively and with a minimum of disturbance to the flow of the presentation. Before the presentation, the presenter should take time to experiment with different room arrangements, set up and check the functioning of any equipment, and place any handouts at each participant's seat. The goal is to shape the setting in ways that will foster interest and participation while minimizing distractions.

d. When should the training occur?

Most people learn best in the morning and worst directly after lunch or dinner. Consulting the participants or their managers for preferred times as well as dates will enhance attendance. The selected date should be advertised well in advance, with multiple reminders. Actual length of the session is dictated by the teaching methods and amount of material to be covered. In general, however, the learning capacity of most people declines steeply after two hours of structured instruction.

e. How can I facilitate accomplishment of the learning objectives?

When teaching skills, a practice-based training method such as the *tell-show-do* method has been found to be most effective.[14] This approach limits lecture time to an initial *tell* component, which includes a brief explanation of the skill and the value of its use. It is particularly important to give a rationale for why the skill is being taught (i.e., how it will benefit residents or employees). The *show* component is a live or videotaped demonstration of correct (and sometimes incorrect) performance of the skill, and the *do* component is an opportunity for the trainee to role-play or practice the skill. Besides its proven effectiveness as a teaching tool, skill practice is important because it gives the teacher and learner a gauge to measure how well the skill has been learned in a neutral setting. Most people enjoy participating in the practice component, especially if it is structured well (e.g., a list of practice steps is provided) and presented enthusiastically. The group facilitator should ensure that corrective *and positive* feedback are provided throughout the practice interval.

Even when the topic is not a procedural skill that can be practiced, teaching methods that require the participant to actually do something other than passively listening to a lecture result in better retention of the information. For example, recognizing infection signs and symptoms could be taught through small group exercises, practica on the units, and even question and answer sessions.

The use of audio-visual aids such as slides, overhead transparencies, videotapes, and flip charts helps to emphasize key points of a presentation and promotes retention. Handouts of main points or steps in an IC practice facilitate learning by providing the participant with a visual structure of material presented through lecture. Participants appreciate having copies of word slides or overheads included in handouts so they don't have to try to take notes in a darkened room. The column labeled "Teaching Method/Aids" in Table 14.3 prompts consideration of various teaching techniques when planning an in-service presentation. Although it is important to vary training techniques for optimal learner interest, each method must relate to the objectives and fit within a logical sequence of the material.

Problem-based learning approaches, increasingly popular in medical education, can be excellent methods for engaging participants in assuming responsibility for their learning experience.[15] Small self- or facilitator-directed groups work together to solve problems posed with "paper cases" of real or semireal residents. With the infection signs and symptoms topic, the cases could include resident diagnoses, risk factors, medications, infection signs, and so on, and the group's problem would be to determine the type of infection and its cause. This teaching method does not need to be restricted to the classroom setting. It could be used as a monthly "Infection Control Challenge" with self-directed groups on each resident unit competing with each other to solve a number of cases.

f. How will I know if the participants have learned the objectives?

A critical element of in-service presentations is a method to evaluate how well participants learned the initial objectives. When a training objective involves being able to "list" or "state" information, a paper and pencil or verbal "quiz" method can be used. If the objective is learning how to perform a procedure, the best evaluation method is observation of the participant actually performing the skill. Trainees may be able to answer questions about the skill but not to put the pieces together correctly in actual performance. If the training session included a skill-practice component, the presenter will already have had an opportunity to observe participant performance, another advantage to this teaching method. To save the presenter time, participants who have demonstrated clear competence in the skill can assist in observing others' performance.

The presenter should also seek feedback from participants on the effectiveness of the training session. This can be accomplished through brief, anonymous questionnaires using rating scales to rate learner satisfaction with training methods, teaching style, and relevance and usefulness to one's work.

As indicated in the discussion of each training method, measures to evaluate learning and participant satisfaction with the learning experience are essential elements to any staff training effort. The results should be used not only to determine whether or not staff have learned expected IC skills but also to improve the training process. Participant feedback as well as level of success in achieving learning objectives should be used to modify future training sessions. In this sense the development of training programs must be viewed as a continually evolving process.

COMPONENT 3: MANAGING STAFF PERFORMANCE

Columns of the planning chart in Table 14.1 relevant to this section are "On-the-Job Evaluation" and "Feedback Method."

One of the most frequent errors in training is the assumption that learning a skill will automatically translate into using it.[16] Effective training programs only equip participants with new skills; consistent use of the skills depends upon the extent to which they are supported by the work environment. Methods of managing ongoing staff performance require as much attention as initial training efforts, if not more. Although ICPs are not usually in a position to effectively manage on-the-job performance, their consultative advice can help managers focus and align management strategies in ways that will more effectively maintain day-to-day use of IC practices. A knowledge of some basic performance evaluation tools and methods for dealing with performance problems will strengthen the impact of the ICP in this aspect of the role.

Evaluation of IC Practice Performance

All IC practices should be monitored at various times to determine if and how well they are being implemented. By making a point of observing staff use of practices during routine interactions, the ICP and managers can usually discern the performance status of the more obvious practices. When questions arise over the performance of a practice, such as an infection outbreak or other surveillance data, a more formal evaluation process may be called for. Evaluation results separate fact from opinion, help to establish whether or not a performance problem exists, and indicate the direction to follow for a solution. They also provide baseline information that can be used later to assess the effectiveness of any efforts to improve performance. Ideally, the selection of target behaviors, the choice of evaluation method, data collection, and data use should be a collaborative effort involving the ICP, the department managers, and the staff.

Several simple measurement strategies can be used to evaluate IC practices. The simplest and least time-consuming method is the collection of *self-report* data. Staff can be asked to provide information about the occurrence of certain behaviors and indicate whether or not they perceive any performance problems. Concerns about the validity of self-report measures can be partially countered by assuring anonymity of responses. Making it a practice to involve staff in the interpretation of results and any ensuing problem-solving efforts will also promote more valid responses.

Another relatively simple procedure is the use of performance *indicators*, whereby tangible evidence of some kind is used to indicate how well or frequently a behavior occurs. For example, the number of used gloves or improperly capped needles may serve as indicators of the correct or incorrect use of these elements of universal precautions. Noting the condition of cleaning equipment, the presence and rate of hand soap use, and even odors could provide information useful in evaluating IC practices.

Direct *observation* of staff on the job provides the most information about skill use because in addition to rates and quality of performance, the observer also has the opportunity to witness potential obstacles to performance. Typically, this is the most time-consuming measurement procedure, requiring clear definitions of the target behavior, observer training, and sufficient sampling of staff and time periods to produce valid data. However, behaviors such as feeding residents and food preparation practices can be relatively easy to observe because they occur at predictable times. A *Program Evaluation Kit*[17] offers step-by-step guides in nontechnical language on all aspects of evaluation and would be a helpful resource for the ICP.

Whatever method is used, the information collected should be summarized in a report to facilitate its use. Time durations and frequencies of behavior occurrences and ratings are most clearly understood when graphed. Examples of how to graph results from self-report, indicator and direct observation evaluation procedures are shown in Figure 14.1. To help understand changes in performance, it is useful to indicate on the graph key events that may relate to those changes: The arrows in graphs A and B of Figure 14.1 indicate when training and other managerial interventions occurred, permitting

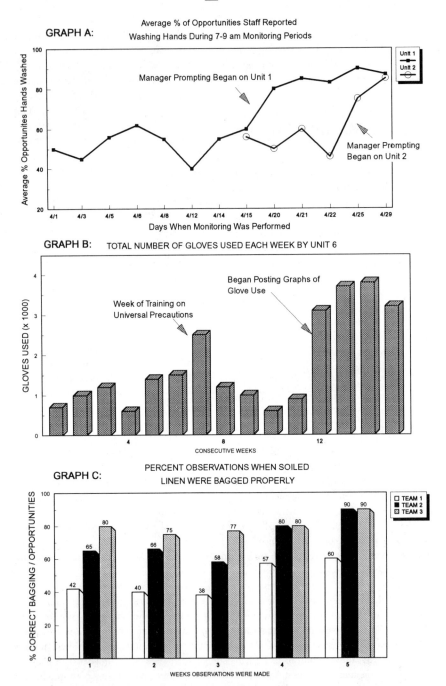

Figure 14.1   *Examples of graphed data to summarize results of staff performance evaluation measures: Graph A: self-report data; Graph B: indicator data; Graph C: direct observation data*

interpretation of their impact on the performance variables. Comments and other qualitative data often provide additional insight into the nature and cause of any performance problem and should be categorized and listed in the summary report.

The value of data depends on the extent to which it leads to actions that improve performance. Managers and staff should set aside time to review data summaries, take credit for favorable results, and brainstorm ways of improving behaviors that are found to be deficient. Posting graphed data of group performance is an effective way of communicating the importance of data and the targeted behaviors, particularly when the data are updated with periodic reassessments. The process of evaluating performance and reviewing results often leads to behavior improvements, especially when the evaluation is initiated from within a department. However, any gains are usually short-lived unless they are paired with other management procedures as discussed here.

Performance Problems

When a performance deficit is identified through monitoring or evaluation activities, a common reaction is to blame individual staff, characterizing them as "resistant" or "difficult." In the vast majority of cases, however, ineffective management methods and obstacles in the work processes are the reasons for poor performance, not the lack of individual desire to perform well. The ICP can help managers to analyze their own behavior and conditions in the work setting that contribute to inadequate use of IC practices. The following sequence of questions can be used to structure this analysis:

1. Have the necessary skills been learned?
2. Have performance expectations been properly communicated?
3. Are there obstacles that interfere with performance?
4. Are there positive consequences for performing as expected?

If the answer to either of the first two questions is no, the course of action is relatively straightforward in terms of training or better communication of expected behaviors. Earlier sections of this chapter deal with these two areas.

To answer the third question, direct observation and flow-charting of each step of the work process involving the problem behavior should be conducted. The objective is to locate conditions in the physical environment, equipment, or sequence of steps needed to accomplish the behavior that might interfere with successful performance. For example, inconveniently located sinks or harsh soaps may be environmental or equipment factors that contribute to poor handwashing practices. The particular kits used for starting IVs may not contain appropriate antiseptics, complicating the steps to perform this procedure. If materials needed to perform frequent IC practices (e.g., gloves) are kept at a central station or supply room rather than close to the resident, the distance and time required to get them will inevitably obstruct their use.

When obstacles are identified, solutions should be sought through problem-solving groups comprised primarily of the staff who are expected to implement the particular IC practice. Some solutions may be too impractical or expensive to implement. The value of the potential improvements in performance and consequent benefit to residents or employees must be weighed against the costs of restructuring the environment or work process.

The fourth question is particularly important in analyzing job performance and requires a basic understanding of positive and negative consequences and their impact on behavior. Consistent performance of a behavior is due to the reinforcing effects of positive events that are associated with the behavior. These may be external events such as praise, internal thoughts/feelings such as "I'm doing a good job," or even the avoidance of an unpleasant event such as getting fired. The effectiveness of a positive event in maintaining a behavior depends on whether or not a "competing" negative event also exists and which one is more powerful. A look at the consequences of handwashing, the most important *and* underused IC practice, helps to illustrate this principle.

The potential positive outcome for handwashing is the belief that one is removing harmful microbes and thereby preventing an infection. For the average health care worker, the strength of this belief is undermined by the lack of observable supporting evidence: Microbes cannot be readily observed, infections do not always occur when hands are not washed; and the "experts" (physicians and nurses) frequently do not wash their own hands. The potential negative consequences for handwashing include loss of time and energy and chapped hands. Because these effects are more observable and immediate, they often are more powerful than the positive outcomes, which must be taken on faith, and serve to control handwashing frequency.

If the positive consequences for performing an IC practice are weaker than the existing negative consequences, it becomes the task of the ICP and managers to *create* more reinforcing outcomes. The following section describes a method for creating performance outcomes that has been proven effective in many work settings including LTCFs.

Performance Feedback

Some of the most consistently effective supervisory procedures are those that entail the delivery of performance consequences in the form of feedback.[18–20] Feedback refers to information provided to employees about the quantity or quality of their performance. Its programmatic simplicity, low cost, and flexibility make it an attractive alternative to other performance consequences. In studies conducted in LTCF settings, both individual and group feedback procedures were found to be effective in increasing appropriate glove use.[21,22]

The method of giving feedback can assume many different forms. Feedback can be delivered privately or publicly, to individuals or groups, by peers or supervisors, and through written, verbal, or graphic means. A number of factors influence the success of feedback procedures. The following list of "ideal" feedback characteristics can be used by ICPs when helping to design a feedback program.

- Feedback should be paired with praise or some other form of recognition for behavior gains.
- Individual feedback is more powerful than group feedback.
- Direct observation or indicators of staff performance (e.g., documentation, number of used gloves, etc.) are the most reliable sources of feedback content. Self-recorded information can be used when it is periodically verified through other means.
- Graphed, numerical feedback (e.g., rates of glove use or handwashing) is more effective than verbal or written feedback.
- Feedback should be given weekly or biweekly.
- Feedback is most effective when delivered by direct su-

pervisors as long as they model the desired practice themselves.

It has also been shown that the person delivering feedback requires recognition and support (their own feedback-gram) to maintain this system, an excellent role for the ICP.[21]

SUMMARY

A staff training and management program that specifies expected IC practices, provides instruction, and reinforces ongoing performance will be effective in achieving high rates of IC practice use. A comprehensive program will take considerable time to develop and will need continuous modifications. These modifications should be based on changes in the field of infection control, data from surveillance activities, and results of evaluation measures that answer the questions, (1) Was training well received? (2) Did staff learn the skills? (3) Are skills performed as expected? Administrators, managers, and all staff members have essential roles to play. The more people who share in both the design and work of this program, the more feasible, acceptable, and effective it will be. The real value of ICPs should be measured not by how well they can teach, but by how well they can create consensus and inspire teamwork so that many people can teach.

Finally, the goal of a program to improve use of IC practices is to reduce nosocomial infections. This chapter has focused on the means or processes intended to achieve this outcome. A training and management program may be effective in terms of staff learning and using IC practices, but its ultimate *value* must be measured in terms of improved health outcomes for residents. To keep this goal in sight, ICPs need to continually look for relationships between infection rates calculated from surveillance data and use of IC practices. Their roles in both of these areas place them in an ideal position to contribute much needed information about the efficacy of IC practices in LTCFs. A well-designed and well-documented program for managing IC practices will help make such efforts possible.

REFERENCES

1. *Federal Register.* 1991; 56:48826–48922.

2. Smith PW, Rusnak PG: APIC guideline for infection prevention and control in the long-term care facility. *Am J Infect Control* 1991; 19:198–215.

3. Seto WH, Org SG, Ching TY, et al: Brief report: The utilization of influencing tactics for the implementation of infection control practices. *Infect Control Hosp Epidemiol* 1990; 11:144–150.

4. Gilbert TF, Gilbert MB: Potential contributions of performance science to education. *J Appl Behav Anal* 1992; 25:43–49.

5. Daniels AC: *Performance Management: Improving Quality Productivity Through Positive Reinforcement.* Tucker, GA, Performance Management Publications, 1989.

6. Malott RW, Garcia ME: A goal directed model approach for the design of human performance systems. *J Organizational Behav Management* 1987; 9:125–159.

7. Berry TH: *Managing the Total Quality Transformation.* New York, McGraw-Hill, 1991.

8. Scholtes PR: *The Team Handbook.* Madison, WI, Joiner Associates, 1988.

9. Byham, WC: *Zapp! The Lightning of Empowerment.* New York, Ballantine Books, 1992.

10. Orsburn JD, Moran L, Musselwhite E, et al: *Self-Directed Work Teams.* Homewood, IL, Business One Irwin, 1990.

11. Smith PW, et al: Consensus conference on nosocomial infections in long-term care facilities. *Am J Infect Control* 1987; 15:97–100.

12. Jackson MM, Lynch P: Education of the adult learner: A practical approach for the infection control practitioner. *Am J Infect Control* 1986; 14:257–271.

13. Latham GP: Behavioral approaches to the training and learning process in organizations, in Goldstein IL (ed.): *Training and Development in Work Organizations, Frontiers of Industrial and Organizational Psychology* San Francisco, Jossey Bass, 1989, pp 256–296.

14. Gardner JM: Teaching behavior modification to nonprofessionals. *J Appl Behav Anal* 1972;5:517–522.

15. Barrows HS: A taxonomy of problem-based learning methods. *Med Educ* 1986;20:481–486.

16. Figa-Talamanca I: Problems in the evaluation of training health personnel. *Health Educ Monographs* 1975;3:232–250.

17. Herman JL (ed.): *Program Evaluation Kit,* 2nd ed. Newbury Park, CA, Sage Publications, 1987.

18. DeVries J, Burnette M, and Redmon W: AIDS prevention: Improving nurses' compliance with glove wearing through performance feedback. *J Appl Behav Anal* 1991;24:705–711.

19. Geller E, Eason S, Phillips J, et al: Interventions to improve sanitation during food preparation. *J Organizational Behav Management* 1980;2:229–241.

20. Mayer J, Dubbert P, Miller M, et al: Increasing handwashing in an intensive care unit. *Infect Control* 1986;7:259–262.

21. Babcock RA, Sulzer-Azaroff B, Sanderson M, et al: Increasing nurses' use of feedback to promote infection-control practices in a head-injury treatment center. *J Appl Behav Anal* 1992;25:621–627.

22. Burgio LD, Engel BT, Hawkins A, et al: Staff management of incontinence in a nursing home. *J Appl Behav Anal* 1989;25:111–118.

HIV INFECTION, AIDS, AND UNIVERSAL PRECAUTIONS

Virginia M. Helget and Jane S. Roccaforte

Discovery of the human immunodeficiency virus (HIV) in the early 1980s changed the delivery of health care. Health care workers (HCWs) are concerned for their own safety as well as that of their patients. Hospitals provide only a portion of care to these people; long-term care facilities (LTCFs) and other agencies have been called upon to help fill the void. The influence of HIV on LTCFs is being felt as they prepare to accept residents and as regulations are made to protect HCWs from exposure to bloodborne pathogens.

HIV INFECTION AND AIDS

The HIV virus is the agent that causes acquired immunodeficiency syndrome (AIDS), a progressive illness that attacks the defense system of the body. It is found worldwide and is fatal in virtually every case. The first U.S. case was reported in 1981. Because of reporting differences, it is difficult to know how many people are infected. It is estimated that the number of those infected with HIV is eight times the number of reported AIDS cases. In the United States, for example, HIV infection is not a universally reportable condition; some states are required to report only the disease, AIDS. Definitions of what constitutes AIDS have changed over time. The current AIDS case definition was published in January 1993 by the CDC.[1]

What Is HIV?

HIV is a virus that attacks the body's immune system, especially the lymphocytes (CD4+ cells, see Chapter 2). HIV enters the CD4+ cells; as the virus reproduces itself, these cells are destroyed. Acute infection with the virus may produce flulike symptoms, which eventually resolve. Six to twelve weeks after infection, blood tests may show the presence of antibody to the virus. The antibody to HIV is not protective but is an indicator that infection has occurred and the body has responded to the infection.

Infection is followed by a latent period during which the person is asymptomatic. This period lasts an average of 5 to 10 years. The person is infectious during this time, even though no symptoms have developed.

Infection progresses to AIDS after a variable period of time. Symptoms begin to develop as the immune system gradually fails. An indicator of the progress of the disease is a measurement of CD4+ lymphocyte counts. As their numbers decrease, the risk of developing an opportunistic infection increases. Numbers below 200/mm^3 become critical.

Associated Infections

Interference with the immune system makes the infected individual prone to a variety of infections as well as certain cancers. Diagnosis of AIDS is based on repeatedly positive HIV blood tests, less than 200 CD4+ T-lymphocytes/mm^3, or the presence of associated clinical conditions.

Table 15.1	*Some Common Infectious Disases Associated with AIDS*

Parasitic infections
Cryptosporidiosis
Isosporiasis
Viral infections
Cytomegalovirus (CMV)
Herpes simplex
Mycobacteria (atypical)
Salmonellosis
Fungal infections
Candidiasis
Coccidioidomycosis
Cryptococcosis
Histoplasmosis
Bacterial infections
Mycobacterium tuberculosis

Common examples of opportunistic infections are *Pneumocystis carinii*, herpes simplex, herpes zoster, and tuberculosis. Other infections such as thrush may be present (see Table 15.1). Effects on the central nervous system may include weakness, confusion, and dementia. Certain cancers are associated with AIDS, such as lymphoma and Kaposi's sarcoma.

Risk Groups

Since its discovery, the risk groups for HIV infection have remained the same over time, but the percentages of infected individuals belonging to each risk group have varied. Those at highest risk are homosexual or bisexual males and injection drug users. Others at risk include sexual partners of homosexuals, bisexuals, or injection drug users; those who received blood or blood products prior to 1985; and children born to those in one of the risk groups. The blood supply has been screened since May 1985, and the risk in blood product recipients has decreased since that time.

Testing

Blood tests most frequently used to diagnose HIV actually look for the presence of antibody. There is a time lag referred to as the window phase, between infec-tion with the virus and the body's production of antibody to HIV during which the blood test will be negative, even though infection has occurred. This is why repeat blood tests are necessary. Screening tests are usually followed by a confirmatory test if the initial results are positive.

Two appropriate reasons to test for HIV infection are to diagnose and treat the condition, and to do appropriate follow-up for exposures to blood or body fluids.

Many issues surround testing for HIV infection. When testing is performed, pre- and post-test counseling should be done by someone who is educated in HIV and its implications.

Informed consent should be obtained, and the test results must be kept confidential. Mandatory routine testing of all residents or staff is not cost effective or advisable. Mandatory testing has not been shown to decrease transmission and may lead to misinterpretation of the results. Testing should not substitute for rigorous use of universal precautions.

Transmission

Transmission of HIV occurs through contact of non-intact skin or mucous membranes with infected blood or body fluids. It is not transmitted by casual contact. The majority of cases occur through sexual contact or blood contact. A few cases have occurred in HCWs.

Table 15.2	*Body Fluids to Which Universal Precautions Apply*

Blood
Body fluids containing visible blood
Semen
Vaginal secretions
Cerebrospinal fluid (CSF)
Pleural fluid
Peritoneal fluid
Pericardial fluid
Amniotic fluid
Synovial fluid

Centers for Disease Control Update: Universal precautions for prevention of transmission of human immunodeficiency virus, hepatitis B virus, and other bloodborne pathogens in health care settings. *MMWR* 1988;37:378–387.

The parenteral route of exposure (e.g., needlesticks, lacerations) carries greater risk of infection than mucous membrane exposure to HIV. Studies show the risk of HIV transmission to a HCW from a needlestick with HIV-infected blood is less than 0.4%.[3,4] Large volumes of infected blood or body fluid carry a greater risk of transferring the infection.[5] Other body fluids may carry a risk of HIV transmission (see Table 15.2).

HIV IN THE LONG-TERM CARE FACILITY

Incidence in Long-Term Care Facilities

The prevalence of HIV in the general population as well as in LTCF residents is unknown. Although most AIDS residents are under 50 years of age, AIDS occurs in every age group, and younger patients with AIDS dementia (which mimics Alzheimer's disease) may be admitted to the LTCF.

The Resident

If possible, residents with HIV should be cared for in the same way as other residents and should be encouraged to participate in facility activities. Their younger age may require some thought and planning by the staff and family or friends to find activities interesting to them.

For infection control purposes, there is no reason to restrict residents to private rooms based solely on the fact that they have AIDS or HIV infection. Restriction of activity, if necessary, should be made on an individual basis. Some facilities place AIDS residents in private rooms for their own privacy and comfort, but those reasons need to be made clear. Residents with HIV, like all other residents, should not share washcloths, towels, razors, or other personal items with others.

There is no need to use disposable items or special dishes for those with HIV. Dishwasher and laundering temperatures or disinfection procedures required in facilities destroy the virus.

A variety of infectious diseases are associated with AIDS. Some of these diseases are indicative of the resident's decreased immune status. Many of them are not a hazard to healthy caregivers and visitors but may lead to significant morbidity for the resident. In any case, HCWs need to know which of these conditions require precautions to prevent transmission (see Chapter 19).

Working with the Family and Support System

There are many fears and doubts to be resolved in caring for residents with HIV. Residents and their families and friends must learn to deal with the facts of the disease, their own fears about it, and each other's needs. While they are struggling with these difficulties, an understanding and compassionate staff can be an asset. Social service workers, counselors, and volunteers may assist in these areas and should be consulted.

Medical information of all residents is privileged and confidential. Medical information should be shared with those who have a need to know, but access to information must be protected. All staff in the facility must protect this right to privacy.

Admission Policies and Screening

A four-state survey of LTCFs found that even though AIDS had been diagnosed in each of the four states and many of the facilities had a policy regarding AIDS, only 9% to 19% said they would definitely accept residents with AIDS.[6]

General policies concerning acceptance of residents with HIV or AIDS should be established, preferably before a need arises. Such policies should take into account the

---

Table 15.3   *Considerations in Accepting HIV-Infected Residents in LTCFs*

Reimbursement sources
Resources
Staffing issues
Skilled care requirements
Infection control practices
Fear
Admission policies
Structural constraints
Knowledge of the staff

Compiled from Bentley DW, Cheney L: AIDS and long-term care facilities. *Infect Control Hosp Epidemiol* 1990;11:202–206.

needs of the resident and the services provided by the facility. Are there adequate handwashing facilities available? Is the facility capable of transporting the resident to another facility for supplemental care if needed? Table 15.3 suggests other factors to consider in this decision.[7]

Economic Issues

Therapy and drugs to treat those with HIV infection are costly, and residents with AIDS may require more intense nursing. An AIDS unit at one LTCF calculated 5.5 nursing care hours per resident-day to provide care.[8] This may be more hours than are typically allotted in LTCFs. Issues such as this must be figured into the resources needed to care for a resident with HIV. Workers' compensation may or may not be available for those who sustained work-related exposure to HIV.

The Staff

Several aspects of caring for residents with HIV in the LTCF relate to the staff. Some issues relate to preparing staff members to care for residents with HIV. One must also consider the HIV-infected HCW who may be employed at the facility. If handled appropriately, most of these issues can be dealt with effectively.

Attitudes and Education

A significant amount of time should be spent preparing the staff to care for residents with HIV. All staff in the facility should be educated according to their duties and types of contact with the residents.

The nursing staff should be taught the general signs and symptoms of the opportunistic infections that may be seen in residents with HIV and should know the drugs (such as zidovudine) used to treat HIV and associated conditions.

Educators must also inform HCWs of the potential for exposure to HIV on the job. All members of the staff should be included in the educational programs that pertain to their duties and potential for exposure. This will be discussed at greater length later.

Risk Factors

The risk of exposure to HIV in the LTCF setting is primarily related to the degree of exposure to infected blood or body fluids. In prevalence studies of HIV in HCWs, those with the highest rates are those who have frequent and prolonged contact with contaminated blood (e.g., laboratory workers, emergency room staff).[9] Those who provide bedside care to patients/residents have approximately the same prevalence of HIV as the general population.

Procedures in the LTCF that increase the risk of staff exposure to body fluids are those that involve starting IVs, drawing blood, or changing dressings. Staff must recognize these and similar procedures as potential hazards and take appropriate precautions to protect themselves. It is advisable to exclude staff members who have open skin lesions from resident contact until the areas are healed. This is for the protection of both residents and staff.

HCWs who have been exposed to body fluids and are awaiting HIV test results should be counseled to use barriers to protect sexual partners during sexual activity and to avoid pregnancy.[10] The exposed employee should be counseled about the risks and implications of the exposure, what actions can be taken, and whether prophylaxis with antiretroviral drugs is indicated.

The Environment

There is no evidence that HIV is transmitted by objects in the environment such as tables, chairs, or telephones. Although HIV may live on these surfaces for a short while, transmission has not occurred. Nonetheless, it is always important to practice good hygiene and frequent handwashing, and to maintain a clean environment.

Disinfection and Equipment

HIV can be transmitted from person to person by equipment that touches mucous membranes or enters sterile body areas if the equipment is not properly cleaned and disinfected. Equipment that is difficult to clean (e.g., endoscopes, biopsy forceps) is especially worrisome. In the LTCF, respiratory therapy and physical therapy equipment may fall into this category.

Standard methods for disinfection, using friction and an effective germicide, are sufficient. If gross soiling is present, the surface or object should be cleaned before it is disinfected.

Needlestick Injuries

Many LTCFs do not have protocols for managing needlestick injuries. Many needlestick injuries in LTCFs are related to the practice of recapping needles.[11] These issues have been addressed by regulatory agencies and will be covered in more detail in the next section.

Because HIV may be transmitted by injury with contaminated sharp objects, HCWs must be educated to prevent this from occurring. To protect staff from HIV and other infections, facilities should have procedures for the proper handling of used sharp equipment. Special handling of regulated or infectious waste is expensive, so care should be taken to exclude regular trash.

Pregnant HCWs

Pregnant HCWs can safely care for those with HIV infection as long as they practice good infection control and universal precautions. It is important that the pregnant HCW be well educated in how to protect herself from HIV transmission and what actions to take if she is exposed. Although the pregnant HCW does not run a greater risk of getting infected with HIV than other staff members, if infection does occur, it may be passed to the fetus.

Health Care Workers with HIV/AIDS

The number of HCWs with HIV infection or AIDS is unknown. HCWs are encouraged to know their own HIV status, but mandatory testing is not usually advised. Those who are infected with HIV should use techniques to prevent exposure of residents or other HCWs to their blood or body fluids.

Employment Issues

Because AIDS is legally a disability, decisions to hire, dismiss, or transfer employees must be made carefully. HIV-infected HCWs should not be discriminated against if they are capable of safely performing their duties. The risk of an HIV-infected HCW transmitting the virus to another HCW or resident is extremely small.

It is important that HIV-infected HCWs who provide resident care consistently comply with universal precautions. They must perform procedures using excellent aseptic technique, as should all HCWs. Consultation with those responsible for infection control and employee health can help determine what, if any, special procedures, restrictions, or instructions are applicable to the infected HCW. By consulting the facility's attorney as well as state and other regulatory agencies, specific policies and procedures can be writ-

ten. Those involved in the decision-making process regarding a HCW infected with HIV must understand the importance of not disclosing information about that HCW to others.

Retraining/Reassignment

Provided the employee complies with the policies and procedures of the institution and does not endanger the safety of others, there should be no reason to reassign an employee because of HIV status. Every reasonable attempt to accommodate the employee should be made. This may require some modification of duties or work schedules.

The physical condition of the HCW and the nature of the work must be considered when making these decisions. Retraining or reassignment to nonresident care may be necessary if the HCW is unable to perform regular duties. One must take care to preserve the HCW's privacy in dealing with these issues.

PREVENTING TRANSMISSION OF BLOODBORNE PATHOGENS

It is important for all HCWs to recognize the potential hazard of contact with HIV, hepatitis B, and other diseases in the workplace and to take appropriate precautions.

The techniques described will help prevent transmission of not only bloodborne pathogens, but other diseases. These techniques have come to be known as universal precautions.

Guidelines and Regulations

In 1987, the CDC published guidelines to protect HCWs from the spread of bloodborne diseases, in particular HIV.[12] It described a system for providing health care based on the assumption that anyone may have an infectious disease. Diseases transmitted by blood exposure were targeted, but many health care facilities extended these rules to apply to all body fluids, hoping to prevent the spread of other diseases as well. In 1988, the guideline was updated to distinguish the body fluids that were specifically associated with HIV and hepatitis B.[13]

The regulations apply to most health care institutions, including LTCFs. HCWs are to assume that most body fluids are potentially infectious and take precautions to

Table 15.4 *Primary Components of the OSHA Standard*

Exposure control plan
Work practices (procedures)
Engineering controls
Personal protective equipment
Housekeeping measures (waste and laundry)
Screening/hepatitis B vaccination
Post-exposure evaluation and treatment
Training and monitoring

Department of Labor: Occupational exposure to bloodborne pathogens; final rule. *Federal Register* 1991;56:64004–64182.

prevent skin or mucous membrane contact with these fluids. Personnel should immediately wash the exposed area with soap and water after contamination with blood or body fluids. Because of the risk broken skin poses, those with open or weeping skin lesions or sores should not have contact with residents or resident care equipment until the condition clears.

The CDC guidelines were utilized by the Occupational Safety and Health Administration (OSHA) to enforce HCW and institutional compliance with universal precautions.[14] Lack of compliance can result in large fines. The federal OSHA standard is in effect unless there is a state OSHA rule that is more stringent. Each facility must have an exposure control plan specifying the definition of an exposure, the methods used to implement universal precautions as described in the regulation, and the procedures used to evaluate exposure incidents to prevent future occurrences. Employees must have access to the plan, and it must be updated at least annually. The OSHA regulation consists of eight general areas (see Table 15.4).

Procedures

One of the primary methods to control exposure of HCWs to blood and body fluids is by modifying work practices. If possible, ways should be found to perform tasks while minimizing the risk of exposure or injury. In each LTCF, procedures should incorporate the use of universal precautions into all resident care practices. These procedures should include not only a description of how to perform a task, but how to protect oneself while performing the task, how to dispose of waste (e.g., sharps or trash) that requires special handling, and what to do with equipment that is used during the procedure. Procedures for all applicable aspects of the OSHA rule should be written and monitored for compliance.

Frequent handwashing should be promoted. Sinks should be conveniently located. If sinks are not readily available, an alternative method of hand disinfection should be provided until the hands can be washed. Education plays an important part in getting people to modify their work practices (see Chapter 14).

Equipment

Equipment and engineering controls are mechanisms to isolate or remove bloodborne pathogens from the workplace. Needleboxes that are puncture resistant and leakproof should be provided in appropriate areas. Most often, this is at the point of use, such as a medication cart, resident room, or medication room. Receptacles should be positioned in other locations where needles may be encountered (e.g., laundry, kitchen). The containers must be labeled or color coded so they can be easily recognized.

Devices that eliminate the need for needles to obtain access to IV systems are useful in reducing needlestick injuries. Since many exposures to blood occur because of needlesticks, this system has great potential to eliminate injuries while working with IVs.

Personal protective equipment is equipment or clothing worn by HCWs to protect themselves from blood or body fluids. Included are items such as gloves, gowns, masks, and protective eyewear. HCWs must know where the apparel is, when to use it, how to put it on, and how to remove it.

Gloves should be worn whenever hands may come in contact with body fluids or when performing invasive procedures, and they must be available in a variety of sizes. Gloves should be removed between procedures, and the hands should be washed. It is a common error for HCWs to wear gloves to protect themselves but not remove them before performing other tasks or touching equipment. The environment becomes contaminated when this occurs, and the potential for cross-contamination between residents increases. Gloves should immediately be removed and replaced if torn or punctured.

Surgical and exam gloves are single-use items and should not be saved and washed for reuse. Washing may destroy the integrity of the glove. Washed and reused gloves may retain organisms on the surface that could be transferred to residents.

As more latex products are used as barriers for protection, skin sensitivities are becoming common. Nonlatex gloves should be obtained for those who have latex allergies. Gloves labeled "hypoallergenic" may not prevent adverse reactions in those who are allergic to latex. Adverse reactions include itchy and watery eyes, sneezing and nasal congestion, dyspnea, wheezing, chest tightness, and hives or rashes. Both residents and HCWs may exhibit signs of allergy; deaths have occurred. It is estimated that 6% to 7% of surgical personnel, 8.8% of dentists and 18% to 40% of spina bifida patients are latex-sensitive.[15,16] Provisions should be made to find substitutes for latex items, both for resident care and employee use.

Gowns should be fluid resistant. They are used to protect clothing from being soiled with body fluids or when splashing or spraying of body fluids is anticipated. Gowns should be removed between tasks and when contaminated. Aprons, jackets, and lab coats may also be worn for protection in some situations.

Masks are worn to protect the mucous membranes of the nose and mouth from exposure to splash and spray of body fluids. Masks should not dangle around the neck to be used again. They should be constructed in a manner appropriate to the degree of protection required.

Protective eyewear, face shields, and other devices are used to protect the eyes from contact with body fluids. It is important that these devices prevent fluids from entering the sides, such as when the face is turned away from the resident. Masks or eyewear may be required during some wound care (e.g., irrigation), when suctioning residents, or when doing arterial punctures for blood gas analysis (e.g., ventilated residents).

Ventilation devices should be used when performing cardiopulmonary resuscitation. They should be placed in convenient locations where they can be quickly located. These include pocket masks, mouthpieces, and resuscitation bags.

Waste Management

There are numerous names for infectious waste (e.g., medical waste, isolation waste, regulated waste). The definition varies somewhat among states and governing agencies. Local, state, and federal regulations should be followed in the facility policy.

Most will agree that liquid or semiliquid blood, items contaminated with blood or infectious material, and items that may cause an infection in others are considered infectious waste. Contaminated sharps are also included.

Procedures to safely handle and dispose of infectious waste should be established. Containers of infectious waste should be labeled or color coded. They should be large enough to contain all the waste and should be closed prior to removal to prevent spilling of the contents. It is essential that they not leak. If the outside of the container is contaminated or has a hole, a second container should be used. Sharps disposal containers or needleboxes should not be overfilled before being closed and discarded. Glass, reusable needles, or other sharp equipment that is contaminated should not be picked up with the hands, but with a tool or piece of equipment. Employees should not reach into containers of contaminated sharps to clean or process them.

Infectious waste may need to be rendered noninfectious before disposal. This can be done using a variety of methods (e.g., autoclaving, incinerating). Some facilities contract this service to others. There are also issues concerning transportation of infectious waste. Local, state, and other regulations should be observed.

Housekeeping Concerns

The facility should be maintained in a clean, sanitary manner. Cleaning schedules and procedures should be used to achieve this. The frequency of cleaning will depend on the item, its use, and its location in the facility. Effective disinfectants should be used that are appropriate to the material to be decontaminated, the type of soil present, and the work environment. Protective apparel should be worn for cleaning when appropriate.

Blood or body fluid spills should be contained as quickly as possible, and the area should be cleaned and disinfected. Sodium hypochlorite in a 1:10 or 1:100 dilution with water is one of the recommended products. Staff should wear protective apparel appropriate to the task. Reusable bins, cans, carts, or other receptacles should be cleaned and disinfected regularly and when overtly soiled.

Laundry

In order to protect themselves when handling laundry, HCWs should handle or agitate linen as little as possible. Laundry should not be sorted or rinsed in resident rooms. Linen should be bagged to contain soiled pieces.

Linen bags should not leak or drip fluids, nor should they be overfilled. Those who have contact with soiled linen should wear protective apparel. If all linen is managed using universal precautions, special marking of potentially infectious linen is not necessary. The temperature and chemicals required for institutional laundry are adequate for killing the HIV virus. Proper procedures in the laundry must be followed, however.

Vaccination Program

Because hepatitis B is one of the bloodborne pathogens that causes work-related illness in HCWs, hepatitis B immunizations should be offered to employees who have the potential for exposure to blood or body fluids in the workplace. Every effort should be made to be sure the employee understands the reasons for the vaccine, its safety, and its effectiveness. It should be offered to employees before tasks are performed that may put them at risk of exposure. If an employee initially declines the hepatitis vaccine, a declination statement should be signed. However, the employee is free to request immunization at a later date.

If the HCW is already immune to hepatitis B (because of prior infection with hepatitis B or prior immunization) or if it is contraindicated, the vaccine should not be given. If an exposure to blood or body fluids occurs after receiving the vaccine, the employee may need to be tested to be sure there is an adequate level of antibody present.

Exposure Evaluation and Follow-up

HCWs must know what to do when an exposure occurs. They should wash the exposed area with soap and water, receive first aid if necessary, and report the incident to an appropriate person.

OSHA requires a confidential medical evaluation and follow-up for the employee exposed to a resident's body fluids. If possible, the resident involved in the incident should be tested for hepatitis B and HIV. The employee should be tested for hepatitis B antibody and HIV to determine baseline values. Periodic testing of the HCW's blood may be indicated in certain circumstances (e.g., significant exposure to the blood or body fluids of an HIV-infected resident). Appropriate consent laws should be observed. Postexposure prophylaxis, testing, and counseling should also be provided.

A record of all employees with occupational exposure must be kept. This record should include results of examinations, laboratory tests, and other pertinent material. The record must be kept confidential and should not be disclosed without the written consent of the employee.

Education and Monitoring

Employees should be educated at the time they are assigned to tasks that may involve exposure to blood or body fluids; educational programs should be repeated at least annually. It is suggested that training be decentralized so that it applies to employees' duties and work areas. Employees must know what bloodborne diseases are, how they are transmitted, and how to protect themselves.

Location of protective apparel, how and when to use it, and how to remove it should be included in the education programs. The presentations should include what employees should do when they are exposed to body fluids or when a spill occurs. Training should be presented at a level that is appropriate for the employee. The date, a summary, the name of the trainer, and a list of attendees must be maintained.

Compliance

Compliance with universal precautions should be monitored periodically to be sure employees are protecting themselves. Monitoring should be department and task specific. Direct observation of personnel is the most accurate method. Both positive and negative feedback to employees can be provided during observation periods. Tools for assessment and monitoring have been developed.[17,18] They can be used as models and adapted to the needs of the facility and the procedures performed. Monitoring compliance with universal precautions is effective in increasing the use of barriers in the facility.[19]

It may be possible to incorporate these checks into the facility quality improvement program. Areas identified as needing improvement can provide topics for educational programs, performance appraisals, or team building projects.

OSHA regulations are designed to protect HCWs from HIV and hepatitis B, small risks in the LTCF. A good infection control program will also address other, more common health risks such as tuberculosis (see Chapter 16). Infection control procedures should apply to all residents so that staff may perform the same way in caring for everyone.

REFERENCES

1. Centers for Disease Control: 1993 revised classification system for HIV infection and expanded surveillance case definition for AIDS among adolescents and adults. *MMWR* 1992;41:1–19.
2. Centers for Disease Control: Revision of the CDC surveillance case definition for acquired immunodeficiency syndrome. *MMWR* 1987;36 (no. S-1).
3. Weber DJ, Rutala WA: Management of HIV-1 infection in the hospital setting. *Infect Control Hosp Epidemiol* 1989;10:3–7.
4. Henderson DK, Fahey BJ, Willy M, et al: Risk for occupational transmission of human immunodeficiency virus type 1 (HIV-1) associated with clinical exposures: a prospective evaluation. *Ann Intern Med* 1990;113:740–746.
5. Shirazian D, Herzlich BC, Mokhtarian, et al: Detection of HIV antibody and antigen (p24) in residual blood on needles and glass. *Infect Control Hosp Epidemiol* 1990;11:180–184.
6. Gwartney DL, Daly PB, Roccaforte JS, et al: PWAs in the long term care facility. *AIDS Patient Care.* 1992;6:15–18.
7. Bentley DW, and Cheney L: AIDS and long-term care facilities. *Infect Control Hosp Epidemiol* 1990;11:202–206.
8. Glatt AE, Risbrook AT. Jenna RW: Successful implementation of a long-term care unit for patients with acquired immunodeficiency syndrome in an underserved suburban area with a high incidence of human immunodeficiency virus. *Arch Intern Med* 1992;152:823–825.
9. Bell DM: Human immunodeficiency virus transmission in health care settings: risk and reduction. *Am J Med* 1991;91:294S–300S.
10. Technical Panel on Infections within Hospitals: American Hospital Association: Management of HIV infection in the hospital. *Am J Infect Control* 1989;17:24A–44A.
11. Crossley K, Willenbring K, Thurn J: Needlestick injuries and needle disposal in Minnesota nursing homes. *J Am Geriatr Soc* 1990;38:793–796.
12. Centers for Disease Control: Recommendations for prevention of HIV transmission in health-care settings. *MMWR* 1987;36(suppl 2S).
13. Centers for Disease Control: Update: Universal precautions for prevention of transmission of human immunodeficiency virus, hepatitis B virus, and other bloodborne pathogens in health-care settings. *MMWR* 1988;37:378–387.
14. Department of Labor, Occupational Safety and Health Administration: Occupational exposure to bloodborne pathogens, final rule. *Federal Register* 56:64004–64182, 1991.
15. U.S. Food and Drug Administration. Allergic reactions to latex-containing medical devices. *FDA Med Alert* 1991;MDA91-1:1–2.
16. Berky ZT, Luciano WJ, James WD: Latex glove allergy. *JAMA* 1992;268:2695–2697.
17. Gauthier DK, Turner JG, Langley LG, et al: Monitoring universal precautions: A new assessment tool. *Infect Control Hosp Epidemiol* 1991;12:597–601.
18. DeFilippo VC, Bowen RW, Ingbar DH: A universal precautions monitoring system adaptable to any health care department. *Am J Infect Control* 1992;20:159–163.
19. Kelen GD, Green GB, Hexter DA, et al: Substantial improvement in compliance with universal precautions in an emergency department following institution of policy. *Arch Intern Med* 1991;151:2051–2056.

INFECTION CONTROL ASPECTS OF THE EMPLOYEE HEALTH PROGRAM

Kent B. Crossley

INTRODUCTION

Importance of Employee Health Issues

For more than a century, it has been recognized that health care workers may spread infections between patients. Health care workers may also transmit their own infections directly to patients and may acquire infections from patients. There are many examples of each of these phenomena. Tuberculosis has been shown to be transmitted from LTCF employees to residents. Widespread concern about infection of health care workers from human immunodeficiency virus (HIV)–positive patients is a reminder that infections may be spread from patients to health care workers.

Unfortunately, there are significant limitations to our knowledge about how to prevent spread of infection between patients and employees and vice versa. Limited resources have often directed attention elsewhere. In many institutions, infection control activities tend to be directed almost exclusively toward patients and patient-related events. Indeed, in many hospitals and LTCFs, little attention is given to efforts to monitor infections in employees. Some aspects of employee health programs in long-term care (e.g., those related to tuberculosis) are defined by regulations established by payors or by federal or state agencies. Other components of employee health programs are not

defined at all by regulation. There are also many common issues that are difficult to address because there are no good relevant studies.

Employee health issues related to infection control often prove to be much more difficult for long-term care institutions than for acute care hospitals. As discussed in Chapter 4, there are less data and resources for LTCF infection control programs.

Major attention in any health care setting needs to be directed toward trying to reduce the frequency of transmission of infection to (and from) that group of individuals with most patient contact. In acute care hospitals, these typically are registered nurses. In long-term care facilities, these individuals are nursing aides. Approximately 80% to 100% of direct care provided to residents in long-term care is provided by nursing aides. Indeed, the amount of skilled nursing time per resident in these facilities averages only about 12 minutes each day.[1]

Employee Turnover and Education

Many people who are employed as nurse's aides in long-term care work in this role for a limited period of time. Because of relatively high turnover, it is difficult to appropriately train these individuals. Moreover, many individuals who work as nursing aides in long-term care are recent immigrants to the United States. The task of educating nursing aides has thus become doubly difficult; the basic level of knowledge of issues related to health may be very limited, and language barriers may make training issues even more complex.

Because registered nurses and licensed practical nurses are often in supervisory roles in LTCFs, they must have a clear understanding of employee health issues. They will often need to decide when employee-related health issues need to be brought to the attention of a physician. But they are clearly less important as vehicles for transmission of infection than are nurse's aides in long-term care.

Although hard to study, benefits provided to employees may also impact the transmission of infection in LTCFs. Paid sick leave is an example. Employees with acute contagious illnesses are presumably more likely to remain away from work for a longer time if they are not being economically penalized for their absence. Influenza immunization is another example of a benefit that is probably valuable to both employees and residents.[2]

The Employee's Role in Cross-Infection

In this chapter, attention will be directed toward observations about the frequency with which infections are spread between residents of LTCFs and facility employees, and vice versa. Most documentation (and regulation) is available in the area of tuberculosis. There has been some interest in HIV infection in long-term care, and a variety of regulations that are designed to prevent transmission of bloodborne pathogens apply to LTCFs as well as to acute care hospitals. These are dealt with in more detail in Chapter 15 and are discussed only briefly here. Prevention of influenza and other viral infections has been studied in long-term care and are reviewed here as well. Information about gastrointestinal infections and streptococcal and staphylococcal infections is included. The chapter ends with a brief discussion of the appropriate evaluation of a newly hired employee from the viewpoint of infection control and with some comments about evaluating an employee with a recent infection for suitability to return to work.

Employee Health Issues

Many of the recommendations made here have been extrapolated and derived from information from studies done in acute care hospitals. Much of what has been written about

Table 16.1	*Infectious Diseases of Concern to the Nursing Home Employee*

Viral hepatitis (Hepatitis B and Hepatitis C)
Human immunodeficiency virus
Tuberculosis
Influenza
Streptococcal and staphylococcal infections
Gastrointestinal infections
Scabies
Herpes zoster/Chickenpox
Pertussis

infections and infection control as related to health care workers provides little, if any, information about long-term care facilities. Indeed, NIOSH's document, *Guidelines for Protecting the Safety and Health of Health Care Workers*,[3] does not address long-term care facilities at all.

The issue for infection control personnel is to make certain that an adequate part of the effort devoted to employee health is related to the prevention of infection. Remember that employee health programs exist for reasons beyond attempting to reduce the risk of infection for residents and for employees. Since the enactment of the Occupational Safety and Health Act in 1970, a variety of standards that relate to injuries, exposure to toxins, and stress have been addressed.[4]

It is important to remember that neither infection control nor employee health can exist in a vacuum. These programs must be coordinated, policies and procedures and educational programs sponsored jointly, and plans for monitoring and controlling potentially serious outbreaks (e.g., influenza) developed together.

A number of infections are of particular concern to LTCF employees (see Table 16.1). These are discussed in the following sections.

BLOODBORNE PATHOGENS, HEPATITIS B, HUMAN IMMUNODEFICIENCY VIRUS

Bloodborne Pathogens in the Nursing Home

A variety of regulations have been put in place recently in an effort to reduce the risk of transmission of bloodborne pathogens to health care workers. It is ironic that, although hepatitis B is more easily transmissible and is associated with more deaths in health care workers, HIV-associated disease is responsible for these new rules. Although issues related to HIV infection are discussed in some length in the previous chapter, a few points that are particularly relevant to the employee health program should be discussed here.

Relatively little data is available about the frequency of infections with bloodborne pathogens among residents of long-term care facilities. It is the general sense, however, that in LTCFs that serve the elderly, HIV infection is quite uncommon (although hepatitis viruses may be seen somewhat more frequently). Simor and colleagues found in a study of a group of 508 residents in a long-term care facility in Toronto that three (0.6%) were positive for hepatitis B surface antigen, seven (1.4%) had antibodies to hepatitis C, and none had evidence of HIV infection.[5]

Details about development of infection control programs that emphasize universal precautions and are intended to reduce the frequency of needlestick injuries are discussed in Chapter 15. References have been published to assist the facility in addressing universal precautions issues.[3,6]

Table 16.2   *Management of Needlestick or Sharp Injury in Long-Term Care*

	HEPATITIS B	HIV
Prevention	Educate employees about universal precautions, bloodborne diseases, and avoidance of injury.	
	Immunize employees potentially exposed to blood.	No vaccine available.
After injury	Assess the significance of the injury and estimate the likelihood that the resident has a bloodborne disease. Obtain informed consent, draw blood, and test for hepatitis B antigen (HBsAg) and HIV antibody. Provide appropriate counseling. Document the testing and results carefully. Protect the confidentiality of the resident and employee.	
	If source is HBsAg-positive and the employee is not immunized, administer one dose of hepatitis B immune globulin (HBIG) and start vaccination series. If employee has been immunized, measure antibody titer (anti-HBs)	If source patient is HIV-positive or refuses testing, evaluate employee for HIV antibody at time of injury and at 6 weeks and 3 and 6 months. Consider use of AZT.
	If source patient is unknown or refuses testing, start vaccination series if not previously given. If the employee has been immunized, measure antibody titer if 5 years since immunization.	Employee should follow guidelines for prevention of transmission for at least 6 to 12 weeks (refrain from blood donation, use appropriate protection during sexual intercourse.)
	If source patient is negative, complete immunization series for employee.	If source is negative, follow exposed worker at worker's request in 3 to 6 months. Source unknown: Individualize. Test and follow up employee.

Adapted from Crossley K, Willenbring K, Thurn J: Needlestick injuries and needle disposal in Minnesota nursing homes. *J Am Geriatr Soc* 1990;38:793–796. Used with permission.

Employee Risks and Protection

The frequency with which health care workers are exposed to blood or other viruses containing fluids in long-term care facilities appears to be low. We studied the prevalence of injuries with needles and other sharps recently in Minnesota nursing homes.[7] Needlestick injuries were usually the result of recapping needles and were seen most often in registered nurses and in licensed practical nurses. However, these injuries were very uncommon; less than one injury per facility per employee-year was reported. Many of the LTCFs in our survey did not have protocols developed for managing needlestick injuries. The process for evaluating needlestick injuries is rather straightforward and is summarized in Table 16.2.

Hepatitis B is transmitted more readily than HIV and has been associated with many more cases in health care workers than has HIV. Moreover, the prevalence of hepatitis B virus carriage by residents appears to be substantially greater than the frequency of HIV carriage. *Note:* This obviously excludes facilities that exist primarily to serve people who are HIV-infected.

Consistent with current Occupational Safety and Health Administration (OSHA) recommendations, individuals who work in long-term care facilities and have exposure to residents should be immunized against hepatitis B. This vaccine has been shown to provide substantial protection against developing infection after exposure to the virus. It is expensive but has clearly been effective in reducing the frequency of this disease.

The hepatitis C virus is rather poorly understood, and there is little agreement about appropriate mechanisms for prevention of its transmission. There are no clear data about the optimal approach to prophylaxis in the event of an exposure to hepatitis C.

It is clear that the costs associated with attempts to prevent HIV infection transmission from residents to employees in long-term care are potentially high. It would be appropriate for those who work in long-term care to be aware that the rules which have been implemented may again be reevaluated.

A variety of other recommendations that have been made for acute care hospitals regarding prevention of transmission of bloodborne infection are also applicable to long-term care facilities. These are discussed in the prior chapter. Even though needle use is dramatically less frequent than in acute care hospitals, attention should be paid to proper disposal of needles and other sharps after use. Contact with blood should be reduced as much as possible through the use of gowns, gloves, and masks.

TUBERCULOSIS

Tuberculosis has been a major issue for patients and employees of health care institutions for many years. Much of the focus in areas of tuberculosis prevention and control in the last several years has switched away from the elderly toward patients who are HIV-infected, recent immigrants, and minorities.

This change in emphasis should not reduce or modify concern about tuberculosis in health care workers or in residents of long-term care facilities. In unpublished studies done in Minnesota, 15% to 20% of elderly residents of long-term care facilities have been tuberculin-positive. The incidence of tuberculosis in residents of nursing homes is approximately twice that observed in people of similar age in the community. Unpublished information from the Centers for Disease Control and Prevention (CDC) suggests that tuberculosis is three times as common in employees of long-term care facilities as it is in individuals of similar age and sex.[8]

Outbreaks of tuberculosis in long-term care institutions may result from infected residents or from infected health care workers. Both have been documented on a number of occasions. Both are obviously of concern to the infection control and employee health efforts in long-term care facilities.

Current recommendations for the prevention of tuberculosis in employees in LTCFs suggest skin testing at the time of employment (using the two-step technique) and repeating tests periodically thereafter. As Bentley has indicated recently, the process of two-step testing is somewhat limited in its utility because of definitions and the meaning of boosted results.[8] Although the multipuncture test is most commonly used in long-term care institutions, intradermal injection (Mantoux technique) is preferred.[2]

Management of tuberculosis and tuberculosis risk in employees is a good example of the bidirectional nature of the relationship between the employee health service and the infection control program. Clearly the process of evaluating exposure by an employee to a resident with tuberculosis requires knowledge about both the nature of the resident's illness and the tuberculin status of the employee.

Similarly, identification of a newly tuberculin-positive resident in a LTCF will make it necessary to look closely for contacts and risk factors for the employee.

A health care worker who has a documented skin test conversion should have a chest x-ray and follow-up medical care. Assuming the chest x-ray does not indicate tuberculosis, isoniazid (INH) should be given as preventive therapy for 6 to 12 months. The CDC recommends that information about the proportion of tuberculin-positive staff and their antituberculous therapy should be maintained. Additional helpful information is contained in the CDC publication, and it should be readily available to LTCFs.[9]

It is important to remember that any peculiar or persisting (greater than three weeks) pulmonary infection might well represent tuberculosis, especially in a person who is known to be tuberculin-positive. In these situations, a chest x-ray and sputum culture are appropriate. Tuberculosis in the LTCF is discussed further in Chapter 5.

INFLUENZA AND OTHER RESPIRATORY DISEASES

Influenza

It has been recognized for over two decades that respiratory infections can be transmitted between health care workers and patients. This has been particularly well established for influenza, and it seems likely that similar transmission will be documented for other types of viral infections, including respiratory syncytial virus. Again, the pivotal two-way role of the employee is obvious. It is necessary to control acquisition of these infections by employees from residents and at the same time make certain that employees who are infected elsewhere reduce as much as possible the probability that they will transmit their infection to residents.

Although it is clear that influenza immunization is not 100% effective, it is also evident that it significantly reduces the frequency of transmission of influenza virus infection. The CDC has recommended for several years that health care workers who have contact with residents be immunized against influenza.[10] This should be an important part of every facility's employee health program.

If an influenza outbreak is underway, administration of amantadine, 100 mg each day, may be ordered for individuals who have not been immunized. This drug may be initiated, influenza immunization given, and the drug discontinued after a period of two weeks. Amantadine is only effective for influenza A.[11]

The experience within acute care hospitals has been that offering influenza vaccine in an employee health service office has not been particularly successful. In many hospitals, employee health service nurses are sent to patient care areas at shift changes in order to offer influenza immunization in a more convenient way. Similar programs have been useful in LTCFs. Targeting physicians at a staff meeting would also be a useful approach.

Other Respiratory Viruses

Often measures for control of the spread of respiratory infection that are basically common sense are ignored. It is reasonable for health care workers who have upper respiratory symptoms to wear masks while working (although this is rarely done). Because many rhinovirus colds are transmitted primarily by contact with infected nasal secretions, handwashing or use of a hand disinfectant (if handwashing facilities are not readily available) is a good idea.

Pertussis

In recent years, pertussis has been documented as an increasingly frequent problem among adults. An outbreak has recently been described in a nursing home.[12] Although there are not yet formal recommendations for use of acellular pertussis vaccine in adults, in an outbreak situation this may be necessary. In the outbreak just noted, none of the employees was found to have a positive throat culture for pertussis but a number had serologic evidence of recent infection. Employees with unusual or persisting paroxysmal cough should be evaluated by a physician, especially if pertussis has been documented in the facility.

STREPTOCOCCAL AND STAPHYLOCOCCAL INFECTIONS

Infections caused by group A beta-hemolytic streptococci and by *Staphylococcus aureus* may be acquired and brought to the LTCF by employees. Employees may also acquire these infections from residents.

Staphylococcus aureus infections are often associated with minor trauma or dermatitis in healthy individuals. Because lesions may be present at sites where they are not readily obvious (and still be a cause of transmissible infection), employees should be told to report any skin infections and promptly see a physician for care. It is usually recommended that employees who have infected lacerations, felons, and so on, not care for residents with open wounds and consider wearing gloves during direct resident contact. If these measures are not possible, these individuals should not provide care until they have received appropriate antibiotic therapy and medical attention.

At the present time, methicillin-resistant *Staphylococcus aureus* (MRSA) is not a major risk for staff of LTCFs. Routine screening of employees for colonization with this organism is not recommended. Occasionally, staff members may be found to be colonized with MRSA. In that event, it is most appropriate to make certain that the employee does not have a reason for being a carrier (e.g., an unreported chronic skin condition, chronic antibiotic use, etc.). Although there is still no certainty about the appropriateness of attempts to "decolonize" employees using multiple antibiotic regimens, generally these have not proven to be of value nor are the drugs that are used (e.g., trimethoprim/sulfamethoxazole and rifampin) necessarily benign.[13] MRSA is discussed further in Chapter 12.

Transmission of group A beta-hemolytic streptococci has been documented between residents and personnel, and streptococci have been transmitted by colonized or infected health care workers to residents as well. Spread from cutaneous infection can be limited by the use of gloves. Respiratory transmission (for example, from residents with pharyngitis) does not occur after they have received antibiotics for about 24 hours.[14,15]

GASTROINTESTINAL INFECTIONS

Although gastrointestinal infections are particularly common among residents, there is relatively little information available about the prevalence of various causative organisms or about the mechanisms of transmission. Presumably, these infections are spread by contamination of hands of health care workers or residents. Many of these infections are viral, and it is difficult to be certain of their etiology.

Outbreaks of *Salmonella* infection have been reported in LTCFs and may be transmitted by individuals who are carriers.[16] Infections with viruses that resemble the Norwalk

agent have also been reported in LTCFs and may infect employees.[17]

Careful handwashing—so important to limiting transmission of many institutionally transmissible infections—is key to preventing spread of these infections.

SCABIES

Scabies may be seen in long-term care facilities, and employees may play a major role in introducing this infestation or in propagating it within an institution. Available data would suggest that scabies is not an infrequent problem in long-term care institutions.[18]

Scabies in LTCF residents may be atypical because lesions are often located in the perineal area and on the back. Eruptions may be impressive and hyperkeratotic. These rashes may be erroneously thought to represent psoriasis or eczema.

Treatment requires use of a drug such as permethrin. Once an outbreak has been identified, all of the residents and staff may need to be treated. Individuals with extensive lesions may need to be treated twice at one-week intervals. An effort should be made to treat everyone within a one- or two-day period (see Chapter 4).

EVALUATION AT THE TIME OF EMPLOYMENT

Employee History and Screening

In a study of infection control practices in nursing homes in the mid-1980s, the variety of employee evaluations done at the time of employment was impressive.[19] Many of the facilities did nothing, others had questionnaires for new employees, some required physical examinations, and a significant number required one or more laboratory tests such as a urinalysis or a complete blood count.

Most of the information that needs to be collected from employees at the time of hire can be obtained through a questionnaire (see Table 16.3). Although there may be other reasons to do a physical examination at the time of employment (e.g., to establish a baseline for individuals who might sustain injury in their work), this is not necessarily a component of an evaluation for infection control purposes.

Table 16.3 *Components of an Employment Evaluation Relevant to Infection Control*

History of chronic skin disease
Medications
Immunizations
History of chickenpox
Tuberculin skin testing

A newly hired employee should be asked about chronic skin conditions, medication use, and any underlying medical problems. The first question will help to identify those who may be at risk for infection (and thus for transmission to residents) by staphylococci or streptococci. The other two questions will help identify individuals who might have significant underlying diseases and who could potentially acquire infections from residents more easily than their healthier peers.

Because of its high level of contagion and increasing incidence, tuberculosis needs to remain a major concern. The recommendations regarding evaluation of a newly hired employee would include skin testing and, if the test is positive, a follow-up chest x-ray. (These recommendations are discussed in detail earlier in this chapter.)

Immunization Status

At the time of employment, an individual should be asked about immunization status. Adults who have not been immunized against *diphtheria* and *tetanus* in the prior ten years should receive a booster immunization or be referred to a physician for this purpose.[20] This vaccine should be repeated every ten years.

Individuals who are hired during the fall and winter should be immunized against *influenza*, and those who are hired at other times of the year should be encouraged to participate in the next influenza immunization program. Whether or not a program for influenza immunization should be mandatory for employees needs to be determined by each facility after consultation with its medical director and administration.

Hepatitis B immunization must be administered to health care workers under current OSHA regulations. These regulations define those individuals who should receive vaccine as employees who are exposed or potentially exposed to blood or body fluids. It is thus certainly not nec-

essary that clerical workers and other individuals who have essentially no resident contact be immunized (see Chapter 15).

Although *rubella* and *measles* immunizations are widely recommended for employees of acute care hospitals, most residents in nursing homes that primarily serve the elderly are presumed to be immune to these diseases, so this recommendation is less important .

It is useful to ask an employee about a history of chickenpox because occasionally visitors to long-term care facilities may develop this disease. When this occurs, it is necessary to determine who has been exposed to the case, for what period of time, and if these individuals (whether residents or employees) are immune to *varicella zoster*.

Both chickenpox and zoster may be easily transmissible to individuals who are not immune; employees with either disease need to be restricted from resident contact, particularly during the early stages when transmission is most likely. Individuals who have not had chickenpox may acquire this disease after being infected with the varicella-zoster virus from a resident who has zoster.

Although extensive information about all of these vaccines is beyond the scope of this book, two appropriate references are the CDC's "Update on adult immunizations"[21] and the American College of Physicians *Guide for Adult Immunization.*[20]

EVALUATION OF AN EMPLOYEE'S SUITABILITY FOR WORK DURING OR AFTER AN EPISODE OF INFECTION

Surprisingly little information is available to help with decisions regarding employees who may have infections that can potentially be transmitted to residents.

Employees who have cutaneous infection should be restricted from resident contact or should wear gloves if they must work. Prompt physician evaluation and antibiotic therapy is appropriate. Individuals with documented streptococcal pharyngitis should not work with residents. Prompt antibiotic therapy rapidly (within 24 hours) reduces the likelihood of transmitting this infection. Employees with acute gastroenteritis should be restricted from work because of a high probability that, no matter what the etiologic organism, it may be transmitted to residents.

An employee with a herpetic lesion of the finger (which usually occurs around the nailbed) should be restricted from work until the lesion has healed. Data are not available to determine whether or not wearing gloves will prevent transmission of these infections. Employees who have oral herpetic lesions may be restricted from taking care of individuals who are immunocompromised but may be assigned other work until these lesions have healed.

Individuals who have had viral hepatitis should be restricted from resident contact depending on the type of infection that has occurred. Individuals who have had acute hepatitis A should not have resident contact for one week after the clinical onset of infection. Employees who have had hepatitis B infection and are carriers of the virus (i.e., are antigen-positive) do not need to be restricted from resi-

dent contact, but they should be taught that in situations where there is a potential of blood exposure for a resident (e.g., an exposure-prone invasive procedure in which their fingers or hands may be lacerated), they need to use particular precautions.

A great many situations are beyond the scope of this chapter, and detailed recommendations for many of the infections mentioned here cannot be provided because of space limitations. *Control of Communicable Diseases in Man* by Abraham Benenson is an excellent source of information about specific situations.[22] City, county, and state health departments are able to provide advice about these types of questions, and infection control practitioners in acute care hospitals and other LTCFs may also prove to be a valuable resource.

REFERENCES

1. Bowers B, Becker M: Nurse's aides in nursing homes: The relationship between organization and quality. *Gerontologist* 1992;32:360–366.
2. Pearson DA, Checko PJ, Hierholzer WJ Jr, et al: Infection control practices in Connecticut's skilled nursing facilities. *Am J Infect Control* 1990;18:269–276.
3. National Institute for Occupational Safety and Health: *Guidelines for Protecting the Safety and Health of Health Care Workers.* Washington, DC, U.S. Department of Health and Human Services, 1988.
4. Moore RM Jr, Kaczmarek RG: Occupational hazards to health care workers: Diverse, ill-defined, and not fully appreciated. *Am J Infect Control* 1991;18:316–327.
5. Simor AE, Gordon M, Bishai FR: Prevalence of hepatitis B surface antigen, hepatitis C antibody, and HIV-1 antibody among residents of a long-term-care facility. *J Am Geriatr Soc* 1992;40:218–220.
6. Centers for Disease Control: Recommendations for prevention of HIV transmission in health-care settings. *MMWR* 1987;36(suppl 2S):1–18S.
7. Crossley K, Willenbring K, Thurn J: Needlestick injuries and needle disposal in Minnesota nursing homes. *J Am Geriatr Soc* 1990;38:793–796.
8. Bentley DW: Tuberculosis in long-term care facilities. *Infect Control Hosp Epidemiol* 1990;11:42–46.
9. Centers for Disease Control: Prevention and control of tuberculosis in facilities providing long-term care to the elderly: Recommendations of the Advisory Committee for Elimination of Tuberculosis. *MMWR* 1990;39:7–20.
10. Centers for Disease Control: Prevention and control of influenza: Recommendations of the Immunization Practice Advisory Committee. *MMWR* 1992;41:1–17.
11. Fedson DS: Prevention and control of influenza in institutional settings. *Hosp Pract* 1989;24:87–96.
12. Addiss DG, David JP, Meade BD, et al: A pertussis outbreak in a Wisconsin nursing home. *J Infect Dis* 1991;164:704–710.
13. Boyce JM: Methicillin-resistant *Staphylococcus aureus* in hospitals and long-term care facilities: Microbiology, epidemiology, and preventive measures. *Infect Control Hosp Epidemiol* 1992;13:725–727.
14. Schwartz B, Elliott JA, Butler JC, et al: Clusters of invasive group A streptococcal infections in family, hospital, and nursing home settings. *Clin Infect Dis* 1992;15:277–284.
15. Ruben FL, Norden CW, Heisler B, et al: An outbreak of *Streptococcus pyogenes* infections in a nursing home. *Ann Intern Med* 1984;101:494–496.
16. Choi M, Yoshikawa TT, Bridge J, et al: Salmonella outbreak in a nursing home. *J Am Geriatr Soc* 1990;38:531–534.
17. Gellert GA, Waterman SH, Ewert D, et al: An outbreak of acute gastroenteritis caused by a small round structured virus in a geriatric convalescent facility. *Infect Control Hosp Epidemiol* 1990;11:459–464.
18. Degelau J: Scabies in long-term care facilities. *Infect Control Hosp Epidemiol* 1992;13:421–425.
19. Crossley KB, Irvine P, Kaszar DJ, et al: Infection control practices in Minnesota nursing homes. *JAMA* 1985;254:2918–2921.
20. ACP Task Force on Adult Immunization and Infectious Diseases Society of America: *Guide for Adult Immunization,* 2nd ed. Philadelphia, American College of Physicians, PA, 1990.
21. Centers for Disease Control: Update on adult immunization. *MMWR* 1991;40:RR-12.
22. Benenson AS (ed): *Control of Communicable Diseases in Man,* 15th ed. Washington, DC, American Public Health Association, 1990.

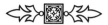

SECTION FOUR

SPECIFIC CONTROL MEASURES

CHAPTER

INFECTION CONTROL MEASURES: THE RESIDENT

Judith K. Stern and Philip W. Smith

To prevent infection in the LTCF setting, efforts must be directed at one or more of the three points in the infection sequence (see Fig. 4.1): optimizing the resistance of the resident to infection, controlling the reservoir of infection, and limiting the transmission of infectious agents. This chapter reviews methods for improving the intrinsic resistance of the host to infection (see Fig. 9.3); the other techniques for control of LTCF infections are discussed in the two subsequent chapters. A number of areas must be addressed by the LTCF to maximize host resistance in the resident (see Table 17.1).

Table 17.1. *Measures to Improve Host Resistance*

Treatment of underlying diseases (e.g., diabetes, heart failure)
Evaluation of medical problems (e.g., incontinence)
Treatment of established infections
Minimization of antibiotic usage
Minimization of other medications
Attention to nutrition and hydration
Skin care/decubitus prevention
Bladder training/catheter care
Aspiration precautions
General cleanliness of resident
Identification of specific immune problems
Resident immunizations

IMPROVING GENERAL HOST RESISTANCE

Underlying Medical Illnesses

Underlying medical illness often predisposes to nosocomial infection in the LTCF. Treatment of these underlying diseases can be expected to improve the resistance of the host. Cardiac and circulatory disorders are common in the elderly. Congestive heart failure and arteriosclerotic vascular disease may impair circulation to the extremities, thereby increasing the possibility of skin ulceration and soft tissue infection.

Residents with poorly controlled diabetes mellitus have an increased incidence of certain infections, including nonclostridial gas gangrene, urinary tract infection, respiratory tract infection, and skin infection.[1] Infections occur in diabetics for a number of reasons, including peripheral vascular disease (extremity infection), diabetic neuropathy with neurogenic bladder and urine retention (urinary tract infection), and glycosuria (recurrent *Candida* vaginitis). There is also a general correlation between poor control of blood sugar in diabetics and susceptibility to infection. This is partly due to the fact that white blood cells in hyperglycemic diabetics do not function normally. A complete discussion of the impact of systemic diseases on immunity to infection can be found in Chapter 2.

Host resistance to pneumonia may be improved by avoidance of cigarette smoke and proper pulmonary toilet in the chronic bronchitis patient. Overhydration may cause pulmonary edema, which impairs lung defenses, and underhydration impairs clearance of pulmonary bacteria by the mucociliary system. Many cases of nursing home pneumonia follow aspiration, which is most common in residents with altered states of consciousness, seizure disorders, or dysphagia.[2] Feeding a clear liquid diet temporarily or elevating the head of the bed after feeding may decrease the chance of aspiration in the high-risk resident. The prevention of pneumonia is discussed in detail in Chapter 5.

The cancer patient is at risk of infection because of local effects of the tumor (e.g., lung cancer causing postobstructive pneumonia). In addition, the cancer itself or administered treatments (chemotherapy, radiation) often cause breaks in local defenses, general immune impairment, and malnutrition.

Finally, it is important to treat established infections in the LTCF resident to prevent secondary infectious complications. For instance, chronic purulent sinusitis may lead to aspiration of the infected sinus drainage with secondary bacterial pneumonia. Recurrent bacterial prostatitis may be the source of relapsing urinary tract infection. An infected decubitus ulcer may spread to involve underlying bone. Any uncontrolled local infection carries the risk of a secondary septic complication, such as bacteremia.

Medication

Antibiotics have the potential disadvantages of toxic side effects, allergic reactions, disturbance of normal bacterial flora, selection of antibiotic-resistant bacteria, superinfection, and expense. Hence, rational prescription of antibiotics is important to the preservation of health in LTCF residents.

The normal flora is an important defense mechanism in the host. It has been shown that antibiotics disturb normal flora and facilitate colonization of the pharynx by potentially pathogenic gram-negative bacilli.[3] Antibiotics may also lead to overgrowth of organisms such as *Clostridium difficile*, the cause of antibiotic-associated enterocolitis. Antibiotic usage is the primary determinant in the selection of antibiotic-resistant bacteria that can cause epidemics in LTCFs (see Chapter 12).

Other medications also have potential adverse effects. Anticholinergics may predispose to urinary retention and increase the risk of urinary tract infection. Sedatives and tranquilizers decrease the cough reflex, thereby preventing

effective clearance of respiratory tract pathogens and predisposing to aspiration pneumonia. Antacids decrease gastric acid, an important antibacterial defense mechanism. Steroids may impair immune function. Finally, drugs many interact with antibiotics in a variety of ways. The chance of an adverse effect due to medication is significant in nursing homes, where residents tend to be on multiple medications.[4]

Nutrition

Malnutrition has an impact on host resistance to infection in a number of areas, including general immunity and wound healing. The nutritional requirements of the elderly differ from those of young people,[5] and the incidence of protein-calorie undernutrition in the LTCF is as high as 30% to 60%.[6]

To meet the nutritional needs of nursing home residents, foods must be edible and enticing, taking into consideration the resident's ethnic background and preferences. Elderly residents often have a diminished sense of taste and smell, making it all the more important that foods be adequately seasoned.

Meals should be served in attractive, uncrowded surroundings with proper lighting and temperature control. Residents who become agitated during meals should be kept separated from others who might be disturbed by this behavior.

The demented resident will require assistance and a longer period of time to eat and may need to be reminded to swallow. A special feeding session and use of volunteers to assist with feeding may help ensure adequate nutrition for these residents.

Each resident should be continually monitored for early signs of protein-calorie undernutrition. These signs may include a decline in the amount of food consumed, weight loss, or a fall in serum albumin or cholesterol levels.

At the first sign of a decline in nutritional status, a search for the cause should be undertaken and the problem corrected. A dental evaluation may be necessary because poor dentition can lead to poor dietary intake. Psychotropic medications and digoxin may cause anorexia. The attending physician should be contacted if a resident on these medications complains of loss of appetite and is eating poorly.

Dietary supplements should be offered as soon as it becomes apparent that a resident is ingesting inadequate amounts of food at regular meals. A multiple vitamin supplement is also advisable. Diuretics can cause zinc deficiency, suppressing immune function and leading to poor wound healing. A supplement of 220 mg of zinc twice a day is recommended in the presence of decubiti or peripheral vascular disease.

In addition, maintaining adequate hydration in the elderly resident is very important. Dehydration may diminish urinary flow and mucous production in the respiratory tract, thereby predisposing to infection in these organ systems. Many nursing home residents have a reduced sense of thirst or are unable to serve themselves water. The resident should be offered at least one liter of fluid per day.

IMPROVING LOCAL DEFENSES
The Skin

Local defenses are the first line of protection against invasive organisms. The skin, for instance, forms an excellent barrier to infection in most individuals. With aging, there is loss of subcutaneous fat and thinning of the skin,[7] which along with immobilization predispose to decubitus ulcers.[8] Intravenous catheters, when present, also violate the skin barrier.

Control measures designed to maintain this first line of protection, discussed in depth in Chapter 7, include frequent change of position of the immobilized resident and the judicious use of devices to relieve the pressure on bony prominences. Skin care programs should address bathing and avoidance of skin maceration or trauma; skin lotion is indicated for dry skin. Areas that are already ulcerated should be kept clean and dry. Ascorbic acid 500 mg twice a day has been demonstrated to improve the rate of healing. Ambulation and activity should be encouraged within the resident's limits. A program for regular skin assessment and clinical staging of pressure ulcers is advisable.

A number of LTCFs administer intravenous (IV) fluids, and residents may have long-term, indwelling IVs such as the subcutaneous Hickman catheter. Policies and procedures dealing with insertion and care of these IVs are needed, and an indwelling venous catheter should always be considered as a possible cause of occult fever.

Gastrointestinal Tract

The elderly resident may have gastric achlorhydria, which negates the potent antibacterial effect of gastric acid,

in turn predisposing to a variety of gastrointestinal infections. Antacids and H-2 receptor antagonists accentuate this problem.

Nasogastric tubes and gastrostomies are seen in the LTCF and require policies and procedures dealing with care of the tube sites, as well as preparation, storage, and administration of alimentation solutions. Feeding tubes predispose to aspiration, and local complications such as nasal erosions, sinusitis, and gastrostomy site infections are a potential concern.

Attention to oral care in the elderly resident should include gingival hygiene, oral hydration, dental status, dentures, and detection of any oral lesions.

Urinary Tract

The most important predisposing factor for nursing home–acquired urinary tract infections is placement of indwelling bladder catheters. Control of urinary tract infections is discussed in Chapter 6. In general, the use of bladder catheters should be minimized.

Urinary incontinence is reported in about 50% of LTCF residents and contributes to the incidence of maceration of perineal skin and urinary tract infection, especially if an indwelling urinary catheter is required.[9,10] Treatable causes of incontinence, such as urologic disease (cystocele), immobility, diabetes, and drugs adversely affecting continence, may be detected by a brief evaluation.[11]

Incontinence can often be managed by timed or prompted toileting, bladder training, reduction of diuretic use, avoidance of oversedation, and removal of mechanical barriers to toileting. Toilet facilities should be prominently identified and easily accessible. The use of siderails and restraints should be minimized. Fecal impactions can cause outlet obstruction with overflow incontinence; impactions should be sought and removed. Muscle relaxers may cause sphincter weakness and should be avoided in the presence of urinary incontinence. An incontinence chart can often assist in developing a plan to maintain continence. If incontinence suddenly worsens, a urinalysis should be obtained to assess for infection.

If a bladder catheter is required, it should be inserted aseptically by trained personnel, and a closed system should be maintained in order to minimize entry of bacteria. Adequate hydration is important, as is treatment of underlying medical diseases predisposing to urinary obstruction (e.g., prostatic hypertrophy).

Respiratory Tract

Local defenses of the upper airway include the cough reflex and the mucociliary system. Factors that interfere with normal upper airway defenses such as cigarette smoking, dehydration, and oversedation are potentially avoidable. Special care of residents receiving gastric tube feedings is recommended to minimize aspiration. This should include elevating the head of the bed during and for one hour after feeding, monitoring gastric residuals, and avoiding agents that slow gastric emptying.[12] Good oral hygiene is also vital to local defenses. The prevention of pneumonia is discussed further in Chapter 5.

General Care

General measures of importance include hydration, ambulation, and documentation of skin and catheter care. Residents should have their own supplies and equipment and wear fresh clothing. Fecal incontinence is a common problem in the LTCF; incontinent residents should be diapered. The resident should receive several complete baths per week. During this time, the staff is afforded an opportunity to visualize a number of problems that could lead to nosocomial infections, such as distended bladders, areas of skin erythema that may presage decubitus ulcers, and draining wounds.[13]

Good skin care and timely bathing can be expected to delay colonization with resistant gram-negative bacteria. There is some evidence, however, that even meticulous bathing will not eliminate such organisms as *Pseudomonas aeruginosa* from the perineal area once this area has become colonized.[14] If the resident's perineum is not kept dry and clean, excoriation of the perineal skin will result.

IMPROVING SPECIFIC IMMUNITY

White Blood Cells

A number of medical conditions cause qualitative deficiencies of the white blood cell. Malnutrition, alcoholism, and diabetes are examples of potentially reversible causes of abnormal white blood cell function. A great many drugs have also been identified that adversely affect white blood cell function. Various bone marrow stimulating factors provide temporary increases in the numbers of white blood cells but are quite expensive.

Antibodies

Antibodies coat bacteria to facilitate their destruction by white blood cells. Other functions include agglutination of organisms, lysis of bacteria, and virus neutralization. IgG is the most important antibody, comprising about 70% of serum immunoglobulin. IgM is the earliest antibody produced in response to infection but is short-lived. IgA is the local antibody of respiratory and gastrointestinal tracts.

IgA deficiency is associated with severe and recurrent respiratory and gastrointestinal tract infection, whereas IgG deficiency is complicated by severe *Streptococcus pneumoniae* and *Hemophilus influenzae* infections. Elderly persons who have undergone splenectomy also have an increased susceptibility to pneumococcal and *H. influenzae* infections.

A high index of suspicion needs to be maintained in patients with IgA deficiency for possible gastrointestinal or respiratory tract infections. For patients with IgG deficiency, monthly IV injections of pooled gammaglobulin (antibody harvested from donors) provides some protection against recurrent infection.

Cellular Immunity

Cellular immunity, or delayed hypersensitivity, involves lymphocytes and is the part of the immune system most responsible for fighting tuberculosis and fungal and viral infections. Residents with lymphoma or AIDS or who are receiving corticosteroid therapy have impaired cell-mediated immunity and are at risk of these infections. The dose of corticosteroids should be minimized to decrease the risk of infection. Patients with impaired cellular immunity should have a baseline tuberculosis skin test.

IMMUNIZATION AND VACCINATION

Passive Immunization

The injection of antibody from an immune donor (see Chapter 2) is passive immunization and provides temporary protection. Passive immunity is useful prophylaxis for those exposed to hepatitis A and hepatitis B. Although passive prophylaxis of nursing home residents on a routine basis against hepatitis A is not recommended, pooled immune globulin may be indicated for residents or personnel who have a significant exposure to hepatitis A or if there is an outbreak of hepatitis A in the institution. The dose is 0.02 ml/kg by the intramuscular (IM) route.

Active Immunization

Active immunity is preferable to passive immunity because it is generally long-lasting, involving production of antibody to the vaccine. The routine immunization schedule that begins in childhood involves administration of the diphtheria-pertussis-tetanus (DPT), oral poliomyelitis (OPV), *Hemophilus influenzae B* (HIB) and measles-mumps-rubella (MMR) vaccines. Adults should receive a standard-dose tetanus/reduced-dose diphtheria (Td) vaccine every 10 years throughout adulthood.[15] Pertussis, HIB, and polio vaccines are not recommended for adults.

Mumps, measles, rubella, and oral polio vaccines are live viruses that are attenuated (made less pathogenic in the laboratory). Attenuated viruses cause mild disease but induce appropriate immunity. They should not be given to the immunodeficient host, such as a patient on steroid therapy.

Influenza vaccine is an inactivated agent. The pneumococcal and HIB vaccines consist of cell wall extracts of the organisms, and hepatitis B vaccine is composed of surface antigen components of the virus. These vaccines, and inactivated virus vaccines, are safe in the immunodeficient host.

Some vaccination preparations (e.g., influenza) contain egg products and should therefore be avoided in those allergic to eggs. Active immunization should be avoided during febrile illness or within three months of passive immunization, when it is less likely to be effective.

Vaccination for the Nursing Home Resident

Several immunizations are of importance for the LTCF resident (see Table 17.2).

Tetanus/Diphtheria

Tetanus/diphtheria immunization is important because of increased risk of acquisition of tetanus in the elderly, especially in the setting of vascular insufficiency, skin ulcers of the extremities, or diabetes mellitus.[16] The highest risk of tetanus is in persons over 60 years of age, and virtually all tetanus cases occur in unimmunized or inadequately immunized persons. Diphtheria still occurs in the United States, and diphtheria vaccination should also be maintained in all elderly persons.

Table 17.2.   *Vaccines of Importance for the Elderly*

Vaccine	Recommended Frequency
Tetanus	Every 10 years
Diphtheria	Every 10 years
Influenza	Yearly
Pneumococcal	One time only

Tetanus and diphtheria vaccines consist of toxoids, substances that resemble the toxins produced by *Clostridium tetani* and *Corynebacterium diphtheriae*, respectively. The resemblance is close enough to induce immunity, yet the toxoid does not have the detrimental effects of the toxin. Immunization with these toxoids induces an effective antibody response 90% of the time for diphtheria and nearly 100% of the time for tetanus. Adequate antibody levels persist for 10 years after effective immunization.

Giving tetanus and diphtheria vaccinations more often than every 10 years may be associated with increased incidence and severity of local reactions and has no benefit. The resident who is fully and currently immunized against diphtheria should be safe even during a diphtheria outbreak. The resident who is fully and currently immunized against tetanus is protected from tetanus even with a dirty wound. Hence, the elderly should receive Td vaccination IM every 10 years.[15] If immunization status is in doubt, an initial series of three immunizations should be given.

Influenza

During influenza epidemics, there is a significant increase in mortality, especially among the elderly and debilitated residents. The development of influenza vaccine is complicated by the fact that antigenic variations of the influenza virus occur frequently. Minor antigenic variations occur every 2 to 4 years and major variations every 10 years, approximately. As a result, previous immunity to influenza becomes obsolete. In addition, the protection induced by the influenza vaccine is short-lived, making annual revaccination with current strains necessary.

The influenza vaccine strain recommended for 1992–1993 (influenza season is primarily in the winter) was a trivalent vaccine with the three prevalent influenza types.[17] The vaccine contained influenza A/Texas (H1N1), A/Beijing/ (H3N2), and B/Panama viruses in a 0.5-ml dose given IM in the deltoid muscle. Adults require only one dose, usually in the late fall. The vaccine is recommended for high-risk groups, including all persons over the age of 65 and persons with underlying disease such as acquired or congenital heart disease, chronic pulmonary disease, chronic renal disease, diabetes mellitus, and immunosuppressive disorders, including malignancies. Side effects are relatively few, even in the elderly.[18] About one third of vaccines have been reported to have local redness and induration for one to two days at the site of injection. Occasionally, residents will have fever, malaise, myalgia, or other systemic symptoms. Allergic reaction to an egg compound in the vaccine may occur.

It appears that those at greatest risk from influenza, including the elderly, may not respond as well to the influenza vaccine as younger persons.[19] Others have suggested that vaccine will at least lessen the severity of clinical influenza and decrease morbidity and mortality during an outbreak in an elderly population.[20–22]

Influenza is a highly contagious disease that causes severe nursing home outbreaks (see Chapter 11). Even though the elderly do not respond as well as desired to influenza vaccination, the vaccine is felt to be efficacious in preventing influenza outbreaks in the LTCF setting.[20–23] In view of the extreme susceptibility of the elderly to influenza, the increased morbidity and mortality of influenza in the elderly, and the relative safety of the influenza vaccine, LTCF residents should be vaccinated annually.[24] A guideline for establishing an influenza vaccination program is available.[25]

Occasionally, during an epidemic in a LTCF, the antiviral drug amantadine hydrochloride can play a supplementary role in preventing influenza A. Amantadine protects only against influenza A, not influenza B, and is not a substitute for vaccination. The duration of protection of amantadine lasts only while the individual is receiving the drug. It is thus recommended that amantadine be used only until vaccination can be performed and has taken effect (about 10 to 14 days after vaccination). Amantadine will not interfere with the efficacy of influenza vaccination. The dose of amantadine recommended for the elderly is 100 mg a day. In the presence of chronic renal failure, the dose should be reduced.

Pneumococcal Vaccine

Streptococcus pneumoniae is the leading cause of pneumonia in the community and has an especially high mortality rate in the elderly,[26] even though the organism remains quite sensitive to penicillin. Residents with certain underlying conditions such as antibody deficiency or the postsplenectomy state are at increased risk of contracting this disease.

There are nearly 100 serotypes of the pneumococcus, and immunity is serotype-specific. A vaccine consisting of a polysaccharide extract of the pneumococcal cell wall from each of the 23 leading types in the United States is available. These 23 types represent 90% of bacteremic pneumococcal disease in the United States. The vaccine is given as a single dose (0.5 ml) by the IM route. The majority of residents vaccinated develop an antibody response, and antibodies can be detected for three to five years. The vaccine appears to be quite safe. About half of those given pneumococcal vaccine develop side effects such as erythema and mild pain at the site of the injection, but severe reactions are extremely rare. The vaccine is currently recommended for persons over the age of two years with splenic dysfunction or anatomic asplenia and for those with chronic diseases that may be associated with an increased risk of pneumococcal disease. These diseases include sickle cell anemia, multiple myeloma, cirrhosis, renal failure, diabetes mellitus, congestive heart failure, chronic lung disease, and immunosuppressive diseases, including malignancies.[26]

It should be remembered that the vaccine is far from 100% effective for those serotypes included in the vaccine, and there are many serotypes not included in the vaccine that cause pneumonia. The efficacy of the pneumococcal vaccine in the elderly has been questioned,[27,28] although it can be effective and cost effective if administered to high-risk groups.[29–32]

Although the efficacy and cost-effectiveness of pneumococcal vaccine in the elderly continue to be studied, at the present time there is a consensus to vaccinate all persons over the age of 55 years or with underlying chronic diseases in the LTCF.[26,33] The vaccine is quite safe. Simultaneous administration of influenza and pneumococcal vaccines is as safe and effective as giving either vaccine alone.[34] The vaccine is currently recommended on a one-time basis only, but boosters may later be recom-

Table 17.3   *The Resident Health Program*

Baseline history (emphasizing infectious diseases)
Baseline physical examination
Baseline chest x-ray
Immunization history
Currently recommended immunizations
Initial and periodic TB skin testing
Effective policies for resident care practices

mended. It is safe to vaccinate a resident whose vaccine status is unknown.

Hepatitis Vaccine

Hepatitis B vaccine is available for high-risk populations. Although the incidence of hepatitis B in LTCFs is low, regulations mandate vaccination of certain staff members (see Chapters 15 and 16). A resident or staff member carrying hepatitis B surface antigen could pose a hazard for those who have contact with that person's blood or secretions.

The Immunosuppressed Resident

All of the vaccines routinely recommended for the LTCF resident (see Table 17.2) and hepatitis B vaccine are safe for the immunosuppressed resident, even HIV infected residents.

THE RESIDENT HEALTH PROGRAM

A resident health program at the institutional level is recommended,[35] and the components are listed in Table 17.3. The baseline resident evaluation and chest x-ray are usually available from the resident's primary physician, as is the immunization history. These should be documented in the medical record.

Certain immunizations are appropriate for LTCF residents (see above), as is tuberculosis (TB) screening. It is recommended that all newly admitted residents have TB screening by the intradermal PPD method unless the resident is known to be positive.[35] Repeat PPD tests should be obtained periodically or after a new TB case is discovered in the LTCF.

Finally, effective policies for appropriate resident care practices will help to protect the resident from infectious complications. Areas to be addressed by these policies include resident bathing, skin care, pressure ulcer assessment, feeding, turning, ambulation, oral care, bladder catheter insertion/care, and intravenous catheter care.

REFERENCES

1. Rayfield EJ, Ault MJ, Keusch GT, et al: Infection and diabetes: The case for glucose control. *Am J Med* 1982;72:439–449.
2. Harkness GA, Bentley DW, Roghmann KJ: Risk factors for nosocomial infection in the elderly. *Am J Med* 1990;89:457–463.
3. Mackowiak PA: The normal microbial flora. *N Engl J Med* 1982;307:83–93.
4. Kalchthaler T, Coccard E, Lightiger S: Incidence of polypharmacy in a long-term care facility. *J Am Geriatr Soc* 1977;25:308–313.
5. Munro HN: Nutritional requirements in the elderly. *Hosp Pract* 1982;17:143–154.
6. Rudman D, Feller AG: Protein-calorie undernutrition in the nursing home. *J Am Geriatr Soc* 1989;37:173–183.
7. Gilchrist BA: Age associated changes in the skin. *J Am Geriatr Soc* 1982;30:139–143.
8. Allman RM: Pressure ulcers among the elderly. *N Engl J Med* 1989;320:850–853.
9. Ouslander JG, Kane RL, Abrass IB: Urinary incontinence in elderly nursing home patients. *JAMA* 1982;248:1194–1198.
10. Williams M, Pannill F: Urinary incontinence in the elderly: Physiology, pathophysiology, diagnosis and treatment. *Ann Intern Med* 1982;97:895–907.
11. Pannill FC, Williams TF, Davis R: Evaluation and treatment of urinary incontinence in long-term care. *J Am Geriatr Soc* 1988;36:902–910.
12. Fisher RL: Indications and complications of enteral and parenteral therapy. *Contemp Intern Med* 1992;4:39–52.
13. Campbell DG: Prevention of infection in extended care facilities. *Nurs Clin North Am* 1980;15:857–868.

14. Gilmore DS, Jiminez EM, Aeilts GD, et al: Effects of bathing on *Pseudomonas* and *Klebsiella* colonization in patients with spinal cord injuries. *J Clin Microbiol* 1981;14:404–407.

15. Centers for Disease Control: Update on adult immunization: Recommendations of the Immunization Practices Advisory Committee. *MMWR* 1991;40:1–94.

16. Irvine P, Crossley K: Tetanus and the institutionalized elderly. *JAMA* 1980;244:2159–2160.

17. Centers for Disease Control: Influenza vaccines, 1992–1993. *MMWR* 1992;9:1.

18. Margolis KL, Nichol KL, Poland GA, et al: Frequency of adverse reactions to influenza vaccine in the elderly: A randomized, placebo-controlled trial. *JAMA* 1990;264:239–1141.

19. Levine M. Beattie BL, McLean DM, et al: Characterization of the immune response to trivalent influenza vaccine in elderly men. *J Am Geriatr Soc* 1987;35:609–615.

20. Barker WH, Mullooly JP: Influenza vaccination of elderly persons: Reduction in pneumonia and influenza hospitalizations and deaths. *JAMA* 1980;224:2547–2549.

21. Gross PA, Quinnan GV, Rodstein M, et al: Association of influenza immunization with reduction in mortality in an elderly population: A prospective study. Arch Intern Med 1988;148:562–565.

22. Foster DA, Talsma A, Furumoto-Dawson A, et al: Influenza vaccine effectiveness in preventing hospitalization for pneumonia in the elderly. *Am J Epidemiol* 1992;136:296–307.

23. Goodman RA, Orenstein WA, Munro TF, et al: Impact of influenza in a nursing home. *JAMA* 1982;247:1451–1453.

24. Gravenstein S, Miller BA, Drinka P: Prevention and control of influenza A outbreaks in long-term care facilities. *Infect Control Hosp Epidemiol* 1992;13:49–54.

25. Centers for Disease Control: *Managing an Influenza Vaccina tion Program in the Nursing Home.* Washington, DC, U.S. Department of Health and Human Services, 1987.

26. Centers for Disease Control: Pneumococcal polysaccharide vaccine. *MMWR* 1989;38:64–75.

27. Simberkoff MS, Cross AP, Al-Ibrahim M, et al: Efficacy of pneumococcal vaccine in high risk patients: Results of a Veteran's Administration cooperative study. *N Engl J Med* 1986;315:1318–1327.

28. Forrester HL, Jahnigen DW, LaForce FM: Inefficiency of pneumococcal vaccine in a high risk population. *Am J Med* 1987;83:425–430.

29. Sisk JE, Riegelman RK: Cost effectiveness of vaccination against pneumococcal pneumonia: An update. *Ann Intern Med* 1986;104:79–86.

30. Sims RV, Steinmann WC, McConville JH, et al: The clinical effectiveness of pneumococcal vaccine in the elderly. *Ann Intern Med* 1988;108:653–657.

31. Gable CB, Holzer SS, Engelhart L, et al: Pneumococcal vaccine: Efficacy and associated cost savings. *JAMA* 1990;264:2910–2915.

32. Shapiro ED, Berg AT, Austrian R, et al: The protective efficacy of polyvalent pneumococcal polysaccharide vaccine. *N Engl J Med* 1991;325:1453–1460.

33. LaForce FM, Eickhoff TC: Pneumococcal vaccine: An emerging consensus. *Ann Intern Med* 1988;108:757–758.

34. DeStefano F, Goodman RA, Noble GR, et al: Simultaneous administration of influenza and pneumococcal vaccines. *JAMA* 1982;247:2551–2554.

35. Smith PW, Rusnak PG: APIC guideline for infection prevention and control in the long-term care facility. *Am J Infect Control* 1991;19:198–215.

CHAPTER

INFECTION CONTROL MEASURES: THE ENVIRONMENTAL RESERVOIR

Nancy J. Haberstich

A long-term care facility (LTCF) must be a healthy environment for both residents and employees. A commitment by the institution to provide a clean and sanitary building is the mainstay of the infection prevention and control program. The primary goal is to eliminate reservoirs of microorganisms in the environment. These reservoirs can be animate or inanimate. This chapter outlines the basic measures for environmental sanitation and the disinfection and sterilization of equipment in the inanimate environment. Control measures relating to animate reservoirs such as residents, visitors, employees, and pets are also discussed. Some of the elements of the environmental reservoir are shown in Figure 9.1.

Microbiologic sampling of the inanimate environment on a routine basis is not indicated in LTCFs, although it is often done.[1] Routine cultures of floors, walls, sinks, air, and equipment are expensive and often provide information that has little correlation with nosocomial infections; environmental cultures should be performed only as part of an epidemic investigation (see Chapter 11). Environmental sanitation is more appropriately assured by having policies and procedures for environmental cleanliness (see Chapter 13) and periodic inspections of laundry, kitchen, physical therapy, and other areas to detect problems. After any inspection, a written report that contains the date, the area inspected, deviations from existing policies and procedures,

potential health hazards, and proposed remedies should be completed and retained.

PREVENTION AND CONTROL MEASURES RELATED TO INANIMATE ENVIRONMENT

Building Design and Construction

The design and construction of the facility is not generally alterable but remains an aspect of infection control that must be considered. The behavior of residents and the work patterns of employees must be assessed and evaluated in light of the building design. The location of sinks, "hoppers," needle disposal containers, and waste receptacles is important. Handwashing recommendations should be developed and communicated to employees. The flow of traffic into and within the building must be considered. Visitors should enter the facility from a central location to permit screening for infectious disease and for security reasons.

Clean and soiled materials should be kept separate. The use of conveyors and chutes to move materials, linens, and waste within the facility will require planning and evaluation of systems to determine if microbial contamination is a risk. The flow of clean and soiled linen should be mapped through the facility and not be allowed to mingle. The waste stream must be evaluated both within the facility and in the community. Separate clean and soiled *utility rooms* are preferred to eliminate mixing of clean and soiled equipment and supplies.

Materials used for walls, floors, furniture, and countertops should be selected for ease of maintenance, cleaning, and disinfection. Many factors such as fire resistance and cost must be considered; the ability of these materials to resist deterioration and cracking will make cleaning easier and prevent them from becoming environmental reservoirs of microorganisms. The use of *carpeting* in health care facilities, especially LTCFs, is controversial. There are advantages in addition to the homelike atmosphere carpet creates. Falls are less injurious, noise is muffled, and maintenance is easier. However, difficulty pushing equipment, difficulty removing soil and stains, and increased static electricity present disadvantages. Decisions regarding the use of carpet must be made considering all these factors along with factors unique to the institution. Short-looped carpets are easier to clean. Cleaning spills promptly helps ensure complete removal.

General Building Maintenance

Building engineering and maintenance must be considered in the prevention of infection in a LTCF. In addition to good building design and construction, preventive care of the building and prompt attention to repairs is essential to an effective infection control program.

Plumbing

In general, plumbing and sewer systems in the facility must be in good repair and undergo routine preventive maintenance work. Poorly functioning floor drains can permit water to accumulate and become stagnant. This creates a reservoir of microorganisms such as *Pseudomonas* and *Aeromonas*. When floors are mopped this contamination can be picked up and spread over the floor surface. Capping of floor drains may be the solution to this problem if the floor drain is no longer needed. Pipes that leak or "sweat" in areas of food preparation and clean storage areas can contaminate food, linen, and supplies. Water

leaks that involve acoustical ceiling tile can facilitate the growth of fungus, especially *Aspergillus*. Wet and water-stained ceiling tiles should be replaced promptly.

Faucet aerators are beneficial for conserving water and preventiing splashing. These devices have some disadvantages, however. Aerators can become blocked with mineral deposits over time. Due to the inherent contamination of tap water and the presence of debris, the aerator can become a reservoir of microorganisms. Thus, aerators contribute to the contamination of tap water. Removal of the aerators, cleaning of the screens, and disinfection with a bleach solution regularly will eliminate this reservoir. If this maintenance cannot be provided, the aerators should be removed permanently.[2]

Plumbing tools and equipment will usually become contaminated, especially with work involving sewer lines. Gross debris should be rinsed off under clean running water and disinfection of the tools attempted. Detergents and disinfectants can damage some tools. Tools should be stored dry.

Regular inspection and preventive maintenance of plumbing is important for eliminating environmental contamination as well as to control repair costs. Inspection and maintenance should include water supply and drainage pipes, vacuum breakers, floor drains, flushing devices, and sinks in resident rooms and kitchen and utility areas.

In some institutions *Legionella* has been shown to contaminate showerheads. If an outbreak of Legionnaires' disease occurs, this contaminant may have to be purged from the system. There are two primary methods for eliminating this problem, hyperchlorination and superheating; both have limitations.[3] It is appropriate to consult with the local health department if this problem is suspected.

Ventilation

The sharing of air by many individuals inside a closed building can contribute to the risk of transmission of airborne infections. Most residents of LTCFs are elderly and may have chronic respiratory conditions and compromised immune systems that make them especially vulnerable to infection with organisms either residing in the ventilation system or moved about by it. Attention to the ventilation system is important to infection prevention and control and also to the comfort of residents and employ-

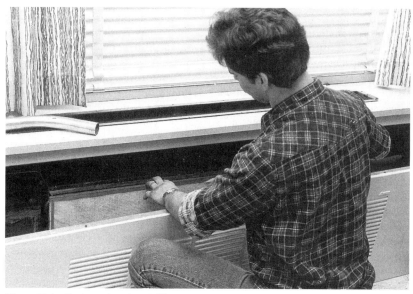

Figure 18.1 *Engineer changing air filter*

ees. Institutional outbreaks of tuberculosis reinforce the necessity for this engineering control.

The relative humidity and the temperature inside the building will determine whether plumbing pipes "sweat" and potentially contaminate clean supplies and food. The humidity and temperature in the facility should be monitored and controlled either electronically or manually.[2]

Positive and negative air pressure determine the direction of airflow in the building. Air should flow from least contaminated areas to areas with more contamination so that potential airborne pathogens pass by the least number of individuals before being exhausted to the outside of the building. Positive pressure is created by supplying more air into an area than is being removed from it by the ventilation system. Negative pressure is created by supplying less air to the area than is being removed by the ventilation system. Positive air pressure is recommended for clean linen areas and storage. Negative pressure is recommended for contaminated areas such as soiled linen areas and soiled utility rooms. Resident rooms should be under negative pressure. Isolation rooms must have negative pressure and be exhausted directly to the outdoors to prevent cross-contamination of airborne infections such as tuberculosis.

Fresh air that is properly filtered will achieve dilution and removal of bacterial airborne contamination and odor. The rate of ventilation is expressed in air exchanges per hour. The minimum air exchanges per hour for a given area or room depends upon the potential contamination of the area. The requirements for LTCFs concerning heating and ventilation systems include specifications for ventilation system design, filter efficiencies, and minimum air exchanges per hour.[4] Two air exchanges are recommended for resident rooms and clean linen storage areas. Corridors and clean utility rooms should have four exchanges per hour. Six exchanges per hour are recommended for physical therapy and occupational therapy areas. Six air exchanges per hour are required for rooms used for tuberculosis isolation. Ten air exchanges are suggested for laundry and soiled utility and bathroom areas.

Verification of negative pressure and the number of air exchanges per hour should be done annually and upon completion of construction projects involving the facility.

Outside air inlets for supplying fresh air should be located as far above the ground as possible and away from exhaust outlets, dumpsters, and other sources of contamination such as incinerators.[5] Filters on the ventilation system should be in place and changed or rotated (if continuous roller type used) regularly. Filters will catch bacteria and fungi to decrease microbial contamination. Pollen, dust, and other allergens are also filtered out of air, which can help prevent irritation of the respiratory tract of residents. If filters are allowed to become blocked, they are not able to filter and the volume of air exchanged is limited. Filters in resident rooms should be changed (see Fig. 18.1) and the area vacuumed (when the resident is out of the room, if possible, because this activity will temporarily increase the number of particles in the immediate environment). Employees changing the filter should consider wearing a face mask for this task, especially those who have a chronic lung disease.[2]

The location of air inlets and exhaust outlets in a room will influence the movement of air in the area. Clean air should be moved downward through the room toward the floor, where it can be removed by the low exhaust vent.[5]

The air-conditioning system in a LTCF can contribute to the risk of airborne infection if attention is not given to routine maintenance and disinfection of cooling systems and cooling tower water. Contaminated air-conditioning systems, for instance, have served as the source for epidemics of Legionnaires' disease in institutions.[3]

Pest Control

Insects and rodents must be eliminated and prevented from gaining access to the LTCF. The primary rationale is aesthetic, but pests and insects can contribute to transmission of infection. They can contaminate food, supplies, environmental surfaces, and even infest a resident (e.g., maggots in pressure ulcers).

Pests are generally controlled with spray or granular chemical insecticides and traps. Insecticides are often needed inside the building as well as outside around the foundation of the building. The chemicals should be nontoxic to humans. Insecticides have a strong odor, which could cause nausea and anorexia in residents who inhale the fumes. Trapping insects and rodents can be an effective process in eliminating them. Mousetraps are aesthetically undesirable but effective. Some trapping devices permit roaches and rodents to enter the trap but not exit. They can become malodorous if not emptied frequently. The use of adhesive insect traps are appropriate outside entrances, but these are not permitted inside facilities by most public health regulations.

Responsibility for pest control may be designated to a contract service. Supervision of the service must be the responsibility of a facility employee. Elimination of observed insects and selection of the appropriate chemical and treatment technique depends upon accurate identification of the species present. Insects found in the building should be placed in a tight-fitting jar and provided to the pest control company employee for identification.

FACILITY SERVICES: LAUNDRY, CLEANING, AND FOOD SERVICES

Laundry

Despite the emphasis given to infection control in the laundry by regulatory agencies, infections associated with linen are quite rare in health care facilities. Linen that is soaked with blood or other body fluids may permit transmission of bloodborne pathogens (like HIV and hepatitis B) as well as other bacterial and viral agents. However, cases of bloodborne infection are not generally traced to this fomite. Soiled linen can become a reservoir of microbes and increase the overall risk of infection to residents. There are numerous opportunities during the laundry cycle for dissemination of microorganisms.

According to the Centers for Disease Control and Prevention (CDC), linens should be handled as little as possible and with a minimum of agitation.[6] This message should be conveyed to the long-term care staff. Stripping linen from a bed can quadruple the number of airborne bacteria in the resident's room and double the count in the adjoining hallway. Linen should be removed from the bed by rolling the soiled sheets and keeping the contaminated surfaces inside the roll. Soiled linen should be bagged at the site of use and transported in bags that adequately contain body fluids.[7]

The soiled linen can be removed from resident care areas by carts or laundry chutes. Design and infection control considerations are important with both mechanisms. Chutes tend to control odor and require less manual effort to move linen a great distance. However, the piston effect of falling linen can disseminate microbes into the environment unless the chute is properly designed. Moving linen in carts or tubs is an effective, sanitary method of transporting soiled linen but can increase the dispersal of odors. A soiled holding area would be required for temporary storage of soiled linen. This room or area must be ventilated under negative pressure and should have a sink for handwashing.

Once soiled linen has reached the laundry receiving area, it is either presorted or weighed and loaded into a washer/extractor unit. The presorting method protects laundry machines and the linen from items left in hampers. The primary advantage to sorting linen after washing is that it minimizes the exposure of laundry personnel to infectious materials by reducing handling of soiled linen. Weighing of linen provides a means for loading appropriate quantities of linen into washer units. If washing machines are overloaded, incomplete rinsing can occur. If insufficient quantities of linen are washed in a load, then water, chemicals, and energy are wasted.

There are five important elements of the normal laundry process. The first action is dilution. Diluting the quantity of microorganisms in the wash water is effective in decontaminating linen. A standard of 4.5 gallons of water per pound of linen will sufficiently dilute and diminish the number of microorganisms. The second action involves the addition of soaps and detergents, which will loosen soil and help remove it. Third, hot water (71°C/160°F) provides the most effective means of destroying microorganisms. However, for the conservation of energy, current recommendations permit decreases in water temperature to 22°C to 50°C. Fourth, bleach added to the washer cycle serves as a disinfectant and removes stains. The fifth and last action performed during the washing process is the addition of a mild acid to neutralize the alkalinity that is present in the water supply and solutions of soaps and detergents. The acid or "sour" will eliminate and minimize yellowing of fabrics due to the alkali residue. The sour will also significantly alter the pH in the washer and destroy microorganisms.[2] Additional chemicals added to the laundry rinses have not been shown to make a difference in the microbial count of the linen and could contribute to skin irritation in the elderly due to residues left in the linen after processing.

In addition to the wash cycle, disinfection of the linens is enhanced with the heat of the dryers and in pressing with flat ironers.

Clean linen must be stored and transported in covered containers or shelves. Ventilation in clean linen storage areas should be maintained with positive pressure to eliminate recontamination. Microbial sampling of linen is not necessary.

Housekeeping and Cleaning

Housekeeping refers to the business of keeping a facility clean. Cleaning is simply the removal of all visible foreign material such as dust and soil. There are three types of cleaning methods used in a health care institution: sanitation, decontamination, and disinfection. These terms refer to the level or extent of antimicrobial activity utilized by the process or the chemical. Environmental cleaning procedures involve at least one of these methods. *Sanitation* refers to the simple reduction in the number of microorganisms to a safe level. A sanitized surface is clean and free of gross soil. Most environmental surfaces in the LTCF require only sanitizing. Kitchen surfaces, dishes, and cooking utensils should be sanitized. *Decontamination* refers to the process of removing disease-producing organisms (pathogens) to make the surface or item safe for handling. Cleaning a blood spill with a bleach solution is an example of the decontamination method. *Disinfection* is the process of killing most disease-producing organisms but not necessarily eliminating all organisms such as spores. Spores are the reproductive element of a microorganism; they have a thick cell wall, enabling the microbe to survive in adverse environments. *Sterilization* is a process that kills all organisms; it is generally applied to surgical equipment and not to environmental surfaces.

Some basic principles of cleaning must be addressed regardless of the level of antimicrobial activity to be accomplished by a procedure:[2]

1. Clean from the least contaminated to the most contaminated surfaces or areas.
2. Work from top to bottom of a room or an object.
3. Remove loose debris before mopping or washing the surface with water.
4. Cleaning solutions, cloths, and mopheads should be changed frequently. The interval for change is determined by the degree of contamination of the surfaces being cleaned. Obviously, the dirtier the cleaning project, the more frequently the solution and mophead will need to be changed.
5. Action should be taken to prevent the growth of microbes on cleaning equipment. Wash and rinse containers prior to refilling. Wash and dry mopheads and cleaning cloths after use. Store buckets dry when not in use.
6. Floor cleaning is best accomplished with a two-bucket system. An alternative system involves spraying the cleaning solution on the floor, with the mop being

Table 18.1 *Commonly Used Disinfectants*

CLASS OF AGENT	LEVEL OF ACTIVITY	EXAMPLES
Formaldehyde	High	Bard-Parker Germicide
Glutaraldehyde (acid)	High	Sonacide
Glutaraldehyde (alkaline)	High	Cidex
Phenolic	Intermediate	Lysol, Phenol
Chlorine	Intermediate	Clorox
Alcohol	Intermediate	70% Ethanol
Quaternary ammonium	Low	Sparquat

used to pick up the solution along with dirt and debris.

7. Use damp dusting and wet mopping methods to eliminate aerosols of dust that can be generated during cleaning with dry methods.

8. All housekeeping equipment should be stored clean at the end of the day.

Schedules should be established for each area of the facility. Frequency of cleaning should be determined by the facility infection control committee (ICC) or the infection control practitioner (ICP) and the housekeeping director based on the nature of the area, the use and critical nature of the environmental surfaces, and the potential risk for infection transmission.

Chemical Disinfection and Sanitation

Chemicals are used to accomplish environmental sanitation and disinfection. *Detergents* are used to help remove soil and are often combined with a disinfectant or sanitizer. The action of a detergent is to decrease the surface tension and to help loosen debris from surfaces for easier removal. They also emulsify the soil so that it can be held in solution. *Sanitizers* are chemical agents used to remove bacterial contamination and generally reduce the numbers of microorganisms. Sanitizers are used primarily in the kitchen and dietary areas and also in the restrooms. *Disinfectants* are used in direct care areas such as the resident rooms and indirect care areas such as physical therapy (see Table 18.1). The two major categories of disinfectants used in LTCFs are quaternary ammonium and phenolic compounds. Special sanitizers and disinfectants that are tasteless and safe if ingested are used in the dietary department.

Quaternary ammonium disinfectants are relatively weak disinfectants used to kill staphylococci and streptococci or other common environmental microbes. Quaternary disinfectants are effective for most routine cleaning procedures in resident care areas. These agents have occasionally become contaminated with gram-negative bacteria and have caused outbreaks.[8]

Phenolic disinfectants are used when contamination with tuberculosis and bloodborne pathogens is suspected. These powerful chemicals can corrode environmental surfaces and irritate the hands of health care workers.

Chlorine is an inexpensive environmental disinfectant used primarily for decontamination and disinfection of blood and body fluid spills. A chlorine bleach solution (0.5%) diluted 1:10 effectively kills the bloodborne pathogens HIV and HBV. Chlorine is also used to disinfect bathroom floors and ceramic fixtures.

Alcohol is a good antiseptic and a disinfectant. Seventy percent alcohol is more effective than 95% alcohol. Seventy percent ethanol or 95% isopropanol are the most commonly used alcohols. Alcohol is used to clean surfaces such as stainless steel.

The use of chemicals for environmental sanitation, decontamination, and disinfection involves some general but important guidelines:

1. Read the label correctly and use the chemical for the appropriate purpose and surfaces.

2. Use cool water for solutions. Chemicals are formulated to be most effective within a given temperature range.

3. Dilute cleaning chemicals according to the manufacturer's directions, accurately measuring all ingredients. Overdilution will result in defective destruction

Table 18.2   *Sample Partial Facility Listing of Disinfectants*

NAME	CHEMICAL	CLASSIFICATION	LOCATION/USE
1. Clorox (Household bleach)	Sodium Hypochlorite	Disinfectant	Blood and body fluid spills on noncorrosive, color-fast surfaces
2. Chlorazene	Chloramine-T	Disinfectant	Physcal therapy as an additive for whirlpool water
3. —	—	—	—
4. —	—	—	—

The chemical agents listed here are approved for use by the given departments and areas to maintain a clean and sanitary environment. These agents are approved for their given use and should be diluted according to the manufacturer's directions.

of microbes. Underdilution can cause damage to environmental surfaces from the more concentrated solution and result in undesirable residue.

4. The presence of organic material on the surface will increase the bioburden in the solution and limit the effectiveness of the chemical agent. Use a trigger sprayer of properly diluted disinfectant and disposable towels to pick up gross soilage and organic matter first. Then general cleaning with the solution can be more effectively accomplished.

A list of approved disinfectants and sanitation chemicals should be maintained for the facility (see Table 18.2). The ICC or ICP should approve specific chemicals after evaluation of the appropriate literature and data. The APIC guideline for selection and use of disinfectants provides an excellent resource for selection and approval of disinfectants in a facility.[8] The specific areas where a chemical is to be used should also be defined. Only approved agents are to be used in the facility. This policy prevents ineffective agents being purchased by individual departments. It also limits confusion among housekeepers about which chemical is appropriate for a specific job or area.

Equipment Cleaning

Equipment and supplies for resident care can become sources of infection if preventive actions are not taken. All equipment and supplies used for resident care should be considered contaminated with potentially infectious material. Handwashing is essential after handling these items, and gloves should be worn if gross soiling with body fluids is possible.

Guidelines for cleaning, disinfection, and sterilization of patient care equipment have been published by the CDC.[9] The recommendations address critical care objects such as surgical instruments and catheters, which must be *sterile*, items that require *high-level disinfection* such as respiratory care equipment, and items for which *cleaning* is sufficient such as bedpans, crutches, water glasses, and food utensils. *Disposable* equipment and supplies may prove appropriate and cost effective when compared with the proper disinfection and sterilization of reusable items. Disposable items (often labeled "single use only") must never be processed and reused. A policy should be in place in the facility to ensure this. Although they may look no different than reusable ones, disposable products are made of materials with a quality that does not permit them to be reprocessed and reused without potentially destroying the integrity of the materials.

Wheelchairs, carts, walkers, beds, and mattresses should be disinfected routinely with a trigger sprayer of an approved quaternary ammonium disinfectant solution. Resident mattresses must be covered with an impermeable material which permits appropriate surface disinfection.

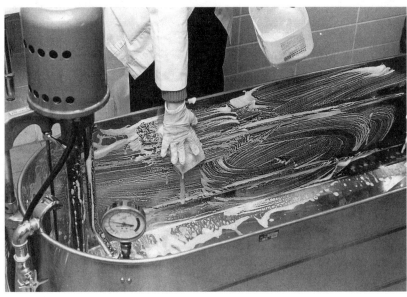

Figure 18.2 *Cleaning the hydrotherapy tank*

Bedpans and urinals should be cleaned after use and routinely. Machines for washing these items are used in many facilities.

Physical Therapy

Physical therapy equipment should be disinfected regularly and any time there is visible soiling with body fluids. Procedures should be in place within the LTCF for the cleaning and disinfection of hydrotherapy equipment (see Figure 18.2). Hubbard tanks and whirlpools can become contaminated with secretions and drainage from open wounds during use. These items should be thoroughly dried after cleaning and disinfection so that tap water contaminants such as *Pseudomonas* are prevented from multiplying. The drain and the agitator are the most common sources of microbial contamination in hydrotherapy equipment, and should be cleaned and disinfected accordingly.

Other items such as orthopedic appliances and occupational therapy tools should be disinfected following soiling with body fluids. Wooden items present problems for appropriate cleaning because their surface is so porous. Usually these items do not have intimate contact with the resident and require only simple cleaning. Care should be taken that these items do not become reservoirs of microorganisms and odors. Environmental cultures are necessary only if equipment is implicated in an outbreak of nosocomial infections.

Respiratory Therapy

Respiratory therapy equipment may be used in some LTCFs and should be processed according to the CDC guidelines.[10] There is significant risk of infection to residents if recommendations are not followed. Cool mist vaporizers are devices that utilize a plastic wheel which spins rapidly in a water reservoir to create aerosols of water droplets. This equipment, used to hydrate respiratory mucous membranes, has safety advantages over hot steamers in preventing accidental burns to residents and employees. However, the devices are not without risk for infection transmission and are generally ineffective in increasing humidity due to the rate of air exchanges in the resident's room. If the water reservoir is filled with contaminated tap water or if sterile water is left in the reservoir for prolonged periods, waterborne bacteria (especially *Pseudomonas* and *Acinetobacter*) will multiply; the device can then expel large quantities of bacteria into the environment and the resident's airway.[11] Central humidification of heated air is preferred.

If room humidifiers are used in the long-term care setting, preventive actions must be taken to minimize the risk of respiratory infection. The water reservoir should be filled immediately before use and refilled only after the reservoir is empty, clean, and dry. Sterile water should be used.

Long-term ventilator patients comprise a select population in a growing number of LTCFs. Ventilators present a definite risk of infection unless steps are taken to prevent their contamination. Only employees skilled in use of the ventilator should handle equipment, and they should practice meticulous handwashing. Manipulating the tubing and opening the system should be minimized in order to avoid introduction of bacteria. Sterile disposable equipment is recommended unless appropriate high-level disinfection can be accomplished in the facility. Guidelines for respiratory therapy equipment have been published.[12]

Thermometers

The measurement of body temperature can be a useful assessment in the elderly. Thermometers are widely used in health-care institutions and require careful attention to asepsis.[13] Hands should be washed before employees take residents' temperatures. A separate glass thermometer should be provided for each resident unless electronic or tympanic devices are used. Between uses, the glass thermometer should be cleansed with soap and water or 70% alcohol and stored dry at the bedside. Terminal cleaning of thermometers can be accomplished with ethylene oxide sterilization or exposure to 90% isopropyl alcohol, glutaraldehyde, or 3% phenolic germicide detergent for at least 30 minutes.

Many institutions have rented or purchased electronic or tympanic thermometers to reduce the time needed to take temperatures and facilitate the aseptic management of the bedside thermometer. This equipment has disposable sheaths or covers to prevent cross-contamination of residents. The hands of the employee should still be washed between residents and before this activity. The external surfaces of the equipment should be disinfected according to the manufacturer's recommendations at regular intervals and if it becomes contaminated with body fluids.

Food Services

The risk of foodborne illness is always present in a LTCF. The consequences of foodborne illness are greater in elderly populations. Outbreaks of foodborne illness have occurred in many facilities across the nation. Inadequate cooking and handwashing facilities and preparation of food by employees with infectious diarrhea have been implicated in various outbreaks in institutions (see Chapters 8 and 11). Salmonellosis is an endemic disease in poultry; the most common vehicle for transmission to humans is through ingestion of undercooked chicken, turkey, or egg products. Incorrect defrosting of frozen poultry and contamination after cooking also present risk. The increasing incidence of community epidemics of diarrheal illness caused by *Shigella* across the country reinforces the need for appropriate handwashing by food handlers. Contaminated ice has caused outbreaks of nosocomial infection. For these reasons, it is important that the food preparation and service environment be clean and that strict attention be given to correct food-handling activities. Control measures should also address hygiene in food handlers and the proper preparation and storage of food.

Food Handlers

Any employee who prepares food should adhere to appropriate procedures for handwashing and sanitation. Food service employees should be in good health and practice good personal hygiene. A food handler's permit should be obtained according to local health department requirements. Hairnets should be worn by all kitchen employees. The food handler should avoid touching food directly and should utilize cooking utensils whenever possible. Nonsterile disposable gloves are often worn for serving food to prevent touch contamination of food items. However, gloves do not replace handwashing. These gloves should be removed and discarded before moving to a personal activity or another food preparation activity that would contaminate the gloves. The employee should take care not to touch the face or contaminated environmental surfaces with gloved hands.

Food Preparation and Storage

Local public health departments determine specific requirements for food service in the LTCF. The intent of regulations is to prevent the introduction of bacteria into food and to prevent the multiplication of any bacteria present in the food. These regulations vary from one community to another but generally include the following:[2,5,14]

1. Refrigeration temperatures should be maintained below 40°F. The capacity of the refrigerator should be sufficient so that large quantities of warm food can be cooled quickly.
2. Foods should not be thawed and refrozen.
3. Meats should not be precooked and held for final cooking.
4. Ice should not be handled by employees with their hands. The ice storage bins should be routinely cleaned with fresh detergent solution and rinsed well. The compartment should be disinfected with a solution of sodium hypochlorite (bleach) at a concentration of 100 ppm. The ice machines should have routine maintenance and internal cleaning to remove mineral deposits, which harbor water contaminants such as *Pseudomonas*.
5. Hot foods should be held at temperatures of at least 140°F, and periodic monitoring of holding temperatures is recommended.
6. Food should be transported to the resident in carts that are temperature controlled.
7. Fruits and vegetables should be thoroughly washed before use.
8. Dry food storage should be clean, dry, off the floor, protected from pests, and at temperatures below 70°F and relative humidity less than 40%.
9. Separation of clean and dirty functions is important. Food storage should be separated from garbage collection areas.
10. Eggs should be purchased from a USDA-approved source, which requires washing of the eggs, does not distribute cracked eggs, and requires that egg products be pasteurized.
11. Adequate dishwashing facilities should be available. It is recommended that dishes be machine-washed at 140°F for 20 seconds and rinsed at 180°F or higher for 10 seconds.
12. All food preparation equipment should be cleaned between uses. Equipment should be easily disassembled to clean.
13. Separate cutting boards should be used for meat/poultry and fruits/vegetables. Cutting boards should be made of hard rubber, plastic, or nonabsorbent wood and should be cleaned promptly after use with hot soapy water.
14. Garbage from the kitchen should be placed in leak-proof containers with tight-fitting lids and should not be allowed to accumulate.

WASTE MANAGEMENT

Definition of Infectious Waste

The waste generated in a health care facility must be safely and effectively managed within the facility to protect employees and residents. Avoiding contamination of the physical environment with waste is a primary concern. Compliance with state and local regulations for disposal of waste will prevent risks to the community. The management of waste is fairly simple if attention is given to each step in the process.

A determination must be made regarding which segments of the waste stream have the potential for causing infection in anyone in the building or in the community. In general, due to the sanitation practices in most communities, solid waste disposal does not constitute significant means of infection transmission. Sanitary landfill operations attempt to reduce access to vectors such as rodents, which could potentially transmit disease to humans. There is currently very little evidence in the literature to support a direct causal relationship between waste disposal and disease transmission in the absence of rodent or insect vectors. With the exception of sharps there have been few reported incidents of disease from biomedical waste. Most waste simply does not provide either an environment conducive to growth and survival of infectious agents or a means by which the infectious agent can enter the body.[15]

The key to facility waste management lies with the definitions of infectious waste. These definitions must be developed for the individual facility but are derived from the CDC recommendations,[16] the EPA,[17,18] and state and local regulations. Definitions should be based on principles of disease transmission.

Unfortunately, current definitions of medical waste are conflicting, and current regulations require greater control measures than appear to be indicated by scientific data.[15] It is to be hoped that a uniform and scientifically based definition of medical waste will be developed. Any definition used by the LTCF must be congruent with federal, state, and local regulations, including OSHA regulations (see Chapter 15). The following are recommended:

Blood and Body Fluids

Blood, blood products, and body fluids should be classified as infectious. The term *human blood and blood products* includes serum plasma and other blood components. The term *body fluid* should include semen, vaginal secretions, cerebrospinal fluid, synovial fluid, pleural fluid, peritoneal fluid, pericardial fluid, amniotic fluid, and any other body fluid visibly contaminated with blood.

Contaminated Sharps Waste

Contaminated sharps waste should be defined as all discarded items derived from human diagnosis, care, or treatment that could potentially transmit disease via direct subdermal inoculation. Infectious sharps include, but are not limited to, hypodermic needles, scalpels, blades, pipettes, and broken glass.

Miscellaneous Contaminated Waste

This is an "optional" infectious waste category. Although there is no uniform opinion regarding the hazards posed by these wastes, the EPA currently believes that the decision whether to handle these wastes as "infectious" should be made by a responsible, authorized person or committee at the individual facility. Examples provided by the EPA include wastes from patients known to be infected with bloodborne diseases and laboratory wastes such as slides and cover slips.

Controversy exists regarding classification of containers and other items contaminated with blood or body fluids. Some resources address this dilemma by considering these items as infectious only when a pourable quantity of blood or body fluid is present. Pourable quantity is further defined as the capacity of a liquid or a semisolid form to drip or flow. Applying this further definition means that a Band-

Aid with a spot of dried blood is not considered infectious waste, and a suction canister with bloody sputum is not considered infectious after the fluid is flushed down a hopper or toilet. The empty soiled container can then be placed in the general waste stream. Without a pourable quantity of body fluid, transmission of infection cannot occur, and routine waste management by the facility and the sanitary landfill will be satisfactory.

Packaging of Waste

Handling infectious waste is the next step in infectious waste management. Handling involves packaging and storage. The ultimate goal is to protect individuals handling or coming in contact with the infectious waste. Personnel should observe universal blood and body fluid precautions at all times with any waste defined as infectious (see Chapter 15).

Infectious waste should be contained in leak-proof plastic bags or containers that are of sufficient strength to resist ripping, tearing, or bursting under normal conditions of use. The bag should be properly labeled. Disposable sharps should be packaged or maintained in puncture-resistant, leak-proof containers that are labeled either with a red color or a "biohazard" label. The container should not be allowed to overfill. Tape can be used to secure the lid of sharps containers for storage, handling, and transport. Infectious waste should not be compacted.

Waste Storage

Infectious waste should be stored in a manner and location that protects the waste from unauthorized personnel,

Table 18.3 *Treatment Methods for Infectious Waste*

WASTE	INCINERATION	STEAM STERILIZATION	SEWER DISPOSAL
Blood, blood products	X	X	X (pourable)
Body fluids	X	X	X (pourable)
Contaminated sharps	X	X	

vectors and environmental elements. Storage time should be minimized; the waste and storage area should be labeled with a "biohazard" symbol.

Waste Treatment

Only waste defined as infectious needs to be treated as infectious. Infectious waste should be appropriately treated prior to disposal. Several methods can be used to treat infectious waste (see Table 18.3). The method chosen for treatment must be based on local regulations.

Blood, blood products, and body fluids can be poured into an approved sewer disposal system as a method of treatment. Other treatment methods include incineration and steam sterilization. The choice of treatment should be based on practicality and cost.

Transporting Waste

Transporting waste within the facility requires frequent disinfection of carts used to transfer waste. Transporting infectious waste from the LTCF to the landfill must be accomplished by individuals with the proper credentials (permits) acceptable to public health authorities.

Garbage, especially from the kitchen, should be removed from the building and stored as far from the entrances to the building as possible, and should be placed on a concrete surface. Plastic bags of garbage should be placed in a rigid container with a cover and garbage containers should have tight-fitting lids.

PREVENTION AND CONTROL MEASURES RELATED TO ANIMATE ENVIRONMENT

Residents

Residents can be reservoirs of pathogens and can introduce a significant risk to others who work or reside in the building. To reduce the risk of infection transmission from the resident, the following areas of control should be addressed:[19]

1. Personal hygiene of residents including bathing, skin care, nail care, oral hygiene, and denture care
2. Individual personal care supplies and equipment of the resident
3. Urinary catheter care and bladder training (see Chapter 6)

4. Care of pressure ulcers (see Chapter 7)
5. Universal precautions and isolation of infected residents (see Chapter 19)
6. Disposal of resident's body wastes and discharges, especially with disoriented or incontinent residents
7. Appropriate treatment of established infections in residents.
8. Screening programs for tuberculosis (see Chapter 5)
9. Influenza vaccination programs

The resident health program is discussed further in Chapter 17.

Visitors

Visitors span the age spectrum and can introduce a wide variety of infectious diseases from the community into the facility. The family member or visitor who understands the unique risks and problems of the institutionalized elderly will be better able to participate in effective control measures. Visitors should be instructed in proper handwashing techniques and the use of protective equipment and apparel such as masks and gloves because they often become involved in direct care of residents.

Policies should address the number of visitors, times of open visitation, and restriction of visitors. Readily visible signs and instructions concerning visitation placed at entrances to the building will facilitate compliance by the visitor. Community epidemics of infection such as shigellosis, as well as seasonal epidemics of influenza, may necessitate prompt action regarding visitation restriction by the administration of the facility. The local public health department is a resource for decision making in these situations.

Employees

The employee in a LTCF has close contact with residents on a daily basis and can both transmit infection to the resident and develop occupationally acquired infection. Both employees and residents are frequently involved in institutional outbreaks of influenza, tuberculosis, and gastroenteritis. For these reasons a comprehensive infection control program and employee health program must be in place in the LTCF (see Chapter 16).

Handwashing

The hands of health care workers are constantly moving from one resident to the other and touching many environmental surfaces. Hands can become reservoirs of microbes and contribute to the transmission of nosocomial infections. Two types of microorganisms colonize the hands of healthcare workers: resident flora and transient flora. *Resident* flora consists of microbes that reside without harm on the skin surface and are considered normal, such as *Staphylococcus epidermidis*, diphtheroids, micrococci, and *Propionibacterium acnes*. Resident flora cannot be totally eliminated by handwashing without destroying skin integrity. *Transient* flora includes nosocomial pathogens such as *Staphylococcus aureus*, *Streptococcus*, and *Pseudomonas*. As the term implies, these microorganisms are transient inhabitants of the skin. They accumulate easily on the hands of health-care workers after resident contact. Frequent handwashing using correct technique will remove most transient microbes and should be done by everyone in the facility. Handwashing is the single most effective method of preventing and controlling infection. The ICP must not assume that individuals know the proper technique and will practice it without reminders. Employees will need repeated instruction and reinforcement of the necessity and procedure for effective handwashing (see Fig. 18.3). Adaptations can be made for instruction of residents and visitors. A handwashing policy and procedure are shown in Chapter 19. The three elements of effective handwashing are soap, running water, and friction.

Soap

Soap can be provided in a variety of forms, each with features and limitations. Bar soap can be an effective form, but it must be maintained in a clean soap dish that allows the bar to drain between uses. When the bar is allowed to sit in a puddle of water, contamination is possible. Liquid soap in a dispenser is generally preferred by institutions because it is more easily managed. The formulation of commercially available soaps varies. Antibacterial formulations are recommended for isolation and before performing invasive procedures; they are rarely needed in the LTCF. Selection of handwashing agents for a facility should be made after reviewing appropriate guidelines.[20]

The method of dispensing liquid soap should be considered. Dispensers with a prefilled cartridge are preferred because they prevent contamination of the liquid. If liquid is added manually to other liquid reservoirs, the dispenser should first be drained and washed. Continually "topping" a dispenser with fresh liquid soap will permit continued growth of bacteria introduced into the dispenser.

Powdered or granular soap is dispensed dry and has less risk of contamination in the dispenser but also has disadvantages. It takes longer to make a lather because the granules must soften with the application of water. This prolongs handwashing time. The granules are rough until fully hydrated, which could become a deterrent to the user, especially those with chapped hands. The health care worker

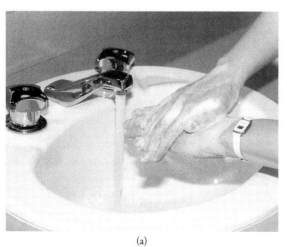

(a)

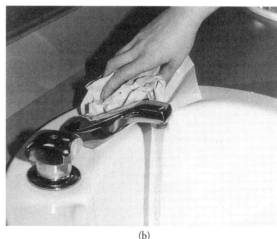

(b)

Figure 18.3 *Correct handwashing technique, demonstrating (a) washing with soap and (b) turning off faucet with paper towel.*

may consciously or unconsciously avoid handwashing because of these materials. Leaf soap is another product for handwashing. Thin leaves of soap are dispensed individually. They quickly hydrate and produce a lather. Humidity can alter the dispensability and limit the use of this soap form. Adequate supplies of soap and paper towels for handwashing are important to ensure employee compliance.

Antiseptics

Antiseptics are agents that can be applied to the skin for their antimicrobial effect.[20] A number of agents are used as antiseptics (see Table 18.4). Antiseptic agents can be used to prepare the resident's skin for insertion of an intravascular device or a urinary catheter. These chemicals can also be added to handwashing agents or to compounds created to replace soap-and-water washing. These compounds are referred to as hand degermers and are dispensed as liquids, foams or gels.

A one- to three-minute wash with 70% to 90% *alcohol* will decrease skin bacteria by more than 90%. The use of alcohol is limited because of the tendency to dry and irritate the skin. Alcohol is volatile and flammable and must be stored and used appropriately.

Iodine is an effective antiseptic. Iodine (0.5%) and alcohol (70%) combine to form tincture of iodine. This combination of agents will kill 80% to 90% of the bacteria on hands with a two-minute wash. Iodophors, which are made up of iodine and surfactants, permit slow release of the iodine. They are generally tolerated well, although they can cause allergy.

Hexachlorophene is an antiseptic that is especially effective against gram-positive bacteria when used in a 1% to 3% solution. The lack of activity against gram-negative bacteria and fungi limits the usefulness of this agent. Hexachlorophene is not recommended for regular use in pregnant women.

Chlorhexidine is an antiseptic agent that is not widely used in LTCFs despite its effectiveness. It may be used as an aqueous solution or as chlorhexidine gluconate emulsion in a detergent. Mild skin irritation may occur in employees who use the chemical for hand antisepsis.

Sinks

Sinks should be conveniently located to facilitate employee compliance with handwashing. The behaviors of caregivers should be evaluated to determine the appropriate location for handwashing in the course of giving care. Sinks that are intended for handwashing should have a deep well and an open drain. Sinks with a shallow well located near medication preparation areas are less desirable for routine handwashing; their purpose is primarily for medication preparation. A barrier can be created between a sink and a clean area in order to prevent splash or splatter onto clean surfaces during handwashing. This might be more effective than trying to divert handwashing to a different location.

Running Water

The temperature of the water at a handwashing sink is important. Employees must learn to adjust the water temperature before starting the procedure. If the water is too hot, the procedure may be abruptly discontinued. Tepid water is recommended for handwashing because it is most comfortable for the individual washing and also because hot water will coagulate some of the surface proteins on the hands and contribute further to chapping and irritation.

Table 18.4 *Commonly Used Antiseptics*

CLASS OF AGENT	LEVEL OF ACTIVITY	EXAMPLES
Alcohol	Intermediate	70% Ethanol
Iodine/alcohol	Intermediate	Tincture of iodine
Iodophor	Intermediate	Betadine, Wescodyne
Hexachlorophene	Low	pHisohex
Chlorhexidine	Low	Hibiclens
Mercurials	Low	Mercurochrome

Paper Towels

The paper towel dispensers should dispense towels easily. Towels should not be left open and stacked next to the sink. This leads to contaminated water dripping onto the towels. If towels do not fit properly into the dispenser they will come out in bunches and then be unavailable when needed; this is expensive and wasteful. The size of the paper towel should be exactly matched to the dispenser to facilitate single-towel dispensing. Proper placement of the dispensers so that hands will not drip onto clean areas or surfaces is important.

The quality of towels is important. A natural towel is probably better than a bleached white towel. The bleaching process leaves residue in the towels that can act as an irritant to hands during drying. The softness of towels is another consideration that will either enhance or deter handwashing. Stiff towels will be abrasive to hands and will inevitably limit employee compliance with handwashing. However, paper towels that are so soft that they deteriorate with use when they become wet are not desirable. The quality of the towel must be evaluated by employees and found acceptable. Linen towels can be utilized by residents for handwashing, but disposable towels should always be used by employees.

Pets

Pets are part of the animate environment, and pet therapy programs are growing in popularity in LTCFs. The benefits to the elderly can be outweighed by the infection risks unless appropriate preventive actions are taken. The local health department must permit such a program, and compliance with specific regulations is essential. Written guidelines for a pet therapy program should include appropriate documentation of vaccination of the pet, careful choice of the pet based on the temperament of the animal, and screening of pets for infections. The role and responsibilities of the person(s) who bring, handle, and take responsibility for the animals should be clearly defined; they must be knowledgeable about the nature of the facility and infection control guidelines. The pet should be clean, and the pet's body functions should be attended to prior to the visit. Pets should be taken outside to void or defecate. A barrier such as a clean linen sheet should be used if the pet is permitted on the resident's bed or furniture. This sheet should be removed and treated as soiled linen after the pet visits. The resident should always wash hands after handling pets. Reported outbreaks demonstrate that pet-associated infections may spread to the LTCF resident.[21]

REFERENCES

1. Khabbaz RF, Tenney JH: Infection control in Maryland nursing homes. *Infect Control Hosp Epidemiol* 1988;9:159–162.
2. Soule BM, Berg R: *The APIC Curriculum for Infection Control Practice*, Vol. I, II, III. Dubuque, IA, Kendall Hunt, 1983–1988.
3. Muraca PW, Yu VL, Goetz A: Disinfection of water distribution systems for Legionella: A review of application procedures and methodologies. *Infect Control Hosp Epidemiol* 1990;11:79–88
4. *Minimum Requirements of Construction and Equipment for Hospital and Medical Facilities.* Publication No.76-4000, Bethesda, MD, U.S. Department of Health, Education and Welfare, 1975.
5. *Infection Control in the Hospital,* 4th ed. Chicago, American Hospital Association, 1979.
6. Centers for Disease Control: *CDC guidelines: Nosocomial infections—laundry services,* Atlanta, GA, 1981.
7. Joint Committee on Healthcare Laundry Guidelines: 1993 guidelines for healthcare linen service. Textile Rental Services Association of America, Hallandale, FL, 1993.
8. Rutala WA: APIC guideline for selection and use of disinfectants. *Am J Infect Control* 1990;18:99–117.
9. Centers for Disease Control: Cleaning, disinfection, and sterilization of hospital equipment. *Infect Control* 1981;2:138–144.
10. Centers for Disease Control. *Recommendations for the Decontamination and Maintenance of Inhalation Therapy Equipment,* Altanta, GA, 1976.
11. Smith PW, Massanari RM: Room humidifiers as a source of *Acinetobacter* infections. *JAMA* 1977;237:795–797.
12. Simmons BP, Wong ES: Guideline for prevention of nosocomial pneumonia. *Infect Control Hosp Epidemiol* 1982;327–333.
13. Centers for Disease Control: *Aseptic Handling of Thermometers*

and Other Equipment for Measuring Patient Temperatures. Atlanta, GA, 1978.

14. Jopke WH: Food hygiene, in Bond RB, Michaelson GS, De Roos RL: *Environmental Health and Safety in Health-Care Facilities,* 1st ed. New York, Macmillan, 1973.

15. Rutala WA: Medical waste. *Infect Control Hosp Epidemiol* 1992;13:38–48.

16. Garner JS, Favero MS: *Infective Waste, Guideline for Hand-washing and Hospital Environmental Control.* Atlanta, GA, Centers for Disease Control, 1985.

17. US Environmental Protection Agency: Guideline for infectious waste management. EPA/530-SW-86-014, Washington DC, 1986.

18. Environmental Protection Agency: Standards for the tracking and management of medical waste. *Federal Register* 1989;54:12326–95

19. Campbell DG: Prevention of infection in extended care facilities. *Nurs Clin North Am* 1980;15:857–868.

20. Larson E: Guideline for use of topical antimicrobial agents, *Am J Infect Control* 1988:16:253–266.

21. Robson D, Frederick H, Spearman G, et al: Avian psittacosis outbreak in a geriatric wing of a tertiary care hospital (abstract). Presented at Association for Practitioners in Infection Control Annual Conference, Reno, NV, 1989.

CHAPTER

INFECTION CONTROL MEASURES TO BLOCK TRANSMISSION: ISOLATION AND BEYOND

Vicki G. Pritchard

INTRODUCTION

Long-term care facilities (LTCFs) today are faced with the need to receive and care for many residents who in the past would have been viewed as unacceptable for admission because of infectious disease problems. Others enter with conditions severely compromising their ability to combat infection. In addition, risk factors related to multiple system diseases in the frail elderly and staffing problems can interact to spread infections in the LTCF. Colonized caregivers and contaminated environments can also play a role in the spread of infection. Isolation procedures reduce this spread by blocking the mode of transmission for the infectious agent (see Fig. 9.2).

Traditional isolation practices (category or disease-specific isolation) as recommended by the Centers for Disease Control and Prevention (CDC) have relied on diagnosis driven systems. That is, the diagnosis of a contagious disease causes caregivers to implement special barrier measures to prevent the spread of the specific disease. This has been shown to be an imperfect system because of the presence of unknown and undiagnosed diseases, and colonized and carrier states that exist outside the isolation room.

The concept of universal precautions (UP) is intended to prevent parenteral, mucous membrane, and nonintact skin exposures of health-care workers to bloodborne pathogens such as human immunodeficiency virus (HIV) and hepatitis B (HBV) from the blood of all patients, regardless of their diagnosis.[1] The use of UP for all hospitalized patients has included a no-touch philosophy for all potential contacts with body fluids and nonintact skin. The overall goal is to change the behavior of health-care workers toward safe protective practices for preventing the transmission or acquisition of infections among both patients and employees.[2]

An isolation system is an important and traditional aspect of the overall infection control program. In adapting an isolation system, the LTCF must consider the available options (see below) and current regulations. Any system needs to be simple, realistic and practical, recognizing the unique problems of the LTCF resident and the modest resources available for care as compared to hospitals.

EVALUATION ON ADMISSION TO THE LONG-TERM CARE FACILITY

Screening New Admissions

All new admissions to the LTCF should be considered potential risks for introducing and transmitting infections within the facility. This is a particular problem when a patient with a nosocomial infection is transferred to the institution from a hospital. Some will have unknown or undiagnosed infectious diseases.

Not only do these patients present a risk of transmitting infections in LTCFs, they may also introduce antibiotic-resistant pathogens into the environment of the facility (see Chapter 12). To reduce the risks of such transmission, preadmission screening for clinical or occult infections should be provided by the referring physician or by the acute care institution before admission to the LTCF. The primary purpose of preadmission screening is to identify individuals who harbor communicable diseases and to identify factors that place the resident at high risk for nosocomial events. In addition, the screening procedure should identify residents who carry resistant organisms that may be transmitted to other residents. Because information obtained from preadmission screens may be incomplete, protocols for evaluation at the time of admission may also be instituted.

If UP are followed, it is no longer a matter of such concern that new residents be housed in a private room (segregated) during the first few days of their admission. Good routine procedures, such as not placing a resident who has a bladder catheter in the same room with another catheterized resident, are wise and do seem to help prevent cross-infection.[3] During the first three to five days of admission, a routine of monitoring the resident's temperature and other vital signs more often than daily (three to four times during the day) seems effective for helping to identify occult infections.

The admission evaluation should include the collection and recording of pertinent historical information, physical findings, and a modest laboratory screen in order to identify active infections. For infection control purposes, the subjective inquiry should focus on a history of active infection with particular emphasis on infections of the urinary tract, skin, respiratory tract, and gastrointestinal tract. Where it can be documented, inquiry regarding the etiologic agent is important.

Whenever possible, a history of bloodborne diseases such as hepatitis B or C and HIV can be elicited, keeping in mind the importance of confidentiality regarding the diagnosis of HIV.[4] This history should not be intended as the primary mechanism for ensuring employee safety because universal precautions must be practiced with every resident.

Information regarding ongoing therapy with antibiotics should also be ascertained and assessed. It is important to determine from where the resident is being admitted—that is, community or hospital. Inquiries should be made into underlying diseases, particularly those that may predispose to infection, such as low level of activity, diabetes mellitus, or dysphagia. Finally, a complete immunization history should be obtained in order to determine what additional immunizations may be necessary, and recommended vaccinations should be given (see Chapter 17).

The admission physical examination should include a thorough review of all organ systems, with particular infection control attention devoted to skin, lungs, and urinary tract. Existing pressure ulcers should be noted, staged, and measured (see Chapter 7).

Laboratory screening procedures can be kept to a minimum, particularly when information is available from previous hospitalizations or visits to the physician's office. When there is a previous history of urinary tract infection or when the resident is admitted with a bladder catheter, a standard urinalysis should be obtained and urine cultures and sensitivities requested. Stool cultures may be helpful if the resident presents with diarrhea. If the resident has open wounds or drainage sites, it is prudent to determine the predominant organisms and identify any multiply resistant organisms that may be a risk to other residents. Whenever possible, such cultures should be obtained within one week prior to admission to the LTCF so that the organisms are known immediately.

Admission Criteria and Data

The early institution of isolation methods is extremely important for preventing the spread of infections. States may not allow LTCFs to refuse to accept a resident because of the presence of an infectious disease, and most LTCFs are required by law to have adequate facilities for appropriate isolation. Seven states define those communicable diseases that are allowed to be admitted, and several others allow patients with communicable diseases to be admitted as long as certain conditions are met.[5] The local or state health department should be consulted for policy development.

The admission data base should include information about resident factors that may facilitate spread of an infection in the institution (e.g., cough or incontinence) as well as especially hazardous bacteria such as methicillin-resistant *Staphylococcus aureus* (MRSA). It is important to identify MRSA colonized or infected residents at admission so that isolation or special precautions can be put into place.[6–8] MRSA is discussed further in Chapter 12.

Tuberculosis (TB) Screening

Because the risk of TB exposure is greater in a LTCF than in the community, prevention of the occurrence and spread of this disease is a major part of all infection control programs. Screening at admission to the LTCF is the first component of the facility's tuberculosis surveillance and control program. A written protocol should be adopted to ensure that all residents and employees have a baseline TB screening prior to or at the time of admission/ hiring. TB screening is discussed in Chapter 5.

HANDWASHING AND ASEPSIS

Handwashing

Handwashing is a component of isolation because handwashing helps prevent transporting of microorganisms from resident/environment to others via the hands of the caregiver, housekeeper, food worker, other employee, resident, or visitor. Handwashing is the single most important procedure for preventing nosocomial infections.[9] An infection control program that relies on gloving and handwashing can minimize persistent hand colonization in health care workers by endemic nosocomial pathogens (such as MRSA) and can contribute to the limitation of cross-infection.[10] The collective evidence from observational and experimental studies is very consistent with the hypothesis that handwashing is associated with a reduction in the risk of infection.[11]

Handwashing with plain soap is effective in removing transient microbial flora. Antimicrobial handwashing agents may be indicated in certain situations, but their efficacy may only be due to better compliance by health care workers who perceive the situation requiring handwashing to be serious.[12]

Alcohol impregnated wipes can be utilized in areas where running water is not available. They have been shown to be an acceptable alternative to soap-and-water handwashing in nonacute health care settings,[13] but regular handwashing with running water should be performed as soon as possible because alcohol wipes are not a substitute for handwashing.

Each LTCF should have a handwashing policy and procedure. The procedure for handwashing (see Table 19.1) should be in writing and should be a regular focus of orientation and in-service education for all health care workers. Handwashing is usually recommended for 10 to 15 seconds.[9]

In the absence of a true emergency, personnel should always wash their hands

- after taking care of any resident.
- before gloving to perform sterile procedures and after removing gloves (regardless of what the gloves were used for). This is because glove integrity is not always optimum and because normal microbial flora of the hands tends to overgrow in the warm moist environment of the gloved hands.
- after any situation in which microbial contamination was likely to have occurred, especially those involving contact with body fluids or mucous membranes, or with inanimate sources likely to be contaminated, such as body fluid/secretion measuring or collecting devices, or dirty laundry.
- before preparing medications or handling food items.
- before going to lunch or break.
- after toileting.
- before beginning duty and before leaving for home.

The convenient placement of sinks, handwashing products, and paper towels encourages frequent and appropriate handwashing. Administrators responsible for planning new construction should consult with the infection control practitioner so that the placement of sinks and bathrooms relative to work activities of staff are taken into account. Placement of the faucet and size of the sink should be adequate to allow rinsing without recontamination. Even though employee handwashing is well documented as a method of infection control, professionals engaged in infection control do not always consider the importance of resident handwashing.[14] Residents should wash their hands before eating, before performing self-care (such as tracheostomy care), and after toileting, if they are able.

Frequent monitoring for compliance with handwashing is important to the LTCF infection control program. How this is accomplished can be as simple as assigning one staff member to keep a checklist of observed instances when another employee or a resident did or did not handwash appropriately. This can be used as a routine monitor and the basis for educational efforts regarding handwashing. The percentage of compliance can be graphed and posted to show improvement and to encourage the participants.

Asepsis

The role of disinfection, sterilization, and sanitation for isolation is no more and no less important than it is for the entire LTCF. Cleaning the rooms, care of linen, and handling food trays is rarely different for the isolated resident than for any other resident.[15] Disinfectants and antiseptics are discussed in Chapter 18.

Table 19.1   *Handwashing: Sample LTCF Procedure*

PURPOSE

To prevent the spread of bacteria

EQUIPMENT

Hot and cold running water
Soap or soap solution
Paper towels

PROCEDURE

1. Remove jewelry.
2. Adjust running water to comfortable force and temperature to prevent contamination of surrounding area by splashing water.
3. Wet hands and lather well with soap or other agent. Wash hands thoroughly using an interlacing motion and friction, paying particular attention to the medial areas of the fingers.
4. Rinse well, keeping hands slightly lower than elbows.
5. Dry hands, using paper towel.
6. Turn off water, using a paper towel to protect hands from contaminated faucets.

NOTES

A. Depending on the activity having been performed it may be necessary also to wash the forearm and elbow before proceeding to the next activity.
B. Skin should be kept soft and intact. Hand lotion or creams may be used after handwashing only if the next activity does not involve direct resident contact, as lotions and creams are potential media for bacterial growth. Do not apply oil-based lotions before donning gloves.
C. If during the handwashing procedure your hands become contaminated, the complete procedure must be repeated.

CONTROL OF INFECTION BY ISOLATION

Interrupting the transmission of pathogenic organisms, that is, breaking the chain of transmission, requires the use of barrier techniques. Conventional isolation schemes rely on the ability of LTCF caregivers to quickly suspect and identify an infectious disease. Isolation must begin at first suspicion in order to prevent spread to others. Thus, authority for implementing isolation procedures resides with nursing personnel as well as physicians. It is essential that nursing staff be granted the authority to make these decisions because they are most intimately acquainted with the resident and will probably be the first to identify an infection. This authority must be in writing and acknowledged by the professional staff and the administration.

Implementation of isolation procedures should be considered for any resident whose condition suggests a possible transmissible infection. The decision to isolate the resident should take into account all of the following factors: the site of the infection (for example, open draining wound versus urinary tract infection); the etiologic agent, if known; the usual modes of transmission (based upon a knowledge of the etiologic agent or site of the infection); availability and access to susceptible hosts; and the coherence and mobility of the infected resident.[16]

The LTCF has several choices in the type of isolation scheme to be adopted for the facility, but no matter which is chosen, all the policies and procedures pertaining to it must be in writing and available to all staff for orientation, periodic reference, and frequent in-services. The choices for isolation schemes include the standard systems of category-specific isolation and disease-specific isolation.[17] All facilities will have some form of universal precautions. A fourth alternative that is gaining favor in acute care facilities, and in many LTCFs as well, is the body substance isolation system (BSI).[18] Facilities may develop their own particular isolation schemes so long as the basic requirements outlined by the CDC are met.

Category-Specific Isolation

Many institutions employ different levels of isolation based upon the nature of the organism and the source of the infection. This approach may be most practical at larger or skilled nursing facilities. The various levels of isolation precautions are designated by cards placed on the door to the room. Advantages to this system include the fact that it requires little foresight or research in order to quickly institute barrier precautions. Staff education is simplified. One disadvantage is that the barrier techniques are not always tailored to meet the specific needs of the resident; thus, excessive isolation procedures or expense could result if the category strategies do not exactly match the mode of transmission of the organism. The categories are as follows:[17]

1. *Strict isolation* is designed to prevent transmission of highly transmissible or epidemiologically important infections that may be spread by both air and direct contact (e.g., varicella/chickenpox).

2. *Respiratory isolation* is designed to prevent transmission of infectious diseases such as measles primarily over short distances through the air (droplet transmission).

3. *Enteric precautions* are designed to prevent infections transmitted by direct or indirect contact with feces, such as *Salmonella* gastroenteritis.

4. *Contact isolation* is designed to prevent transmission of highly transmissible or epidemiologically important infections that do not warrant strict isolation. They are not spread by the airborne route. An example would be a major pressure ulcer infection caused by *S. aureus*.

5. *Drainage/secretion precautions* are less stringent, involving the spread of infections that are transmitted by direct or indirect contact with infectious body fluids, such as conjunctivitis or a minor pressure ulcer infection.

6. *AFB isolation*, or acid-fast bacillus/tuberculosis isolation, for residents with suspected or contagious pulmonary or laryngeal tuberculosis is similar to respiratory isolation. A private room with special ventilation is indicated. These residents have positive sputum smears for AFB or suspicious x-rays.

7. A seventh category, blood/body fluid precautions, as suggested for hepatitis B, HIV, and other blood-borne diseases, is no longer in use as a standard isolation type because of the recent mandate for the use of universal precautions. Now, in all LTCFs all residents are considered to require blood/body fluid precautions. Obviously, there is no need for this

special designation or sign-posting for residents who are known to have a bloodborne disease. Indeed, because of the laws governing confidentiality, it is no longer prudent to post such a sign outside the door of any resident because of the stigma that may be associated with HIV.

Isolation cards have been suggested for use with the category-specific type of isolation. The front of the card lists the name of the category and apparel needed to enter the room, and diseases requiring that category of isolation are listed on the back of the card.[17]

A private room is required for strict isolation, respiratory/AFB isolation and contact isolation. A private room used for airborne diseases should have minimum ventilation (supply and exhaust) of six air changes per hour, and two of the changes should be from outside, not recirculated air. Such areas should be constructed so that there is no cross-circulation or recirculation of air between the isolation room and other sections of the LTCF unless the air is passed through high-efficiency filters. The room should be under slightly negative pressure with regard to the hall; it is preferable for the room to have its own supply and exhaust for ventilation air.[19]

Strict isolation requires that masks, gloves, and gowns be worn by all who enter the room—and could be used for a disease such as MRSA pneumonia. In respiratory and AFB isolation, masks are worn by all entering the room. A resident requiring enteric precautions may be in a room with others as long as they are cooperative, and do not have such severe diarrhea or fecal incontinence that either roommates or objects used by them become contaminated. In contact isolation (e.g., a resident with a major pressure ulcer infection caused by *S. aureus*), gowns and gloves are worn by those having direct contact with the infected material.

Sources are available that discuss gown, mask, and glove use; disposition of contaminated articles, linen, and dishes; and terminal cleaning after the room is vacated.[17] Standard laundry and dishwashing cycles are adequate for isolation room materials, and neither routine nor terminal cleaning of isolation rooms is usually different from the cleaning of other resident rooms. It involves emptying all receptacles, discarding disposable items, wet-vacuuming or mopping floors, and washing visibly soiled areas on walls. Equipment, furniture, and mattress covers should be washed with a germicidal detergent solution. Personal effects require no special attention unless visibly contaminated by infective secretions. All visitors entering an isolation room should be instructed regarding necessary measures for preventing transmission of infection. Finally, handwashing after leaving an isolation room needs to be emphasized.

Disease-Specific Isolation

To simplify isolation procedures for LTCFs, an approach to isolation based on the specific disease (disease-specific isolation) may be used. Minor alterations in the basic procedure may be instituted in accordance with the nature of the infecting organism and the site of the infection. One drawback with this system is that the required level of precautions is difficult to determine for residents whose diagnosis has not been confirmed. Also, extensive education of the staff may be needed to ensure correct implementation of precautions. Using this approach, the infection precautions recommended for reducing the risk of transmitting infectious diseases in nursing homes are outlined in a single *isolation card* (see Fig. 19.1).

In general, private rooms are not necessary; however, several exceptions should be noted. Residents with respiratory infections that are spread by aerosolization should be confined to a private room. This includes residents with presumptive or active tuberculosis and residents with lower respiratory infections due to antibiotic-resistant organisms (e.g., MRSA). Residents with disseminated herpes zoster infections—that is, involvement of more than one dermatome—should also be placed in a private room. Finally, residents with diarrhea or draining skin infections who are incoherent or unable to care for themselves should be considered for private rooms if diapering or secure dressings cannot be guaranteed.

In general, gowns, masks, and gloves are not necessary unless the health care worker comes in direct contact with drainage or secretions from the infected site. Gloves are necessary for nursing personnel who come in direct contact with blood or potentially bloody body fluids or secretions (universal precautions). In addition, special precautions must be exercised in disposing of syringes and needles that may have been used in the care of residents. Refer to the preceding discussion of category-spe-

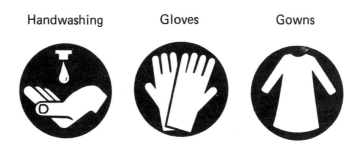

For:_____Stool_____Sputum_____Urine_____Wound/Skin Drainage

1. Private room - Not necessary *
2. Gowns—Only when soiling of clothes likely
3. Mask—Not necessary*
4. Hands—Must be washed on entering, and following resident care
5. Gloves—For contact with infected area, drainage or blood
6. Articles—Special precautions for contaminated instruments and dressings
7. Housekeeping—Routine cleaning
8. Specimens—Place in leak-proof container. Bag if outside is contaminated.

*Unless otherwise indicated by guidelines in Table 19.2

Figure 19.1 *Sample Isolation Card—Disease-Specific System*
Summary of infection precautions for segregating a resident with presumed infection in a nursing care facility. This information can be prepared as a 5x8 card for placement outside the resident's room, above the bed, and on the resident's record in order to indicate need for special precautions.

cific isolation for details that also apply to disease-specific isolation regarding linen, dishes, cleaning, and so on.

To assist in the execution of proper infection precautions, the reader is referred to Table 19.2. The table has a sampling of common diseases organized according to the infectious agent or site of infection. Columns on the right indicate the necessity for private room, gowns, masks, and so on, depending upon the presumed infectious agent. This list is adapted from the CDC isolation guideline, which contains isolation recommendation for many other diseases as well.[17] Information on the necessary duration of isolation is available from Table 19.2 and other sources.[17] Each disease has care requirements that can be transposed onto the isolation card so as to tailor the isolation routines to the specific needs of the resident.

Universal Precautions

The primary intent of universal precautions (UP) is to reduce risks to HCWs from bloodborne pathogens. The CDC guideline[1] emphasizes that blood and body fluid precautions should be used for all residents regardless of known HIV status.

Universal precautions are designed for the protection of the health care worker and mandated by the Occupational Safety and Health Administration (OSHA) for use by all health care workers during the routine care of all residents. They are discussed in more detail in Chapters 15 and 16. Anticipated contact with blood or potentially bloody body fluids from any resident should cue workers to take appropriate precautions.

The apparent simplicity of the approach is appealing, but in the LTCF, intensive physical caring may seem to conflict with the universal precautions ideology. For example, the heavy

Table 19.2 *Disease-Specific Isolation Precautions*

AGENT/SITE OF INFECTION	PRECAUTIONS OR ISOLATION INDICATED? (1 = NO; 2 = YES)	PRIVATE ROOM INDICATED? (1 = NO; 2 = YES FOR RESIDENT WHO CANNOT USE GOOD HYGIENE; 3 = YES; 4 = YES WITH SPECIAL VENTILATION	MASK INDICATED? (1 = NO; 2 = YES FOR THOSE WHO GET CLOSE TO RESIDENT; 3 = YES)	GOWN INDICATED? (1 = NO; 2 = YES WHEN SOILING OF CLOTHES LIKELY; 3 = YES)	GLOVES INDICATED? (1 = NO; 2 = YES FOR CONTACT WITH INFECTED AREA OR DRAINAGE; 3 = YES)	COMMENTS (INCLUDING DURATION OF PRECAUTIONS OR ISOLATION)
Abscess, etiology unknown						
Draining	2	1	1	2	2	Maintain for duration of illness. Emphasize pus (drainage) precautions.
Not draining	1	—	—	—	—	—
Bronchitis	1	—	—	—	—	Maintain respiratory secretion precautions for duration of illness
Candidiasis, all forms, including mucocutaneous (moniliasis, thrush)	1	—	—	—	—	
Cellulitis						
Intact skin	1	—	—	—	—	—
Draining	2	1	1	2	2	Maintain for duration of illness. Emphasize pus (drainage) precautions.
Closed-cavity infection						
Draining	2	1	1	2	2	Maintain for duration of illness. Emphasize pus (drainage) precautions.

Table 19.2 *Continued*

AGENT/SITE OF INFECTION	PRECAUTIONS OR ISOLATION INDICATED? (1 = NO; 2 = YES)	PRIVATE ROOM INDICATED? (1 = NO; 2 = YES FOR RESIDENT WHO CANNOT USE GOOD HYGIENE; 3 = YES; 4 = YES WITH SPECIAL VENTILATION	MASK INDICATED? (1 = NO; 2 = YES FOR THOSE WHO GET CLOSE TO RESIDENT; 3 = YES)	GOWN INDICATED? (1 = NO; 2 = YES WHEN SOILING OF CLOTHES LIKELY; 3 = YES)	GLOVES INDICATED? (1 = NO; 2 = YES FOR CONTACT WITH INFECTED AREA OR DRAINAGE; 3 = YES)	COMMENTS (INCLUDING DURATION OF PRECAUTIONS OR ISOLATION)
Not draining	1	—	—	—	—	—
Common cold	1	—	—	—	—	Maintain respiratory secretion precautions for duration of illness
Conjunctivitis, acute or viral	2	1	1	1	2	Maintain for duration of illness. Emphasize pus (drainage) precautions.
Decubiti (infected)	2	1	1	2	2	Maintain for duration of illness. Emphasize pus (drainage) precautions.
Diarrhea, acute— infective etiology suspected (see Gastroenteritis)	2	2	1	2	2	Maintain for duration of illness. Emphasize stool precautions.
Fever of unknown origin (FUO)	1	—	—	—	—	Patients usually do not need isolation; it is appropriate, however, to isolate patient with signs and symptoms compatible with a disease that calls for isolation.

Table 19.2 *Continued*

AGENT/SITE OF INFECTION	PRECAUTIONS OR ISOLATION INDICATED? (1 = NO; 2 = YES)	PRIVATE ROOM INDICATED? (1 = NO; 2 = YES FOR RESIDENT WHO CANNOT USE GOOD HYGIENE; 3 = YES; 4 = YES WITH SPECIAL VENTILATION	MASK INDICATED? (1 = NO; 2 = YES FOR THOSE WHO GET CLOSE TO RESIDENT; 3 = YES)	GOWN INDICATED? (1 = NO; 2 = YES WHEN SOILING OF CLOTHES LIKELY; 3 = YES)	GLOVES INDICATED? (1 = NO; 2 = YES FOR CONTACT WITH INFECTED AREA OR DRAINAGE; 3 = YES)	COMMENTS (INCLUDING DURATION OF PRECAUTIONS OR ISOLATION)
Furunculosis, staphylococcal	2	1	1	2	2	Maintain for duration of illness. Emphasize pus (drainage) precautions.
Gastroenteritis Unknown etiology	2	2	1	2	2	Maintain for duration of illness. Emphasize stool precautions.
Campylobacter spp.	2	2	1	2	2	Maintain for duration of illness. Emphasize stool precautions.
Clostridium difficile	2	2	1	2	2	Maintain for duration of illness. Emphasize stool precautions.
E.coli (enteropathogenic, enterotoxic, or enteroinvasive)	2	2	1	2	2	Maintain for duration of illness. Emphasize stool precautions.
Giardia	2	2	1	2	2	Maintain for duration of illness. Emphasize stool precautions.
Salmonella spp.	2	2	1	2	2	Maintain for duration of illness. Emphasize stool precautions.

Table 19.2 *Continued*

AGENT/SITE OF INFECTION	PRECAUTIONS OR ISOLATION INDICATED? (1 = NO; 2 = YES)	PRIVATE ROOM INDICATED? (1 = NO; 2 = YES FOR RESIDENT WHO CANNOT USE GOOD HYGIENE; 3 = YES; 4 = YES WITH SPECIAL VENTILATION	MASK INDICATED? (1 = NO; 2 = YES FOR THOSE WHO GET CLOSE TO RESIDENT; 3 = YES)	GOWN INDICATED? (1 = NO; 2 = YES WHEN SOILING OF CLOTHES LIKELY; 3 = YES)	GLOVES INDICATED? (1 = NO; 2 = YES FOR CONTACT WITH INFECTED AREA OR DRAINAGE; 3 = YES)	COMMENTS (INCLUDING DURATION OF PRECAUTIONS OR ISOLATION)
Shigella spp.	2	2	1	2	2	Maintain until 3 consecutive feces cultures taken after ending antimicrobial therapy negative for infecting strain. Emphasize stool precautions.
Viral	2	2	1	2	2	Maintain for duration of illness. Emphasize stool precautions. See also rotavirus.
Hepatitis, viral						
Type A (infectious epidemic hepatitis)	2	2	1	2	2	Maintain for 7 days after onset of jaundice.
Type B including antigen carrier	1	—	—	—	—	Use UP.
Hepatitis C and non-A non B	1	—	—	—	—	Use UP.
Unspecified type, consistent with viral etiology	2	2	1	2	2	Use UP.

Table 19.2 *Continued*

AGENT/SITE OF INFECTION	PRECAUTIONS OR ISOLATION INDICATED? (1 = NO; 2 = YES)	PRIVATE ROOM INDICATED? (1 = NO; 2 = YES FOR RESIDENT WHO CANNOT USE GOOD HYGIENE; 3 = YES; 4 = YES WITH SPECIAL VENTILATION	MASK INDICATED? (1 = NO; 2 = YES FOR THOSE WHO GET CLOSE TO RESIDENT; 3 = YES)	GOWN INDICATED? (1 = NO; 2 = YES WHEN SOILING OF CLOTHES LIKELY; 3 = YES)	GLOVES INDICATED? (1 = NO; 2 = YES FOR CONTACT WITH INFECTED AREA OR DRAINAGE; 3 = YES)	COMMENTS (INCLUDING DURATION OF PRECAUTIONS OR ISOLATION)
Herpesvirus hominis (herpes simplex)						
Mucocutaneous, disseminated or primary, severe (skin, oral, and genital)	2	3	1	2	2	Maintain for duration of illness. Emphasize secretion precautions with lesions.
Mucocutaneous, recurrent (skin, oral, and genital)	2	1	1	1	2	Maintain for duration of illness. Emphasize secretion precautions with lesions.
Herpes zoster						
Localized in immunocompromised patient or disseminated	2	4	3	3	3	Maintain for duration of illness.
Localized in normal patient	2	2	1	1	2	Maintain for duration of illness. Personnel susceptible to herpes zoster (chickenpox) should wear mask.
Influenza	1	—	—	—	—	Respiratory secretions may be infectious.

238

Table 19.2 *Continued*

AGENT/SITE OF INFECTION	PRECAUTIONS OR ISOLATION INDICATED? (1 = NO; 2 = YES)	PRIVATE ROOM INDICATED? (1 = NO; 2 = YES FOR RESIDENT WHO CANNOT USE GOOD HYGIENE; 3 = YES; 4 = YES WITH SPECIAL VENTILATION	MASK INDICATED? (1 = NO; 2 = YES FOR THOSE WHO GET CLOSE TO RESIDENT; 3 = YES)	GOWN INDICATED? (1 = NO; 2 = YES WHEN SOILING OF CLOTHES LIKELY; 3 = YES)	GLOVES INDICATED? (1 = NO; 2 = YES FOR CONTACT WITH INFECTED AREA OR DRAINAGE; 3 = YES)	COMMENTS (INCLUDING DURATION OF PRECAUTIONS OR ISOLATION)
Legionnaires' disease	1	—	—	—	—	
Meningitis						
Bacterial, etiology unknown	2	3	2	1	1	Maintain for 24 hours after start of effective therapy. Emphasize respiratory secretion precautions.
Other diagnosed bacterial	1	—	—	—	—	—
MRSA Multiply resistant organisms, infection or colonization						See multiply resistant organisms
GI	2	3	1	2	2	Maintain until off antibiotics and culture negative twice. Emphasize stool precautions.

Table 19.2 *Continued*

AGENT/SITE OF INFECTION	PRECAUTIONS OR ISOLATION INDICATED? (1 = NO; 2 = YES)	PRIVATE ROOM INDICATED? (1 = NO; 2 = YES FOR RESIDENT WHO CANNOT USE GOOD HYGIENE; 3 = YES; 4 = YES WITH SPECIAL VENTILATION	MASK INDICATED? (1 = NO; 2 = YES FOR THOSE WHO GET CLOSE TO RESIDENT; 3 = YES)	GOWN INDICATED? (1 = NO; 2 = YES WHEN SOILING OF CLOTHES LIKELY; 3 = YES)	GLOVES INDICATED? (1 = NO; 2 = YES FOR CONTACT WITH INFECTED AREA OR DRAINAGE; 3 = YES)	COMMENTS (INCLUDING DURATION OF PRECAUTIONS OR ISOLATION)
Respiratory	2	3	2	2	2	Maintain until off antibiotics and culture negative twice. Emphasize respiratory secretion precautions.
Skin	2	3	1	2	2	Maintain until off antibiotics and culture negative twice. Emphasize pus (drainage) precautions.
Urine	2	3	1	1	2	Maintain until off antibiotics and culture negative twice. Emphasize urine precautions, especially if patient has indwelling urinary catheter.
Mycobacteria, nontuberculous (atypical)						
Pulmonary	1	—	—	—	—	—
Wound	2	1	1	2	2	Maintain for duration of illness. Emphasize pus (drainage) precautions.

Table 19.2 *Continued*

Agent/Site of Infection	Precautions or Isolation Indicated? (1 = no; 2 = yes)	Private Room Indicated? (1 = no; 2 = yes for resident who cannot use good hygiene; 3 = yes; 4 = yes with special ventilation	Mask Indicated? (1 = no; 2 = yes for those who get close to resident; 3 = yes)	Gown Indicated? (1 = no; 2 = yes when soiling of clothes likely; 3 = yes)	Gloves Indicated? (1 = no; 2 = yes for contact with infected area or drainage; 3 = yes)	Comments (Including Duration of Precautions or Isolation)
Pediculosis	2	2	1	1	2	Maintain for duration of illness. Close contact with infected patients or their personal effects can result in transmission; effective treatment of patient rapidly reduces this hazard.
Pharyngitis, etiology unknown	1	—	—	—	—	Maintain oral secretion precautions for duration of illness.
Pneumonia						
Etiology unknown	1	—	—	—	—	Maintain precautions necessary for the infection that is most likely. Use respiratory secretion precautions.

241

Table 19.2 *Continued*

Agent/Site of Infection	Precautions or Isolation Indicated? (1 = NO; 2 = YES)	Private Room Indicated? (1 = NO; 2 = YES FOR RESIDENT WHO CANNOT USE GOOD HYGIENE; 3 = YES; 4 = YES WITH SPECIAL VENTILATION	Mask Indicated? (1 = NO; 2 = YES FOR THOSE WHO GET CLOSE TO RESIDENT; 3 = YES)	Gown Indicated? (1 = NO; 2 = YES WHEN SOILING OF CLOTHES LIKELY; 3 = YES)	Gloves Indicated? (1 = NO; 2 = YES FOR CONTACT WITH INFECTED AREA OR DRAINAGE; 3 = YES)	Comments (Including Duration of Precautions or Isolation)
Bacterial— not listed elsewhere (includes gram-negative bacterial)	1	—	—	—	—	Maintain for duration of illness. Emphasize respiratory secretion precautions.
Mycoplasma (primary atypical pneumonia)	1	—	—	—	—	Maintain for duration of illness. Emphasize respiratory secretion precautions.
Pneumococcal	1	—	—	—	—	Maintain respiratory secretion precautions until 24 hours after start of effective therapy.
Resistant bacteria	2	3	2	2	2	Maintain until off antibiotics and culture negative twice. Emphasize respiratory secretion precautions.
Staphylococcus aureus	2	3	2	2	2	Maintain for duration of illness. Emphasize respiratory secretion precautions.

242

Table 19.2 *Continued*

AGENT/SITE OF INFECTION	PRECAUTIONS OR ISOLATION INDICATED? (1 = NO; 2 = YES)	PRIVATE ROOM INDICATED? (1 = NO; 2 = YES FOR RESIDENT WHO CANNOT USE GOOD HYGIENE; 3 = YES; 4 = YES WITH SPECIAL VENTILATION	MASK INDICATED? (1 = NO; 2 = YES FOR THOSE WHO GET CLOSE TO RESIDENT; 3 = YES)	GOWN INDICATED? (1 = NO; 2 = YES WHEN SOILING OF CLOTHES LIKELY; 3 = YES)	GLOVES INDICATED? (1 = NO; 2 = YES FOR CONTACT WITH INFECTED AREA OR DRAINAGE; 3 = YES)	COMMENTS (INCLUDING DURATION OF PRECAUTIONS OR ISOLATION)
Streptococcus, group A	2	3	2	2	2	Maintain until 24 hours after start of effective therapy. Emphasize respiratory secretion precautions.
Viral	1	—	—	—	—	Maintain sputum precautions for duration of illness.
Ringworm (dermatophytosis, dermatomycosis, tinea)	1	—	—	—	—	—
Rotavirus infection	2	2	1	2	2	Maintain for duration of illness or 7 days, whichever is less. Emphasize stool precautions.
Salmonellosis	2	2	1	2	2	Maintain for duration of illness. Emphasize stool precautions.
Scabies	2	2	1	2	2	Maintain for duration of illness. Gowns and gloves should be worn for close contact.

243

Table 19.2 *Continued*

Agent/Site of Infection	Precautions or Isolation Indicated? (1 = no; 2 = yes)	Private Room Indicated? (1 = no; 2 = yes for resident who cannot use good hygiene; 3 = yes; 4 = yes with special ventilation	Mask Indicated? (1 = no; 2 = yes for those who get close to resident; 3 = yes)	Gown Indicated? (1 = no; 2 = yes when soiling of clothes likely; 3 = yes)	Gloves Indicated? (1 = no; 2 = yes for contact with infected area or drainage; 3 = yes)	Comments (Including Duration of Precautions or Isolation)
Staphylococcal disease (*S. aureus*)						
Pneumonia or draining lung abscess	2	3	2	2	2	Maintain for duration of illness. Emphasize respiratory secretion precautions.
Skin, wound, or burn infection—limited or minor lesions	2	1	1	2	2	Maintain for duration of illness. Emphasize pus (drainage) precautions.
Skin, wound, or burn infection—major lesions	2	3	1	2	2	Maintain for duration of illness. Emphasize pus (drainage) precautions. Major lesions are those not covered by dressings or for which dressings do not adequately contain pus (drainage).
Streptococcal disease (group A streptococcus)						

Table 19.2   *Continued*

AGENT/SITE OF INFECTION	PRECAUTIONS OR ISOLATION INDICATED? (1 = NO; 2 = YES)	PRIVATE ROOM INDICATED? (1 = NO; 2 = YES FOR RESIDENT WHO CANNOT USE GOOD HYGIENE; 3 = YES; 4 = YES WITH SPECIAL VENTILATION	MASK INDICATED? (1 = NO; 2 = YES FOR THOSE WHO GET CLOSE TO RESIDENT; 3 = YES)	GOWN INDICATED? (1 = NO; 2 = YES WHEN SOILING OF CLOTHES LIKELY; 3 = YES)	GLOVES INDICATED? (1 = NO; 2 = YES FOR CONTACT WITH INFECTED AREA OR DRAINAGE; 3 = YES)	COMMENTS (INCLUDING DURATION OF PRECAUTIONS OR ISOLATION)
Pharyngitis	2	1	1	1	1	Maintain for 24 hours after start of effective therapy. Emphasize respiratory secretion precautions.
Skin, wound, or burn infection— limited or minor lesions	2	1	1	2	2	Maintain for 24 hours after start of effective therapy. Emphasize pus (drainage) precautions.
Skin, wound, or burn, infection— major lesions	2	3	1	2	2	Maintain for 24 hours after start of effective therapy. Emphasize pus (drainage) precautions. Major lesions are those not covered by dressings or for which dressings do not adequately contain pus (drainage).

Table 19.2 *Continued*

AGENT/SITE OF INFECTION	PRECAUTIONS OR ISOLATION INDICATED? (1 = NO; 2 = YES)	PRIVATE ROOM INDICATED? (1 = NO; 2 = YES FOR RESIDENT WHO CANNOT USE GOOD HYGIENE; 3 = YES; 4 = YES WITH SPECIAL VENTILATION	MASK INDICATED? (1 = NO; 2 = YES FOR THOSE WHO GET CLOSE TO RESIDENT; 3 = YES)	GOWN INDICATED? (1 = NO; 2 = YES WHEN SOILING OF CLOTHES LIKELY; 3 = YES)	GLOVES INDICATED? (1 = NO; 2 = YES FOR CONTACT WITH INFECTED AREA OR DRAINAGE; 3 = YES)	COMMENTS (INCLUDING DURATION OF PRECAUTIONS OR ISOLATION)
Syphilis Latent (tertiary) and seropositivity without lesions	1	—	—	—	—	—
Skin and mucous membrane, including congenital, primary, and secondary.	2	1	1	1	3	Maintain until 24 hours after start of effective therapy. Blood from these patients may be infectious.
Tuberculosis Pulmonary (confirmed or suspected)	2	4	3	1	1	Maintain until patient improving and sputum negative for TB organisms. Prompt use of effective antituberculous drugs is the most effective means to limit transmission.
Skin test positive with no evidence of pulmonary disease	1	—	—	—	—	—

246

Table 19.2 *Continued*

AGENT/SITE OF INFECTION	PRECAUTIONS OR ISOLATION INDICATED? (1 = NO; 2 = YES)	PRIVATE ROOM INDICATED? (1 = NO; 2 = YES FOR RESIDENT WHO CANNOT USE GOOD HYGIENE; 3 = YES; 4 = YES WITH SPECIAL VENTILATION	MASK INDICATED? (1 = NO; 2 = YES FOR THOSE WHO GET CLOSE TO RESIDENT; 3 = YES)	GOWN INDICATED? (1 = NO; 2 = YES WHEN SOILING OF CLOTHES LIKELY;3 = YES)	GLOVES INDICATED? (1 = NO; 2 = YES FOR CONTACT WITH INFECTED AREA OR DRAINAGE; 3 = YES)	COMMENTS (INCLUDING DURATION OF PRECAUTIONS OR ISOLATION)
Urinary tract infection (including pyelonephritis), with or without urinary catheter	1	—	—	—	—	See multiply resistant bacteria if infection is with these bacteria.
Wound infection						
Limited or minor lesions	2	1	1	2	2	Maintain for duration of illness. Emphasize pus (drainage) precautions.
Major lesions	2	3	1	2	2	Maintain for duration of illness. Emphasize pus (drainage) precautions. Major lesions are those not covered by dressings or for which dressings do not adequately contain pus (drainage).

Adapted from Centers for Disease Control Guidelines for Isolation Precautions in Hositals, 1985 focus in gloving can conceivably lead to the inadvertent elimination of handwashing as the primary focus for preventing infection. Nevertheless, LTCFs are mandated by OSHA to adopt universal precautions for the routine care of all residents.[20]

Long-term care facilities must choose how they will utilize universal precautions. They can expand them to encompass all potentially infected body fluids as in "body substance isolation" (BSI),[21] or they can limit their use as an adjunct to traditional diagnosis-driven isolation practices as originally proposed by the CDC.[17]

Body Substance Isolation

Body substance isolation (BSI) is a system that combines the standard isolation goal of resident protection with the employee protection goal of UP.[18] A consensus document from the Missouri Department of Social Services, Division of Aging, gives a good interpretation of BSI for LTCFs.[22] Excerpts are included in this section. Traditional isolation practices that focus on diagnosed cases of infectious diseases provide an incomplete strategy for infection prevention and control. These practices can cause detrimental psychosocial effects in residents and their families and interfere with the homelike atmosphere that nurses try to establish. The body substance system described here is a practical, safe approach that fits well with the extended care environment.

Many infectious organisms are carried without symptoms. This is certainly true for HIV infection and for hepatitis B. Similarly, virulent or antibiotic resistant strains of gram-negative and gram-positive bacteria such as MRSA may colonize moist body surfaces without symptoms. These organisms can easily be transmitted from resident to resident on the hands of personnel. Because medical history and examination cannot reliably identify all persons infected with these or other infectious diseases, it makes far more sense to treat *all* moist body substances as potentially infectious rather than to focus precautions only on the residents who are diagnosed with infectious diseases. The BSI system reduces the risks of such transmissions by the consistent use of barriers whenever any body substances are likely to be in contact with the caregiver's hands.

For these reasons a system has been developed that is called body substance isolation (BSI) because it focuses on keeping all moist body substances (blood, feces, urine, wound drainage, tissues, oral secretions, and other body fluids) from the hands of personnel. This is accomplished primarily by increased glove use and handwashing. The system eliminates many of the ritualistic practices associated with traditional isolation systems while it increases the use of barriers for all contact with body substances.

Body substance isolation is consistent with universal precautions but goes a step further and considers all blood and body fluids as potentially infectious, regardless of the resident's diagnosis. In order to follow these recommendations, the need to use barriers must focus on the care provider's routine *interactions* with the resident. In the past, the resident's *diagnosis* had been the cornerstone of the traditional isolation systems.

The appropriate barrier to be used is selected *after careful consideration of each specific situation for the overall reasonable exposure risk associated with the task*. Risk factors that should be included in the evaluation include

- Type of body fluid with which there is or will be contact
- Volume of blood/body substances likely to be encountered
- Reasonable anticipation of exposure; e.g., "will my hands touch the resident's secretions?"
- Probable route of exposure; e.g., hand contact, airborne, droplet, splashing
- Microbe concentration in fluid or tissue

Many resident care procedures dictate the use of specific barriers for the resident's protection (e.g., sterile gloves for dressing changes). However, when personal protective equipment is selected for protection of the caregiver, use individual judgment in determining when barriers are needed. Individuals must establish their own standards for consistent use of barriers. These personal standards should be based on the individual's skills and interactions with the resident's body substances, nonintact skin, and mucous membranes. The risk factors outlined earlier should be used to assist in the decision-making process.

Implementing the BSI system includes the following elements and should be followed by all personnel at all times regardless of the resident's diagnosis:

1. *Gloves*

   Wear gloves when it can be reasonably anticipated that hands will be in contact with mucous membranes, nonintact skin, and/or moist body substances (blood, urine, feces, wound drainage, oral secretions, sputum, vomitus, or items/surfaces soiled with these substances). Examination gloves are recommended for most indications. Gloves must be changed between residents; do not wash gloves for reuse. Dirty gloves should be changed promptly, and handling medical equipment and devices with contaminated gloves is not acceptable. Always wash hands after removing gloves.

2. *Handwashing*
   Wash hands often and well, paying particular attention to around and under fingernails and between fingers. Wash hands for indications as listed earlier in "Handwashing and Asepsis."

3. *Face and Eye Protection*
   Wear masks and/or eye protection when it is likely that eyes and/or mucous membranes will be splashed with body substances (e.g., when suctioning a resident with copious secretions, emptying fluids, or irrigating a wound).

4. *Apron or Gown*
   Protect clothing with a plastic apron or gown when it is likely that clothing will be soiled with body substances. These items are primarily designed to reduce the soiling of the clothing of personnel with moist body substances.

5. *Sharps Handling and Disposal*
   Do not recap needles, and dispose of them in a puncture resistant container.

6. *Laboratory Specimens*
   Laboratory specimens should be in leak-proof containers and appropriately labeled.

Cleaning and handling of linen and waste are as discussed for earlier isolation systems. Blood spills are discussed in Chapter 15.

The major reasons for use of a private room are diseases transmitted in whole or in part by the airborne route or the resident who extensively soils the environment with body substances. In the absence of culture and sensitivity information, private rooms are generally indicated for residents with uncontrollable excretions (diarrhea) or secretions, excessive coughing, heavy wound drainage and widespread skin disease. Residents should be confined to their rooms while these conditions exist. If a multiply resistant organism (e.g., MRSA) has been identified by culture as colonizing or infecting a resident, a private room is indicated or a room could be shared with another resident having the same organism.

For residents with airborne diseases, a private room is provided with special ventilation (negative pressure), and a *STOP sign* alert should be posted on the door. The door should remain closed except when entering or leaving the room. The airborne diseases include chickenpox, disseminated varicella-zoster and pulmonary tuberculosis. The nurse is responsible for determining whether a mask is indicated for entering the room. For example, all persons entering the room of a resident with active TB would wear a mask, but a person who has had chickenpox (and is immune) could enter the room of a resident with disseminated varicella-zoster without a mask. Personnel should know their chickenpox, measles, and rubella immune status. Decisions to restrict resident activities should be made on the basis of contagious risks and resident behavior.

Concern has been expressed that BSI may "underisolate" some infectious conditions.[23] On the other hand, the BSI approach can prove more costly than simply implementing universal precautions according to the OSHA regulations. More personal protective equipment is required for institutions using the BSI approach rather than one of the traditional isolation types in conjunction with universal precautions. Staffing limitations often encountered in the LTCF and training and monitoring problems are possible considerations for the success of BSI. Additionally, the "caring" requirements for residents are often much more intensively physical than is the care in an acute care facility. Residents are in their home environment in the LTCF. Workers are often much like their own family, with intense emotional ties and physical contacts. These "caring" activities may also make implementation of BSI more difficult. Certainly, more LTCFs are moving toward only BSI as the isolation type of choice. As their experiences are shared, the true success of BSI in LTCFs can be discovered.

Comparing the Isolation Methods

Jackson and Lynch compared the four systems of isolation and discussed the different approach to diseases with each system.[24] Several diseases are compared in Table 19.3. The relative merits and costs of the four systems have yet to be determined.

EDUCATION

Isolation/precautions policies and procedures should be developed, evaluated, and updated, and compliance should

Table 19.3 *Comparison of Four Isolation Precautions Systems*

SITUATION	CATEGORY SPECIFIC	DISEASE SPECIFIC	BODY SUBSTANCE ISOLATION	UNIVERSAL PRECAUTIONS
Resident with salmonellosis (gastroenteritis)	Enteric Precautions: gloves for contact with feces; gown if soiling is likely; private room if personal hygiene is poor; sign on door — "Enteric Precautions".	See named disease. Gloves for contact with feces; gown if soiling likely; private room if hygiene is poor; sign on door listing precautions needed.	Gloves: put on clean gloves immediately before contact with mucous membranes and nonintact skin; gloves for contact with moist body substances; gown or plastic apron if soiling is likely; private room if personal hygiene is poor.	Universal precautions do not apply to feces unless visibly bloody.
Resident infected or colonized with MRSA	Contact Isolation: gloves for touching infective material; mask if close to resident; gown if soiling is likely; private room indicated; sign on door — "Contact Isolation".	See named disease. Gloves for touching infective material; mask if close to resident; gown if soiling is likely; private room with sign on door listing precautions needed.	Same precautions as above for salmonellosis; may select "Stop Sign" for respiratory MRSA.	Universal Precautions do not apply unless secretions are visibly bloody.
Resident with pulmonary TB	AFB isolation: mask when entering room; sign on door "AFB isolation"; private room with special ventilation.	See named disease. Mask when entering room; private room with special ventilation; sign on door listing precautions needed.	Use the CDC recommendations (19): private room with at least 6 air changes per hour; negative pressure relative to the hallway; room air must exhaust to the outdoors; mask for room entry; keep door closed; mask the resident if they must leave the room.	Use reference 19: private room with at least 6 air changes per hour; negative pressure relative to the hallway; room air must exhaust to the outdoors; mask for room entry; keep door closed; mask the resident if they must leave the room.

*Adapted from Jackson MM, Lynch P. An attempt to make an issue less murky: A comparision of four systems for infection precautions. Infect Control Hosp Epidemiol 1991;12:448-450. Used with permission.

be monitored.[25] The educational aspects of an infection control program have been discussed in Chapter 14, but some additional attention could be given to the aspects that have to do with isolation/precautions. Keeping in mind that these must be in writing and readily available to caregivers for reference, the policies and procedures on isolation/precautions must be presented as formal education.

In as much as the orientation of new employees should be tailored to the needs of the particular department based on job tasks and resident exposure, a specific course outline for each department should be developed. The content must include the procedures needed for isolation/precautions in general. For example, the food service worker must have a good understanding of what isolation signs to look for so as to don the appropriate protective clothing for food tray delivery and pickup.

As a rule, in-services regarding isolation and universal precautions must be mandatory for all employees on at least a yearly basis. Additionally, whenever outbreak problems arise (such as scabies exposures, tuberculosis exposures, or the spread of MRSA, for example), immediate classes for caregivers should be given to reinforce their knowledge base and their adherence to the accepted procedures. Their input for problem-solving at these critical times is very helpful.

Visitors can play a role in the introduction or spread of infection. All visitors to dependent physical-care residents should be cautioned about not visiting when they may have a contagious illness. Handwashing must be stressed, and if the visitor is likely to provide direct care where body fluids can be contacted, gloves and other protective clothing must be explained and provided. Visiting children are of special concern because they can sometimes spread or pick up infections with significant consequences. Children therefore need good supervision when visiting the LTCF. Whether or not traditional isolation schemes such as category or disease specific isolation are in use, visitors need education.

Education of residents is also important in reducing transmission of disease. This step in the education process is perhaps more important in LTCFs than in acute care hospitals because residents are more likely to be mingling and moving from room to room. The nursing staff should be assigned the responsibility of disseminating information regarding the risks and steps to be taken in controlling transmission of infectious diseases within a LTCF. Whereas education of the coherent, well-oriented individual should be sufficient, special steps will have to be taken for incoherent persons. For example, if the resident who is infected is also uncooperative, it is reasonable to restrict the activities of that individual to the room. This is particularly important for individuals with readily transmissible respiratory or gastrointestinal diseases. Above all else, teaching simple handwashing will best serve to protect residents from their own bacteria and from the pathogens of others.

EVALUATION

Monitoring is appropriate for all aspects of isolation/precautions. Using the written policy and procedures, a data collection tool can be developed to monitor for compliance. Results of such monitoring can point out the need for new educational strategies or for reevaluation of the procedure i self. Quality improvement activities can attempt to measure either process or outcome. Because some caregivers react negatively to the continuous quality improvement concept, it may be best to stress that the purpose of monitoring is for the presentation of performance data to the caregivers themselves. The caregivers need to see the evidence of their success or failure in order to solve their own problems and in order to have input into the process. Monitoring for the sake of monitoring is useless.

Monitoring for compliance to handwashing, for example, can be a simple check-sheet method that is done by one caregiver who is watching the behavior of co-workers. Results can be posted for review and comment. The results could indicate that some or all of the caregivers need additional education, that handwashing facilities are not in convenient locations, or that supplies are deficient.

Monitoring for knowledge base about universal precautions, for example, would include a questionnaire and the interviewing of several caregivers. The results could indicate, for example, that only a certain group of workers need education regarding some aspect of UP.

Similar visual monitoring of practice and/or questionnaires can be developed (with the criteria derived from written policies and procedures) for resident handwashing, visitors' knowledge, ancillary service workers' performance, understanding of isolation categories, and so on. In all cases, evaluation and monitoring efforts must be directed at assessing and planning for continuous quality improvement.

Certainly, caregivers who have LTCF experience can appreciate the magnitude of the caring task behaviors employed by direct caregivers in the LTCF. Nowhere in nursing is it more evident that caring is the essence of nursing. How does caring interface with the requirements of isolation or universal blood and body fluid precautions? Studies need to be done to measure the outcomes brought about by this interface. It is apparent to LTCF caregivers that isolation/precautions must coexist with caring in order to protect the residents, workers, and visitors who live and interact in the facility.

REFERENCES

1. Centers for Disease Control: Update: Universal precautions for preventing transmission of human immunodeficiency virus, hepatitis B virus, and other bloodborne pathogens in health-care settings. *MMWR* 1988;37:377–388.

2. Pugliese G, Lynch P, Jackson MM: *Universal Precautions: Policies, Procedures and Resources.* Chicago, American Hospital Publishing Co., 1991.

3. Wong ES, Hooten TM: Guideline for prevention of catheter-associated urinary tract infections. *Infect Control* 1981;2:125–130.

4. Dickens BM: Legal limits of AIDS confidentiality. *JAMA* 1988;259:3449–3451.

5. Crossley K, Nelson L, Irvine P: State regulations governing infection control issues in long term care. *J Am Geriatr Soc* 1992; 40:251–254.

6. Goetz AM, Muder RR: The problem of methicillin-resistant *Staphylococcus aureus*: A critical appraisal of the efficacy of infection control procedures with a suggested approach for infection control programs. *Am J Infect Control* 1992;20:80–84.

7. Bennett ME, Thurn JR, Klicker R, et al: Recommendations from a Minnesota task force for the management of persons with methicillin-resistant *Staphylococcus aureus. Am J Infect Control* 1992;20:42–47.

8. Pritchard V, Sanders N: Universal precautions: How effective are they against methicillin-resistant *Staphylococcus aureus*? *J Gerontol Nursing* 1991;17:6–11.

9. Garner JS, Favero MS: Guideline for handwashing and hospital environmental control. *Infect Control* 1986;7:231–243.

10. Larson E, Bobo L, Bennett R, et al: Lack of caregiver hand contamination with endemic bacterial pathogens in a nursing home. *Am J Infect Control* 1992;20:11–15.

11. Larson E: A causal link between handwashing and risk of infection: Examination of the evidence. *Infect Control Hosp Epidemiol* 1988;9:29–36.

12. Doebbeling BN, Stanley GL, Sheetz CT, et al: Comparative efficacy of alternative handwashing agents in reducing nosocomial infections in intensive care units. *N Engl J Med* 1992;327:88–93.

13. Butz AM, Laughon BE, Gullette DL, et al: Alcohol-impregnated wipes in hand hygiene. *Am J Infect Control* 1990;18:70–75.

14. Pritchard V, Hathaway C: Patient handwashing practices. *Nurs Times* 1988;84:68–72.

15. Rutala WA: APIC guideline for selection and use of disinfectants. *Am J Infect Control* 1990;18:99–117.

16. Berg R: *The APIC Curriculum for Infection Control Practice*, Vol. III: Dubuque, IA, Kendall Hunt, 1988; pp 583–593, 1162–1163.

17. Garner JS, Simmons BP: Centers for Disease Control guideline for isolation precautions in hospitals. *Infect Control* 1983;4:245–325.

18. Lynch P, Cummings MJ, Roberts PL, et al: Implementing and evaluating a system of generic infection precautions: Body substance isoloation. *Am J Infect Control* 1990; 18:1–12.

19. Centers for Disease Control: Prevention and control of tuberculosis in facilities providing long-term care to the elderly: Recommendations of the Advisory Committee for Elimination of Tuberculosis. *MMWR* 1990;39 (No. RR-10).

20. Department of Labor, Occupational Safety and Health Administration: Occupational exposure to bloodborne pathogens, final rule, *Federal Register*, 56:64004–64182, 1991.

21. Lynch P, Jackson MM, Cummings MJ, et al: Rethinking the role of isolation practices in the prevention of nosocomial infections. *Ann Intern Med* 1987;107:243–246.

22. Consensus Opinion Document: *Infection Control in Long-Term Care Facilities with an Emphasis on Body Substance Precautions*, Kansas City, MO, Missouri Department of Health, 1992.

23. Garner JS, Hughes JM: Options for isolation precautions. *Ann Intern Med* 1987; 107:248–250.

24. Jackson MM, Lynch P: An attempt to make an issue less murky: A comparison of four systems for infection precautions. *Infect Control Hosp Epidemiol* 1991;12:448–450.

25. Smith PW, Rusnak PG: *APIC Guideline for Infection Prevention and Control in the Long-Term Care Facility.* Mundelein, IL, Association for Practitioners in Infection Control, 1991.

INDEX

Page numbers followed by the letter *t* refer to information in tables.

Teaching. *See* Staff training and management
Testing for HIV, 184
Tetanus/reduced-dose diphtheria (Td)
　　vaccine, 207
Thermometers and infection control
　　measures, 219
Thrombocytopenia, 99
Thrush. *See* Oral candidiasis
Thymus gland, 12, 14
　immune function of, 12, 13*t*
　involution of, 14
Ticks, 6
Tissue hypoxia, 83
T-lymphocytes
　CD4+, and tests for AIDS, 183
　effects of age on, 14
　function of, 12, 13*t*
　　in diabetic patients, 18
　T-cell response, 14
Tobramycin, 147
Tonsils, 12
Toxicity of antibiotics, 148
Tracheobronchitis, 128
Training. *See* Staff training and management
Transmission of infection, control
　　measures, 112–13, 227–52
　asepsis, 230
　education, 249–51
　evaluation, 251
　　on admission to LTCFs, 228–29
　handwashing, 229–30
　isolation systems, 227, 231–50
　　body substance, 248–49
　　category-specific, 231–32
　　comparison of methods, 249, 250*t*
　　disease-specific, 232–33, 234–47*t*
　　universal precautions (UP), 227, 233, 248
Triceps skinfold thickness, 20
Trimethoprim, 74
Trimethoprim/sulfamethoxazole (TMP/SMZ)
　　and MRSA treatment, 153, 198
Tuberculosis, 61–67
　ATS/CDC treatment recommendations, 66
　cause of epidemic outbreaks in nursing
　　homes, 132
　clinical features, 62–63
　converters, 64
　diagnosis, 63
　disease, defined, 61
　dormant lesions, reactivation of, 62
　education/in-service training of staff, 67

　epidemiology of, 61–62
　in HCWs, prevention of, 196–97
　incidence, 61–62
　infection, defined, 61
　infection control guidelines, 65–67
　　assessment, 66–67
　　containment, 66
　　surveillance, 65–66
　isolation precautions for, 66, 246*t*, 250*t*
　isoniazid therapy, 64–65
　multi-drug resistant, 150
　nosocomial infection in nursing homes, 48
　pathogenesis, 62
　prevalence of, in LTCFs, 196
　preventive therapy, 64–65
　resources and support, 67
　rifampin therapy, 65
　screening at admission to LTCFs, 229
　transmission of, 62
　treatment of active TB, 65
　tuberculin skin testing, 62, 63–64
　　booster phenomenon, 64
　　false-negative reactions, 63
Tuberculous disease (TB). *See* Tuberculosis
Two-step PPD (TB) test, 64
Typhoid fever, 97, 133

Ulcerative gingivostomatitis, 47
Ulcers. *See* Pressure ulcers
Universal precautions (UP)
　applicable body fluids, 184*t*
　compliance with, monitoring, 190
　monitoring compliance to, 251
　and waste management, 221
Upper respiratory infection (URI), 48
Urinary tract
　improving local defenses to infection, 205
　and predisposition to infection, 17
　as site of hospital-associated infection, 42
Urinary tract infection (UTI), 71–82
　acute pyelonephritis, 73, 74
　acute uncomplicated UTI and morbidity, 74
　antimicrobial management of, 74
　bacteriuria, 74
　　asymptomatic, 73–74, 77–78
　complicated, 71, 72–73
　control aspects in nursing homes, 79–80
　　antimicrobial use, 80
　　epidemic UTI, 79
　　control measures, 79
　　indwelling catheters, 79–80